Paediatric / 0–5 years

Second edition

This bo

Practical Aspects of Audiology

Series Editor: Michael Martin, OBE, Royal National Institute for the Deaf, London

Audiology is a relatively new discipline, formed over the last 50 years. As with all new disciplines, the pace of research is high and standardisation or acceptance of agreed procedures and norms has been low. Examples of this may be seen in the work of the International Standards Organisation (ISO) which only in recent years has produced standards for basic audiometric test methods and given levels for masking signals in pure-tone audiometry.

While much is written on audiology, a great deal of the material concentrates on research aspects of the work. The aim of this series of books is to emphasise the practical aspects of audiology and to set out clearly current practice and ways in which research might be applied.

Furthermore, an international perspective will be given to the series, in order to spread the information that is available on a world-wide scale. This will bring to the attention of practitioners and students ideas and procedures that may appear novel in their own countries but which are widely used in other parts of the world. Today, audiology is an international subject, and recognition must be given to this fact in our thinking. With the move to international standardisation, particularly in instrumentation, it is essential that we are aware of the different approaches being used.

Speech Audiometry, edited by Michael Martin, Royal National Institute for the Deaf, London.

Paediatric Audiology, 0–5 years, edited by Barry McCormick, Nottingham General Hospital, UK.

Manual of Practical Audiometry, Volume 1, edited by Stig Arlinger, Swedish Audiometry Methods Group.

Manual of Practical Audiometry, Volume 2, edited by Stig Arlinger, Swedish Audiometry Methods Group.

Cochlear Implants: A Practical Guide, edited by Huw Cooper, Royal Ear Hospital, London.

Tactile Aids for the Hearing Impaired, edited by Ian Summers, University of Exeter.

Paediatric Audiology
0–5 years

Second edition

Edited by
Barry McCormick, PhD
Children's Hearing Assessment Centre, Nottingham

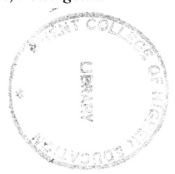

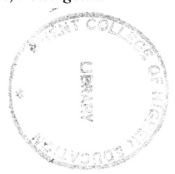

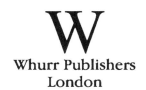

Whurr Publishers
London

© 1993 Whurr Publishers Ltd
First edition 1988 by Taylor & Francis Ltd, London
All rights acquired 1990 by Whurr Publishers Ltd
Second edition published 1993 by Whurr Publishers Ltd,
19b Compton Terrace, London N1 2UN, England
Reprinted 1994

British Library Cataloguing in Publication Data
A catalogue record for this book is available from the
British Library.

ISBN 1-897635-25-7

Singular number 1-565932-39-0

Photoset by Stephen Cary
Printed and bound in the UK by Athenaeum Press Ltd,
Gateshead, Tyne & Wear.

Foreword

The detection of hearing loss at the earliest possible age is of the utmost importance, as the ability to hear from birth provides us with the basis for developing normal speech and language. Hearing loss in the first 5 years of life can have a profound effect on a child if it is not detected, diagnosed and appropriate management provided. Even mild degrees of hearing loss can cause a reduction in the rate of development of speech and language and therefore intellectual and social development. These effects, in many cases, do not stop at childhood and are with the individual for the rest of his or her life. The importance of early detection diagnoses and management cannot, therefore, be overemphasised.

Barry McCormick has therefore quite rightly concentrated on these very important first few years of life. The range of topics has increased in this revised edition and the introduction of a chapter on cochlear implants reflects a very significant change in the treatment of young children and in the attitudes of professionals, parents and others. When the first edition of the book was produced it was not possible to write such a chapter.

Progress in the field of paedo-audiology is undoubtedly taking place and the contents of the revised version reflects this.

M.C. Martin, OBE
Series Editor

To Janet, Fleur and Neil

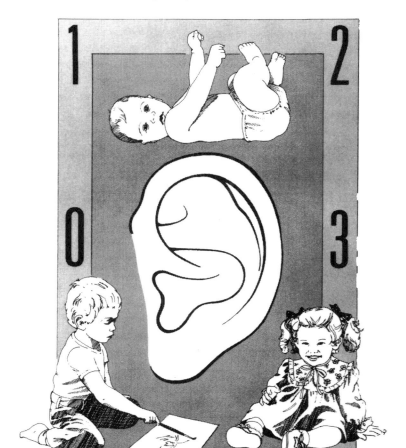

Reproduced from the original cover of the first edition, the illustration above was designed by Fleur McCormick with the assistance of Caroline Archer.

Preface

For this, the second edition of *Paediatric Audiology 0-5 years*, the contributors were invited to address the shortcomings of many texts in paediatric audiology by covering the finer points of detail in their topics and guiding the reader from first principles through to a practical working knowledge of the clinical application of relevant techniques. This shadowed the style of the first edition which, judging by its popularity, succeeded with its objective to fill a significant gap in the literature.

The contributors rose to this challenge and it is hoped that this expanded and updated text will prove to be of value to the student and practitioner in this highly specialized field.

One criticism of the first edition was the absence of coverage of cochlear implantation in young children. The omission of this topic was not surprising given that this was a completely no-go area in the UK at that time. It did, in fact, take the editor and his colleagues nearly 2 years to persuade the powers that be that this was an important development and that the UK lagged behind the rest of the world (or so it seemed) by not introducing this technique into routine clinical service. The situation has changed considerably over the past 4 years and now one of the world's leading centres for paediatric cochlear implantation resides in the heart of England. A chapter on cochlear implantation in children is now proudly contained within the text of this new edition.

As predicted in the first edition, microchip technology has been harnessed with pace and effectiveness to benefit paediatric audiology, and examples of such developments are included throughout the revised text.

The huge topic of otitis media with effusion is given additional space in this edition with a valuable contribution from Professor Haggard following his extensive literature search. The remaining chapters update and expand the knowledge contained in the first edition to give the reader an authoritative coverage of paediatric audiology in the UK.

Barry McCormick
May 1993

Contents

Contributors

John Bamford, PhD, Centre for Audiology, Education of the Deaf and Speech Pathology, University of Manchester, UK

Joan A. Birkin, PhD, Medical Research Council Institute of Hearing Research, University of Nottingham, UK

Denzil N. Brooks, PhD, Regional Audiology Unit, Withington Hospital, Manchester, UK

Yvonne Cope, MSc, Children's Hearing Assessment Centre, Audiology Centre, General Hospital, Nottingham, UK

Adrian R. Davis, PhD, Medical Research Council Institute of Hearing Research, University of Nottingham, UK

Philip I.P. Evans, MSc, The Newcomen Centre, Guy's Hospital, London, UK

Kevin P. Gibbin, FRCS, Department of Otolaryngology, Queen's Medical Centre, University Hospital, Nottingham, UK

Roger Green, PhD, Community Health Unit, King Edward VII Hospital, Windsor, UK

Mark P. Haggard, PhD, Medical Research Council Institute of Hearing Research, University of Nottingham, UK

Mark E. Lutman, PhD, Medical Research Council Institute of Hearing Research, Clinical Outstation, Audiology Centre, General Hospital, Nottingham, UK

Steve Mason, PhD, Evoked Potentials Clinic, Medical Physics Department, Queen's Medical Centre, University Hospital, Nottingham, UK

Barry McCormick, PhD, Children's Hearing Assessment Centre, Audiology Centre, General Hospital, Nottingham, UK

Eileen McSporran, MSc, Centre for Audiology, Education of the Deaf and Speech Pathology, University of Manchester, UK

Michael Nolan, PhD, Starkey Laboratories Ltd, Stockport, UK

Diane P. Pringle, BA (Hons), Medical Research Council Institute of Hearing Research, University of Nottingham, UK

Sarah Sheppard, MSc, Children's Hearing Assessment Centre, Audiology Centre, General Hospital, Nottingham, UK

Sally Wood, MSc, Children's Hearing Assessment Centre, Audiology Centre, General Hospital, Nottingham, UK

Chapter 1
A public health perspective on childhood hearing impairment

ADRIAN DAVIS

Introduction

In this chapter a public health perspective on permanent bilateral hearing impairments in 0–5-year-old children is presented together with epidemiological data relevant to the planning of these children's hearing services. The public health perspective enables an overview of the needs of hearing-disabled children and the types of health, educational and other services that should be purchased to give benefit to these children and their families. It also emphasizes the need to set appropriate targets and quality standards in paediatric audiology, and the need to audit the quality of the outcome from the intervention afforded by these services.

Purchasers and providers alike require an epidemiology appropriate to providing and developing optimal services for childhood hearing impairments. Two important parameters of that appropriate epidemiology are reviewed here: the prevalence of different severities of hearing impairment and the percentage of these attributable to individual aetiologies (or risk factors). The extent to which these epidemiological parameters are stable over time and place allows generalization to settings other than those in which the data were collected. The public health perspective and the epidemiology give an indication of the overall size and balance of services, their appropriate targets and indicators that can be used for audit.

Recent developments

The years since the first edition of this book was published have seen a substantial change in the approach to child health in the UK. The three major influences on this approach as it applies to hearing have been the publication of two editions of *Health for All Children* (Hall, 1991), *Screening Children's Hearing* (Haggard and Hughes, 1991) and the National Health Service and Community Care Act 1990.

In 1989 *Health for All Children*, a report of a joint working party of the British Paediatric Association, the Royal College of General Practitioners, the General Medical Services Committee of the British Medical Association, the Health Visitors' Association and the Royal College of Nursing (Hall, 1991), proposed a 'Programme for Child Health Surveillance'. This report emphasized the central role of health promotion through 'an equal constructive partnership between parents and professionals' (p. 8) in the development of children to their full potential in society. Besides offering an integrated view of child health, and emphasizing the centrality of early detection of impairments, disabilities and handicaps, *Health for All Children* reviews the literature pertaining to 'screening for hearing impairment' (Chapter 10) and makes recommendations for a desired programme of screening and surveillance of hearing impairment within a health promotion context. This programme brought together for the first time (for an interdisciplinary audience) an integrated approach, rather than viewing each aspect in isolation, by tier or speciality of service. A major recommendation of this report that goes beyond the mechanics of testing, facilities and equipment is that 'One person in each (health) district or health board should take responsibility for co-ordinating the programme of hearing screening ...' (p. 76).

The need to develop this co-ordinated approach is further echoed in the Department of Health-commissioned review *Screening Children's Hearing* (Haggard and Hughes, 1991) in which it is stressed that this approach should be backed up by 'a cumulative register of the known moderate, severe and profoundly permanently hearing-impaired children ...' containing all relevant data for use in routine review of a district's screening strategy (p. 323). This publication contains recommendations for such a strategy, including aspects of present practice that should cease; most importantly these present an outline of what further research is required to underpin present practice and to develop new more effective and efficient services. *Screening Children's Hearing* is mainly concerned with the problems of otitis media with effusion (OME, see Chapter 3), but it rightly views this within an integrated programme of screening and surveillance for hearing impairment and disability. The book's major message is to emphasize the need for the development of high-quality services (in all tiers of the health service) that are justified by the appropriate epidemiology and sustained by valid technology and appropriately trained personnel. 'Valid technology' in this context includes information systems as well as equipment that can be used for testing children's hearing. Information on present services is of a very heterogeneous nature, and service development is not always based on valid tried and tested advances. The need for action is not a prescription to do more, but recommends evaluation of what is being done locally before proposing a springboard towards developing new, more integrated services.

The National Health Service and Community Care Act 1990 has introduced many 'new' concepts into health care, which have acted as a focus to renew the commitment to 'effectiveness and efficiency in health services' (Cochrane, 1964). The introduction of a clearer divide between purchasers of health care and its providers has forced a more public debate on the aims, provision and arrangements for assessing the benefits of health care related to hearing impairment. Whilst this has generally had a good effect in reviewing the structure, process and outcomes of primary care services, there is still a lack of clear evidence concerning the benefits of different approaches to hearing screening and of early detection and intervention for some severities and types of hearing disability. Furthermore, in the short term, what may be good changes for one district may be retrograde in another, because the structure and process are markedly different between districts, in both content and quality.

This chapter aims to explore the needs of children in the context of the debate provided by these three major influences. To this aim the 'community health model' presented in the first edition is developed. This model elaborates factors that influence auditory disability and handicap (for a definition of the specialist terms used in this chapter see the glossary on pp. 33–36) and takes on board the new emphases with respect to health promotion. From this model a view of the 'needs of hearing-impaired children' is defined for the purpose of purchasing appropriate services. Some of the inputs to this model from the epidemiology of childhood hearing impairments are discussed, with respect to the prevalence, risk factors (including meningitis) and aetiologies of hearing impairments. Finally the major issues concerning infant hearing screening are reviewed with a consideration of how the needs of hearing-disabled children and their families may best be met in the future.

Model of auditory domains

The processes by which auditory pathology and impairment lead to disability and handicap apply to a wide range of severities and types of pathologies (Davis, 1983, 1987). In this chapter I am predominantly concerned with bilateral sensorineural auditory pathologies and the factors that affect them and influence their consequences. Figure 1.1 illustrates five sets of factors that might influence these processes. The sets are not exhaustive, but give a range of factors that are important.

The first set of factors, marked 1 in Figure 1.1, increases the incidence of auditory pathology. I have adapted the schema outlined by Davidson, Hyde and Alberti (1989) to describe this set. The second set,

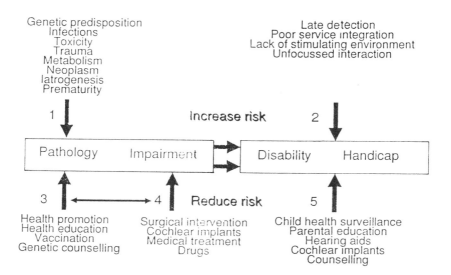

Figure 1.1 A public health model of the five sets of factors that increase or decrease the risk of prevalence or incidence of differential aspects of auditory health problems.

marked 2, increases the prevalence of auditory disability and handicap. The first factor in set 1 is genetic predisposition to auditory pathology. Dominant and recessive modes of inheritance of defects are both important factors that account for a high proportion of hearing impairments (Williamson and Steel, 1990; Morton, 1991). This factor has become the focus of a great deal of research effort to isolate genes that are implicated in certain types of hearing impairment. It is probable that there are many genes involved in congenital genetic hearing pathologies. Tackling some of the major syndromes with associated auditory impairments – Waardenburg's, Usher's and Pendred's account for about one in five of these impairments (Fraser, 1987) – may provide considerable insight into the wider problem.

As well as direct genetic predisposition to auditory pathology, there may be indirect mechanisms by which genetic predispositions affect hearing impairment. External factors such as infections, trauma, toxicity and the problems associated with prematurity do not affect all children adversely. Whilst there is no direct evidence at present, some genetic predispositions may be primed by or act in synergy with these external agents to produce an auditory pathology.

Infections, such as congenital rubella in the prenatal period (Miller, 1991) and bacterial meningitis in the postnatal period (Fortnum, 1992), increase the risk of auditory pathology developing and raise the prevalence of auditory impairments in a birth cohort. These major infections, and a number of others (Gerber, 1990) are associated with a widely varying proportion of the congenital (prenatal) and early acquired hearing impairments. Their impact is very dependent on the prevalence of the infection, which may be highly geographically and temporally determined, and also on the coverage of relevant vaccination and health promotion campaigns.

Trauma, such as that produced by excessive noise immission, is an important factor affecting postnatal acquired auditory impairment in adults, and may also contribute to prenatal acquired impairments (Lalande, Hetu and Lambert, 1986). In Figure 1.1 prematurity and the range of 'risk factors' that place a new-born child in the neonatal intensive care unit (NICU) such as noise and birth events have been added separately to trauma, because this factor will be explored in more detail later in this chapter. Extreme sensitivity to noise may also be a contributory factor to the high incidence of hearing impairments associated with the trauma of prematurity. As discussed with the genetic factor, why some children exposed to a wide range of external noxious factors develop auditory pathology and some do not remains a mystery. The development of the auditory system (Pujol et al., 1991) and its ability to withstand insult between 24 and 36 weeks post-conceptional age may have a wide range of individual variation. This may be one component of interest in establishing reasons for the differential effect of the traumatic risk factors.

In the first set of factors shown in Figure 1.1, prevention of the pathology at several levels may be possible as shown in set 3. Health promotion is the most general of these factors, and may comprise several aspects including health education, child surveillance and screening for impairments. Health promotion may help reduce the incidence of auditory pathology due to trauma, infections, and prematurity by making parents more aware of the factors that may lead to auditory pathology in their children. The role of immunization, for rubella and, more recently, for some types of bacterial meningitis, depends crucially on the take-up of these services. Take-up is dependent in turn on the education of parents and on the organization and education of primary healthcare staff. At a different level, health education, backed up where necessary by informed genetic counselling, has a role to play in preventing genetic auditory pathology. This service is not universal through health districts in the UK.

The weight a purchaser assigns to the factors that reduce pathology and impairment and consequently disability and handicap (set 1) and to the factors that minimize those problems that increase the prevalence of disability (set 2) is crucial to determining the form of audiological services to be provided and the long-term benefit accrued.

The fourth set of factors in Figure 1.1 concern the reduction of the prevalence of impairment, with possible consequent reduction in the risk of disability and handicap. A reduction of impairment is possible by some forms of beneficial surgical intervention. The most common of this sort of intervention (discussed fully in Chapter 2) is the insertion of grommets for persistent OME in children with evident auditory disability (including signs of evident developmental delay), when other 'medical treatment' has not been successful. Whilst this intervention is fairly inexpensive individually, overall expenditure is very large because of the large numbers involved. This has to be contrasted and evaluated with respect to the small amount, in total, spent on interventions to reduce the impairment of children who receive no substantial benefit from hearing aids through individually expensive cochlear implants. For instance, a 10% saving in the budget for treatment of OME could pay for a comprehensive cochlear implant programme.

When it has not been possible to prevent or reduce impairment the fifth set of factors shown in Figure 1.1 work to reduce disability and handicap. Child health surveillance (Hall, 1991), when properly structured, may be aligned with some secondary prevention procedures. The aim of these procedures is to facilitate early detection and intervention by the use of screening programmes, high risk follow-up, opportunistic case finding, and incorporation of observations by relatives and care-workers in routine child health reviews. Appropriate parental education after confirmation of an auditory impairment in a child, before establishing an agreed route for rehabilitation and education, followed by counselling for the parents (and family) play an integral part in the provision of any aids to hearing.

To an extent the factors shown in set 2 can be expressed in a more positive way to supplement those shown in set 5. Early detection enables the potential for normal child development. That potential is best released if there is a seamless service, in partnership with the family, that places an emphasis on providing a stimulating auditory environment with a focus on personal interaction. Positive and negative influences on 'hearing services' are explored further in Figure 1.2. The processes and activities that might facilitate or hamper public health aspects of the management of 'hearing services' will undoubtedly influence the individual rehabilitation of a child with hearing impairment. One key aspect of each arm of influence has been highlighted for attention in Figure 1.2. Screening programmes should facilitate the early management of childhood hearing impairment. They will do so, provided that they are embedded in a good programme of health promotion and education, that knows precisely the aims and objectives it is trying to achieve and has feedback on how well it is achieving those objectives. Screening programmes without this primary care base are likely to cause more problems than they solve. The three most important preconditions for establishing a screening programme were discussed by Davis (1987) and Sancho et al. (1988), and rely on the

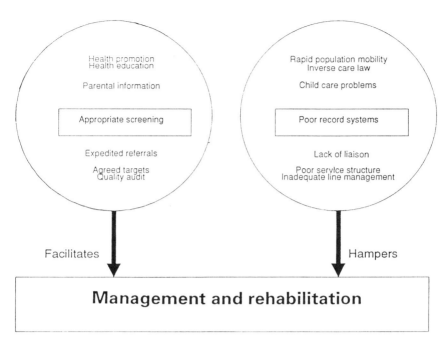

Figure 1.2 Some of the factors that facilitate or hamper the appropriate management and rehabilitation of hearing-impaired children.

principles put forward by Wilson and Jungner (1968) and Cochrane and Holland (1969). They are:

- that the condition addressed by the screen should have important health, social or educational consequences;
- that good audiological services are available for assessment and diagnosis; and finally
- that appropriate rehabilitative opportunity exists.

Thus screening programmes also need to have good and thorough audiological and educational service backup at the secondary and tertiary level.

The key aspect that hampers management is poor record systems, one of the problems highlighted by *Screening Children's Hearing*. The organization of screening programmes and the infrastructure needed for their success in achieving good management of hearing services and appropriate rehabilitation requires the coordination of up to half a dozen separately funded providers (e.g. GP, paediatrician, community medical officer, health visitor, medical physicist, audiologist, speech and language therapist, peripatetic teacher of the deaf, otolaryngologist, social services, genetic counsellor). Furthermore, there is no standard model for the structure and management of these services.

Inadequate record systems will hide the problems in line management. This may affect good practice as it relates to individuals, or policy such as childhood screening. For instance, the coverage of screening and surveillance need to be very high to be worthwhile. The inverse care law operates to an extent here, in that the children with hearing problems tend to be in the minority who are not screened (Johnson and Ashurst, 1990). Hence good record systems are essential to monitor the coverage of any screening or routine checks that are carried out.

Whilst the problems of liaison within a district need to be solved to counter the inverse care law pattern of provision, a great effort is needed in some districts to overcome the low coverage due to very high population mobility. To implement a useful record system based on an agreed database for each sphere of action (primary, secondary, tertiary) using uniform definitions requires a lot of the problems in structure, liaison and management to be solved before its implementation. Many of the problems highlighted in Figure 1.2 that hamper management may be reduced by having a key named individual responsible for co-ordinating the hearing services.

Figures 1.1 and 1.2 show the factors leading to an increased incidence of auditory pathology and increased prevalence of hearing disability, and the factors that can be organized within a public health programme or a specialist department to reduce incidence of auditory pathology and the prevalence of impairment and disability. These factors are mostly general in that they concern the whole population but some concern only the child with a hearing impairment and their family. In the next section the concept of need is explored to focus on what services might be needed and what data are needed to assign a priority to that service.

Audiological health needs for children

Table 1.1 shows three classes or levels of need for audiological health care which might be considered: the population, the sub-population and the individual/family.

The population level concerns the children in each birth cohort. At this level the actions needed to reduce need (e.g. immunization) are similar to those shown in Figure 1.1 (set 1), and are aimed at reaching the whole birth cohort living in a particular district at the appropriate age. Other examples of combating need at the population level are education concerning the factors that promote good auditory health or normal auditory and communicative development, combined with surveillance and screening at critical times.

There may be several sub-populations of children in each age cohort, for example children on an at-risk register or who have failed a primary screen. The need here may be for a very prompt and efficient

Table 1.1 Three levels at which paediatric auditory health needs should be considered and actions that might appropriately reduce need

Class of need	Action to reduce need
Population	Vaccination
	Education
	Surveillance
	Screening
	Elicit concern at key stages
Sub-population	Assessment
	Advice
	Hearing aid provision
Individual	Diagnosis
	Counselling
	Training in use of aid
	Education
	Assessment of benefit from aid and rehabilitation programme

auditory assessment of the child. Advice on why assessment is necessary and an explanation of the results of each assessment are needed. For the sub-population whose hearing is impaired one of the major provisions will be hearing aids. Much of the reduction in need at this level is accomplished by the second or third tier audiology services.

At an individual or family level the consideration of needs is difficult. What are those needs? What place or priority should they have in a properly constructed audiological health service configured to give maximum benefit to society? One of the major needs of an adult with an acquired hearing impairment is to be able to hear and communicate with other people. Therefore it is easy to imply that one of the first steps in providing a service to meet that need is one that supplies an appropriate rehabilitative package, usually including a hearing aid, at the optimum time with the aim of improving hearing and communication.

Consideration of a child's needs along the parallel of adult service provision is not the correct model for several reasons. Not only do the needs of the child depend very much on the age of confirmation of the hearing impairment and its severity, but also the need of a very young child is very different from that of an adult. The hearing-impaired child needs help to develop the skills necessary to learn to communicate with other people, so society has to purchase a service that aims at the population level to eliminate the causes of deafness in children via appropriate vaccination, education and preventive programmes, at the sub-population level to identify the hearing-impaired child as early and efficiently as possible and at the individual level to provide appropriate forms of rehabilitation for the child and its family at different stages of development dependent upon the degree to which the child's 'full potential' is disabled.

There are several important consequences if it is agreed that these aims of a broad paediatric audiological service meet the needs of hearing-impaired children. First, emphasis is placed on enabling an individual child to develop its place in society. Secondly, this emphasis provides a rationale to concentrate on two types of indicators of the potential benefit from these services. What have previously been considered as process indicators (e.g. rubella vaccination coverage, first year screening coverage, age of provision of hearing aids, delay between suspicion to diagnosis) assume a higher profile if measured against the enabling aim (Markides, 1986; White and White, 1987; Davis and Wood, 1992; Ramkalawan and Davis, 1992). Thirdly, the role of the parent(s) in enabling the child to develop (including their role in diagnosis and rehabilitation, that they may or may not decide to include 'aids to hearing', signing, or a combination) becomes central rather than peripheral to the service. This shifts the emphasis of rehabilitation to communication and participation, and consequently there is a requirement to develop outcome indicators that reflect these emphases, rather than rely solely on language/speech measures.

The present services may have most difficulty overcoming the administrative problems at the individual level, because of the variety of services from different sectors needed to sustain a good rehabilitative programme. Not all of the providers are funded by the same agency and so there seem to be no real financial incentives to minimize the overall costs or to maximize the potential of the child in the long term. Savings in the educational budget (albeit in a few years time) cannot be used as a means of funding neonatal screening or better parental and professional education. The factors influencing the funding of neonatal screening will be discussed in more detail later.

Discussion of the public health model of auditory disorders and the need for services at the three levels would not be complete without some attention to the matters raised in Figure 1.2. The heterogeneity of present record systems makes it very difficult to establish basic data on a particular birth cohort concerning the coverage and impact of child health surveillance on hearing services, the distribution of childhood hearing impairments in the UK, the uniformity of risk factors over districts and the distribution of age of detection, confirmation and hearing aid fitting of congenital hearing impairments. One of the major steps forward that could be used as a model for this process is the Recommended Paediatric Hearing Screening Protocol issued by the Welsh Office (1991) in which an element of 'audit of screening for hearing loss in children' is included, with the establishment of an interdisciplinary audit team. However, to be capable of collecting the data required above such an audit would need to be considerably expanded. Whilst it is a mistake to overburden audit with the task of providing a register or being a research activity, such a system might be built on to an audit system at minimal cost.

In Figure 1.2 it was suggested that management and rehabilitation would be facilitated by setting reasonable targets. However, setting targets for each level of need at district, regional or national level is a difficult task. The question of whether such targets should be set regardless of the present performance is difficult to answer. A compromise should perhaps be agreed in which the targets are set regardless of the present service position, but which takes account of present and past performance indicators in the quality audit and notes the change of quality against time.

The public health model, considering matters of need (the potential for groups to benefit from health care), demand (the extent to which groups ask for particular services) and supply (the services provided) has been partly developed by Stevens (1991) in step with the National Health Service and Community Care Act 1990. I have tried to make it relevant to children's hearing services through a discussion of the structure of need in the audiological domain (Figure 1.1) and the way in which need occurs in different levels of the population (Table 1.1). The way in which services ought to meet those needs has also been discussed in Figure 1.2, taking into account the recommendations of *Health for All Children* and *Screening Children's Hearing*. These recommendations may be considered to be one element in the 'demand for services' category. Another element in framing this should be estimates of prevalence of hearing disorders in children and associated risk factors, which follow.

Epidemiology of childhood hearing impairment

Prevalence

Several recent reviews of the incidence and prevalence of childhood hearing impairment (Davidson, Hyde and Alberti, 1989; Dias, 1990; Morton, 1991; Brookhouser, 1993; Mauk and Behrens, 1993) emphasize the many uncertainties that arise in interpreting much of the data gleaned from a variety of methodological and definitional problems. The effect of non-standard definitions, the inaccuracy of retrospective estimates, the difficulty in testing young children and the problems with progressive and fluctuating conditions are some of the problems with interpreting prevalence estimates of severe–profound impairment.

The major problem with respect to mild–moderate sensorineural hearing impairments is that no study has been carried out to reliably ascertain prevalence in this group. This is due to the systematic under-ascertainment of hearing impairments below 40 or 50 dB HL even late into school age.

Population mobility is another problem for estimating prevalence data (Das, 1988; Davis et al., 1993). This has an unpredictable effect on the estimates, and will vary considerably from district to district. It has been suggested that in districts with high population mobility a large number of children are at risk. Districts with low mobility and good health services have reported a drift of hearing-impaired children towards them.

Mauk and Behrens (1993) summarize ten studies that they consider to be the 'most carefully done and most defensible of existing research'. The studies were published over a 14-year period and consider birth cohorts ranging from the mid 1960s to the mid-1980s. These authors remark that there is a considerable scatter among the data points. The problems mentioned above mean that we cannot tell whether these differences are true – due to geography or time – or are artefacts of the methods used. It would not be surprising, however, that comparing birth cohorts in a country such as Israel (Feinmesser, Tell and Levi, 1986) over a decade starting in the mid 1960s with Denmark in the 1970s (Parving, 1988) or with the UK in the 1980s (Davis and Wood, 1992) should lead to some differences. The corollary of this is that great care should be taken before transferring estimates in the literature to a particular district! An awareness of some aspects of the demography and epidemiology of hearing disability is also required.

An illustration of the way in which some confusion can arise by using imprecise terminology and then be propagated is shown by reference to one of the reviews (Brookhouser, 1993), which adapts a table from another review (Morton, 1991). The table gives a range of estimates for 'the incidence of profound childhood deafness per million births' from about 400 to 800. The upper estimate is derived from a study in the UK (Newton, 1985): that study actually gives an estimate of 0.8 per 1000 children with bilateral sensorineural hearing impairment at a threshold level of 25 dB or worse over the mid-frequencies 0.5–4 kHz. An estimate for severe and profound impairments ($\geq$ 80 dB HL) may be made at about 440 per million from that study. A further hindrance to interpretation (Davis, 1993) is the criterion 'deaf' or 'profoundly deaf', used for instance in another of the studies referred to in these reviews (e.g. Morton, 1991; Majumder, Ramesh and Chinnapan, 1989). It is very difficult to maintain the same definitions across studies even for the same child (on one occasion a child's latest audiogram may indicate a mixed impairment but in the next paper the clinical judgement may have changed to a progressive sensorineural; another sibling may be born with a hearing problem, which may change the view of the aetiology of the first child completely). However, the terms 'deaf' or 'profoundly deaf', which seem to refer indiscriminately to mild, moderate or even severe congenital hearing impairment, should be defined very carefully when interpreting the incidence/prevalence estimates. Further problems arise in understanding 'overall' prevalence rates that are quoted from differences in whether all children with a hearing impairment at a criterion level are included, children with a purely conductive impairment are properly excluded, or only children with a true congenital sensorineural impairment are considered. Not all authors make clear what criteria they are using for these purposes.

The nine publications shown in Table 1.2, based on eight sets of data concerning prevalence of childhood hearing impairment and disability, will be considered with respect to the UK; for comparison the

Table 1.2 Prevalence (per 1000) of all hearing impairment in children from several studies

Paper First author	Nation	Date	Cohort	Report	Better ear hearing level average ≥								
					25	30	35	40	50	55	70	80	95
Davis [1]	UK	93	83-88					1.2			0.6		0.4
Davis [2]	UK	92	83-86						1.3				
Davis [3]	UK	92	83-86						1.1			0.5	0.3
Das	UK	88	81-84			1.1						0.6	
Butler	UK	86	70	1.7						(0.7)[5]			
Newton	UK	85	77-80		1.2							0.4	
Taylor	UK	80	75-78									0.5	
Martin	UK	79	69						1.0		0.7	0.6	0.3 (100+)
Sheridan [4]	UK	72	58							2.4 (1.4)[6]			
Parving	DK	93	70-79		1.5								
Parving	DK	93	80-89		1.5								
Feinmesser	Israel	86	67-78						1.7 (41+)	1.4 (56+)	1.2 (71+)		0.8 (91+)
Parving	DK	85	70-79		1.4								
Kankkunen	SW	82	70-80						1.3				
Upfold	Aus	82	?							1.1 (60+)			0.5 (90+)
Martin	EC	79	69						0.9				0.3 (100+)
Schein	US	74	?	1.0 (deaf)									

[1] All sensorineural and mixed impairments
[2] All hearing impaired children
[3] All sensorineural/mixed congenital and progressive impairments

[4] cf Peckham (1986) for detailed analysis
[5] Estimated from p 240-241
[6] Estimated using 'correction factor'

table contains seven publications from other countries. The prevalence severity distribution is given where it can be derived from the paper. This table gives an overall impression of the range of hearing impairments over which prevalence has been reported. The severity quantization may not be equivalent between authors because of the way in which the severity has been reported: in some cases an average of the thresholds over 0.5, 1, 2, 4 kHz has been used (Davis and Wood, 1992; Davis et al., 1993; Parving, 1993), over the range 0.25–4 kHz in others (Newton, 1985; Das, 1988; Taylor, 1980), and in others the range is not defined. The study of the 1958 birth cohort (Sheridan, 1972; Peckham, 1986) used the threshold exceeded at two frequencies at least.

The age at which the children were assessed differed between and within most of the studies, and so there is a further element of doubt about the quantization of severity. Whilst the numeric tag should be treated with caution, it is much preferable to applying verbal tags: as mentioned above, 'profoundly deaf' can mean very different disabilities to different scientists (e.g. Morton, 1991; Schein and Delk, 1974; Butler and Golding, 1986; Peckham, 1986).

At average hearing threshold levels of 55 dB HL or greater, the data reflect hearing impairments with a substantial sensorineural component. Below that, unless specified (as in Davis and Wood, 1992; Davis et al., 1993), there is considerable scope for confusion as to the type of hearing impairment.

All of the studies in Table 1.2, with two exceptions, have ascertained the hearing-impaired population (e.g. from clinic records) and then have gone on to estimate the prevalence of a given level of hearing impairment. The two exceptions are the cohort studies in the UK (Sheridan, 1972; Butler and Golding, 1986) which studied births in the years 1958 ($n = 15\,496$) and 1970 ($n = 12\,629$). These two population studies potentially give the least biased information about the prevalence of hearing impairment at age 7 years for the first cohort and 5 years for the second. However, because of the limitations of the audiometric information they are difficult to interpret.

Peckham (1986) indicates that the 1958 cohort at age 7 years had 11 (0.7 per 1000) children with ≥ 75 dB HL thresholds for at least two thresholds. For children with ≥ 55 dB HL this increases to 1.8 per 1000. However, 11 children had difficulty doing the audiograms, and were suspected to have a similar level of hearing impairment. This leads to the relatively high prevalence of 2.4 per 1000 (cf. Table 1.2). Part of this can be explained by the threshold measure taken to classify the severity, which would emphasize the role of high frequencies. Applying a correction factor derived from a database of adults in a cross-sectional study (Davis, 1989) would imply that about 60% of those exceeding 55 dB HL at two frequencies would have an average of 55 dB HL or greater. This leads to the prevalence 'guesstimate' of 1.4 per 1000 given in Table 1.2. With over 25% of the hearing impaired not undergoing full audiometric tests, this number may be an overestimate.

The Butler and Golding (1986) cohort of 1970 recorded hearing impairment from parental records and questionnaires. The prevalence for 'severe hearing difficulties' (Butler and Golding, 1986) or 'severe hearing loss' (Peckham, 1986) was reported as 23 of 12 629 or 1.7 per 1000, with up to 8% of all children reported as having some hearing difficulty. Interpolating from Table 16.2 in Butler and Golding (1986), this would indicate that up to nine children had hearing difficulties that were not due to conductive problems or were impairments better than about 50 dB HL, a prevalence rate of about 0.7 per 1000 at the nominal 55 dB HL or worse level reported above. The low level of school screening at the time of the study when the cohort was 5 years old, 40% (Butler and Golding, 1986), indicates that this figure might well be an underestimate. This study also enables an estimate of about 1 in 3000 with an ear anomaly associated with hearing difficulty.

The advantage of a population study is that the ascertainment bias (i.e. the tendency for mild–moderate impairments not to get recorded in the audiology/hearing aid system) may be minimized. The Butler and Golding (1986) study of the 1970 cohort may contain bias due to the under-reporting of hearing difficulties, particularly among children with associated handicaps. (A big disadvantage of such a study is that very large samples are needed for stable estimates of prevalence for impairments with a risk in the range 1 in 500 to 1 in 4000.) The advantage of ascertainment studies is that they are usually based on clinical records, which means that substantial audiological investigation has (usually) been done, and each child has been evaluated several times. The estimate of average threshold in the better ear can be more reliable, especially for children who are difficult to test.

The EC study (Martin et al., 1979) gave a prevalence estimate of 1.0 per 1000 for ≥ 50 dB HL averaged over frequencies 0.5, 1 and 2 kHz in the UK, which equates to 0.9 per 1000 in the EC as a whole. The results were compiled by a questionnaire sent to appropriate auditory health care professionals in each country when the children were about 8 years of age. Table 1.2 shows that about 0.3 per 1000 children in the UK had hearing impairments of ≥ 100 dB HL at this age.

The remaining studies in the UK can be divided into two sets: the overlapping studies of the children born and resident in Greater Manchester over the period 1975–1984 (Taylor, 1980; Newton, 1985; Das, 1988); and the studies that focus on collaborative work at the MRC Institute of Hearing Research (Davis and Wood, 1992; Davis et al., 1993). This second set uses a Nottingham birth cohort from 1983 to 1986 (Davis and Wood, 1992) and a multicentre study of overlapping birth cohorts in Nottingham, Sheffield and Oxford district health authorities from 1983 to 1988 (Davis et al., 1993). The first set of studies used average hearing threshold level over the mid-frequencies 0.25–4 kHz, the second over the mid-frequencies 0.5–4 kHz.

The studies in the Greater Manchester area give a unique view of hearing impairment in a region of the UK from the mid-1970s to the mid-1980s. Whilst the low fence used for inclusion in the studies of the 1977–80 and 1981–84 cohorts at 25 and 30 dB HL, respectively, leads to a considerable underestimate of the incidence and cumulative incidence of hearing impairment due to lack of ascertainment of prevalent cases at this level, it may represent a reasonable estimate at higher levels. Thus, at ≥ 80 dB HL an overall estimate of 0.5 per 1000 is obtained from the three individual estimates of 0.4 (cohorts 1977–80), 0.5 (cohorts 1975–78) and 0.6 (cohorts 1981–84), for all congenital and post-natally acquired hearing impairments.

The Nottingham study of the 1983–86 cohort (Davis and Wood, 1992) found that 1.8 (95% confidence interval 1.4–2.3) per 1000 children had been fitted with a hearing aid at the time of study. The prevalence of all hearing impairments greater than 50 dB HL was 1.3 per 1000 (confidence interval 0.9–1.8) at the time of the study, with 1.1 per 1000 (confidence interval 0.8–1.5) having a sensorineural or mixed congenital hearing impairment. Table 1.2 shows that this incidence decreases to 0.5 per 1000 at impairments greater than 80 dB HL, and 0.3 at the level of 90 dB HL or higher.

A later study (Davis et al., 1993) compared three areas in the UK, and the overall results are shown in Table 1.2. Significant differences were seen between areas, especially for moderate hearing impairment, and the authors speculated that this might have been due to differential under ascertainment (e.g. the prevalence of impairment above 40 dB HL was 1.9 per 1000 in Sheffield, 1.5 per 1000 in Nottingham and 1.0 per 1000 in Oxford health authorities). The overall estimate of 1.2 per 1000 (confidence interval 1.1–1.4) was for sensorineural and mixed hearing impairments over all onsets. The estimate excluding impairments acquired after birth was 1.1 per 1000, and 1.0 per 1000 excluding transfer into the areas. The variation between areas was not significant for profound hearing impairments (≥ 95 dB HL), with an overall estimate of 0.4 per 1000 (confidence interval 0.3–0.5).

Parving (1993) updates earlier estimates for the 1971–80 birth cohort in Copenhagen and adds to it the data for Copenhagen County and the 1981–90 data for both areas. She uses the same average of hearing threshold as the MRC studies and shows no difference between the cohorts 1971–80 and 1981–90 or between the two areas, the overall prevalence estimate for 'congenital and early acquired hearing impairments' ≥ 25 dB HL being 1.5 per 1000. Davis and Parving (unpublished results) compare the prevalence estimates between Denmark and the UK for the studies mentioned above and analyse the data in more detail. The prevalence of congenital hearing impairment of sensorineural or mixed type was 1.2 per 1000 (confidence interval 1.0–1.3) for impairment ≥ 40 dB HL and 0.4 (confidence interval 0.3–0.5) for impairment ≥ 95 dB HL over both studies, with the UK estimate being 1.1 (confidence interval 1.1–1.3) and the Danish estimate 1.3 (confidence interval 1.1-1.7) for ≥ 40 dB HL, with similar variation at ≥ 95 dB HL. This similarity was not borne out in terms of the severity distribution of impairment or the risk factors for hearing impairment. This indicates that we must not assume that, because two countries (or two districts in the same country) have the same prevalence rates, the risk factors must be similar. It follows, of course, that appropriate action for one area may not be appropriate for another (e.g. Watkin et al., 1991). A further point about the studies of Parving (1983, 1988, 1993), Das (1988) and Newton (1985) is that if a low criterion is used for entry into the study it does not follow that the prevalence estimate will be unbiased for that low criterion level, unless a population study methodology is used with good audiology.

The study of Schein and Delk (1974) marks an interesting point in studies concerning the demography of hearing disability. Schein and Delk estimated that about 1 per 1000 people in the USA were considered 'deaf'. This study was concerned more with the social and economic consequences of being 'deaf' and, although it was calibrated to hearing impairment for the population concerned, this was not necessarily of prime importance to them in considering rehabilitation. With new technical and educational developments, the planning of future services may depend crucially on the degree of hearing impairment as well as the cultural expectations of the family.

The studies of Feinmesser, Tell and Levi (1986) in Israel and of Upfold and Isepy (1982) in Australia show the highest prevalence of 'profound' hearing impairments (≥ 90 dB HL), possibly due to several methodological or demographic factors. It may be that the denominators being used are inappropriate (i.e. the geographic boundaries and birth rates within those boundaries may be subject to error) or that for some reason (e.g. immigration, rubella epidemics) these countries really do differ.

The study of Kankkunen (1982) in Goteborg, Sweden, gives a similar estimate for ≥ 50 dB HL to the Davis and Wood (1992) study (1.3 per 1000). One of the purposes of Kankkunen's study was to assess the extent to which children could be assessed for hearing impairment at very young ages, before the discovery of evoked otoacoustic emissions (see Chapter 8).

In summary, there is a great need to collect more systematic and accessible data on the occurrence of hearing impairment in children. A register of hearing-impaired children containing a minimum data set specification would greatly assist the present patchy knowledge of the epidemiology of childhood hearing impairments. Such a register would enable study of trends of prevalence and risk factors over time or difference between areas and would highlight the need for changes in particular preventive and rehabilitative programmes.

The papers summarized in Table 1.2 suggest that, over all types and onsets of hearing impairment, there does appear to be some agreement that about 1 in 2000 children in the UK, at about the age of 5 years, have impairment $\geq$ 80 dB HL. This estimate increases to 1 in 770 at $\geq$ 50 dB HL. These estimates are not incompatible with those from the population studies once adjustment is made for the terminological confusion and different metrics used to assess severity of hearing impairment and disability. European data give broadly similar estimates (Parving, Kankkunen, Martin), but those in Israel, Australia and the USA appear to be slightly different for unknown reasons.

The following sections will concentrate on the data in the UK from the studies of Davis and Wood (1992) and Davis et al. (1993).

Risk factors for childhood hearing impairment

Neonatal history

Davis and Wood (1992) reported that babies in a neonatal intensive care unit (NICU) were 10.2 (confidence interval 4.4–23.7) times more likely to have a sensorineural or mixed, congenital or progressive hearing impairment $\geq$ 50 dB HL in the better ear than those who did not undergo intensive care, given that there was neither a family history of impairment nor craniofacial abnormality. Davis et al. (1993) confirmed that children who spent longer than 24 h in NICU had a high risk of hearing impairment, and that the 7% of children with such a history yielded 32% (confidence interval 26–40%) of the congenitally hearing-impaired children with at least 40 dB HL. There appeared to be little variation between the three areas studied, but the Danish data (A.C. Davis and A. Parving, unpublished results) showed a great difference with only 17% of the Copenhagen hearing-impaired children coming from the group who had been in an NICU: we are currently investigating what may lie at the root of this difference. It could be that the criteria for entry into the NICU are different in the two countries, or it may be an ascertainment problem. Such differences are very important, as they could influence the healthcare policy considerably in terms of screening, prevention and rehabilitation. While neonatal medicine continues to improve, it is important to monitor this risk factor, because changes in outcome may affect screening strategy.

In the UK, therefore, a neonatal screening programme targeted on the NICU, using a highly sensitive test such as evoked otoacoustic emissions (see Chapter 8) or abbreviated automated auditory brain stem responses (see Chapter 7), might detect up to one-third of all hearing-impaired children at a cost of about £30–40 per child screened. This is a small cost per child compared with the overall cost of a child's stay in the NICU (Haggard, 1992; A.C. Davis and M.P. Haggard, unpublished results). Over the three areas studied 7% of live births had been treated in an NICU (Davis et al., 1993).

Some clinicians may argue that screening the hearing of children in the NICU should be restricted to the children that fall into specific categories of risk (e.g. as defined by The Joint Committee on Infant Hearing, 1991) but Mauk et al. (1991) have shown that 23% (confidence interval 12–39%) of hearing-impaired children in the NICU would have been missed in the cases reviewed if this restriction had been practised. Reviewing cases seen at the Children's Hearing Assessment Centre in Nottingham we concluded that over the period 1982–1991, 10 children out of a total of 42 congenitally hearing-impaired children of all severities with a NICU history would not have fallen into the JCIH risk categories. The implication for Nottingham is that a very sensitive neonatal screening programme based on screening all NICU children would pick up 31% (18–44%) more children than screening using the JCIH risk criteria. For bilateral ≥ 50 dB HL impairments this reduces to about one-half the previous figure (16 (4–30)%). The theoretical gain depends on the aims of the programme, the sensitivity of the test to mild–moderate hearing impairments and the health gain associated with identifying mild–moderate hearing impairments as early as possible. This last parameter is difficult to quantify. It has been suggested that the NICU group do have more difficulty in developing language and communication, and therefore it would be sensible to note any perceptual problems as early as possible in order to minimize the possibly synergistic effects of delay due to hearing impairment.

Family history of childhood hearing impairments

Davis and Wood (1992) showed that about 16% of children who had not been treated in an NICU with bilateral ≥ 50 dB HL impairment had a family history of childhood hearing impairments. This is similar to the 23% (35/155) reported by Das (1988) and 25% (21–34%) using the data from Davis et al. (1993).

A major problem in using the family history criterion for neonatal screening is the reliability and validity of any questions that try to establish a positive family history during the first antenatal appointment, on the maternity ward, or as part of the health visitor routine for early surveillance of risk factors for hearing problems to supplement the 'Can your baby hear you?' information (see Chapter 4). This issue should be resolved with appropriate training of professionals and parents, clear guidelines on what initial question should be used, and what supplementary questions should be used for those replying positively to the first question. The format of the question used in Nottingham ('Do you or your partner have a close relative who has had a permanent hearing problem from early childhood? If YES, please ask a nurse to make an appointment for your baby to see our hearing screening nurse') on the maternity wards appears to be successful. For wider clinical use (e.g. by health visitors) the question may need revision to eliminate over-referral.

So, apart from the value in helping with aetiological assessment, the presence of a positive family history of hearing impairment could be used as part of a targeted neonatal screening programme, and depending on the efficiency of the questions may detect up to 25% of hearing-impaired children in the UK. However, a significantly greater proportion of children in Copenhagen have a family history of childhood hearing impairment (and of consanguinity): 27% of children in the UK had a positive family history, but in Copenhagen 40% had such a history. This could be due to a proposed higher proportion of children from first-generation immigrant families in Copenhagen, and there may be some difference in the extent to which the family history is elicited. However, as there was no significant difference between different areas within the countries, this methodological explanation is not very likely.

Craniofacial abnormalities

The presence of craniofacial abnormalities at birth is very often associated with syndromes that carry a high risk of hearing impairment, and has been included in the JCIH risk criteria since 1972. Further analysis of the study by Davis et al. (1993) showed that 25% of all hearing-impaired children in the Sheffield and Oxford health authorities had a craniofacial anomaly, with only 11% in the Nottingham area. However, there was considerable overlap between this risk factor and the NICU and family history factors. Overall, 7% of the hearing-impaired children were reported to have a craniofacial anomaly but neither a positive family history nor a NICU history.

Discussion of risk factors in the context of targeted neonatal screening

Taking all three risk criteria into account it may be possible, through targeted neonatal screening with high coverage of the risk factors and an infallible test, to detect up to 64% of hearing-impaired children. However, high coverage of all three risk factors is difficult in practice, and there is no easy way to establish the coverage for craniofacial anomalies or family history. In the Nottingham district health authority, a targeted neonatal screening programme has been in operation for a number of years to capitalise on this potentially cost-effective method for very early identification of hearing-impaired children. As Nottingham is also a regional NICU facility the yield in terms of children with hearing impairment from NICU is far greater (about 66%) than would be predicted on the basis of the statistics presented above, if only children from the Nottingham district health area attended the Nottingham NICUs. This is important when considering the facilities needed at regional centres and district units.

For the period between April 1989 and June 1991 (Davis, 1991, unpublished presentation at BSA annual meeting) of the 894 babies tested in the targeted neonatal screening programme, 83% were from the NICU (coverage of both 'Nottingham DHA babies' and outside referrals amounted to about 90% of babies in NICU). Family history and craniofacial anomaly accounted for the remaining 17%.

Over that period 12 (1.3%) children had diagnostic auditory brainstem response thresholds that were considered to be raised, and were considered to have a sensorineural pathology of some degree from the target group. Six (1 of 127) children were considered for a hearing aid, of whom one declined (family history). A further hearing-impaired child with a NICU history was missed by the screening programme due to lack of cover for the tester. Long-term evaluation of this sort of programme is much needed, but it is inevitable that the data for detailed evaluation of sensitivity is available only over the long term (i.e. when other potential misses are found at ages 1, 3 and 5 years or later). In the short term other indicators of the effectiveness and quality of the programme (e.g. coverage of the target groups, a running average of the yield and the positive predictive value i.e. the number of hearing-impaired children referred onwards as a percentage of the total referred onwards for assessment) have to be used.

If a 50% per annum surcharge on recurrent expenditure was made to cover staffing and funding capital overheads, the cost per child tested during this part of the programme (which contains additional research and teaching components in the job description of the nurse responsible for testing neonates) at 1991 prices, was £46. For a typical at-risk neonatal programme, with fewer teaching and research responsibilities and lower overheads, this figure should be somewhere between £30 and £40. Further discussion of the cost-effectiveness of different hearing screening programmes is needed, but there is a lack of data at present on the comparative cost-effectiveness of different types of screening programme.

Aetiology of childhood hearing impairment

Acquired hearing impairment

Considerable emphasis was placed in the discussion of the public health model of hearing disorders on the factors that contribute to childhood hearing impairment (see Figure 1.1). Acquired hearing impairments in the studies in the UK vary somewhat in terms of the percentage of all sensorineural/mixed hearing-impaired children at a given age. However, Das (1988) and Davis and Wood (1992) both show that 6–7% of all hearing-impaired children at the age of about 5 years may have an acquired impairment. Das (1988) indicates that 8% of the ≥ 80 dB HL children had meningitis; Davis et al. (1993) indicate that, whereas only 3% of the moderately hearing-impaired children (40–69 dB HL) had an acquired impairment, this increased to 12% for severe (70–94 dB HL) and 18% for profound (≥ 95 dB HL) impairments. Of the acquired impairments 90% were attributed to meningitis.

Post-meningitic hearing impairment is an important problem that should contribute substantially to the planning of services for detection and rehabilitation (Fortnum, 1992). The incidence of childhood meningitis has been increasing over the last decade (Fortnum and Davis, 1993a) and its impact on the incidence of hearing impairment seems to vary substantially in the literature (Fortnum, 1992) as a function of birth cohort and country. However, during the last decade in Nottingham the prevalence of hearing impairments in survivors of meningitis who have been assessed for hearing impairments suggests that up to 7.4% (4.5–11.9%) have some degree of permanent hearing impairment, with 4.5% (2.3–8.3%) having bilateral impairment and 2.0% (0.7–5.2%) having profound (≥ 95 dB HL) bilateral impairment (Fortnum and Davis, 1993b).

Although screening is important for congenital hearing impairment, it will not minimize impairment arising from meningitis. Every child who survives meningitis should be formally assessed for auditory function as soon as possible after discharge (target time 2–4 weeks).

Congenital hearing impairment

Assessment of aetiology in congenitally hearing-impaired children is not always straightforward, and the major problem with making comparisons in the literature is that there is a large and variable number of children to whom no aetiology is attributed. In some publications (e.g. Newton, 1985; Das, 1988; Majumder, Ramesh and Chinnapan, 1989; Morton, 1991) it is to some extent presumed that the unknown category is essentially genetic in origin. This presumption needs to be researched in more detail and an agreed protocol implemented at several sites so that this question can be looked at more systematically.

In the children with bilateral sensorineural/mixed ≥ 40 dB HL impairment in the Nottingham district health authority area between 1983 and 1989 (n = 77) an assessment was made of the primary aetiological factor for each child by a team including a physician and audiological scientist. Figure 1.3 shows the percentage for each aetiology in these children. It was not possible to assign an aetiology to 22% of the children; a further 25% had been assigned to autosomal recessive inheritance in the absence of any family history of hearing impairment; 18% of the children had a family history of hearing impairment, of whom 5% had been classified as autosomal recessive; 20% of the children had perinatal factors that may have had primary contributions to the impairment; a further 4% had no obvious perinatal factor associated with the impairment, but were pre-term babies who had a history of treatment in a NICU .

In order to investigate further the factors that might be important for children treated in a NICU alone (20 of the 77 had congenital sensorineural impairments of all severities, and no syndrome associated with sensorineural impairment, or a cleft lip and palate), a logistic regression was performed to determine which risk factors were

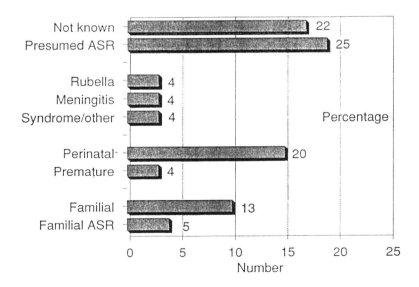

Figure 1.3 The proportion of children with sensorineural/mixed hearing impairment in Nottingham district health authority (birth cohort 1983–89) who had been assigned to different 'aetiological categories' (n = 77).

significantly different between these children and 2470 children who had been in the neonatal screening programme from the NICU during the same period. Three factors were significant:

1. Birth asphyxia (APGAR<5 at 5 min).
2. History of fits.
3. Ototoxic drugs (predominantly gentamicin).

It was statistically impossible to evaluate the contribution of each of these risk factors and their interactions because of the small number of hearing-impaired children and the large degree of collinearity between the risk factors. The best model was a non-specific combination of the risk factors, as shown in Table 1.3. This shows that while only 1.3 per 1000 with none of these risk factors had a hearing impairment, a child with just one factor had a risk of hearing impairment 10.1 times greater, and a child with all three 63.2 times greater, than children with no risk factors.

The majority of the hearing-impaired children had only one of the significant risk factors: however, the small group of children with all three risk factors do have a very substantially raised risk. A larger group of hearing-impaired children would help to establish a better model of the risk factors, but at this stage if targeted screening was to be concentrated on a particular subset of children then these three risk factors could be used to find up to 90% of the hearing-impaired children. It is particularly important to investigate in more detail children with more than one risk factor.

The proportion of children with rubella (4%) was significantly different to that found by Martin et al. (1979) and by Taylor (1980) for earlier cohorts (at about 20%), but it was not significantly different to that found by either Newton (1985) or Das (1988), which was 9–10%.

Profoundly hearing-impaired children

In order to make rational decisions concerning needs and priorities it is necessary to examine the characteristics of those children with pro-

Table 1.3 The prevalence of hearing impairment in the NICU as a function of birth asphyxia, history of fits and administration of ototoxic drugs*

Number of factors	Hearing impaired	Total	Prevalence (%)	Raised risk
0	2	1432	0.13	—
1	11	779	1.4	10.1 (CI 2.2–45.7)
2	4	225	1.7	12.7 (CI 2.3–70.0)
3	3	34	8.8	63.2 (CI 10.2–391.0)

* No child had a syndromal hearing impairment or a cleft lip and palate abnormality.
CI = confidence interval.

found hearing impairments (A.C. Davis and G. O'Donoghue, unpublished results). One of the major factors here is whether the hearing impairment was acquired or congenital. As shown above almost one in five profoundly hearing-impaired children has an acquired impairment, predominantly due to meningitis. The proportion of congenitally profoundly hearing-impaired children who have a history of treatment in a NICU is less than the average in the UK at about 12% (compared with 28% for other severities) and they are less likely to have other handicaps (18% compared with 39%) (A.C. Davis and G. O'Donoghue, unpublished results). The proportion with a family history of hearing problems did not vary with severity.

If the prevalence of profound hearing impairment ($\geq$ 95 dB HL) is taken from Davis et al. (1993), then in a typical birth cohort for the UK in the 1990s we might expect in the region of 220 congenitally profoundly hearing-impaired children, and by the age of 5 years another 70–80 acquired profound impairments. If a cochlear implant is technically and financially available, and all congenitally profoundly hearing-impaired children are considered as potential candidates with the families given appropriate counselling from the outset of rehabilitation, then the uptake of cochlear implants is a major concern. With take-up at 25%, there would be an eventual annual demand in the UK for 75 implants. For current multichannel implant devices, this might mean an annual expenditure in the UK of about £1 million. However, the associated costs of establishing teams and realizing the potential of the implantees through structured rehabilitation programmes will add about £1.5 million to this, in terms of both cost and trained personnel.

The development of this service to meet the needs of the hearing impaired depends on a number of factors, some undoubtedly local and others perhaps more universal. In some ways, if we consider a model of human need such as that proposed by Doyal and Gough (1991) there are strong arguments for arguing that meeting the needs of the profoundly deaf child should have first priority in an audiology/otolaryngology service. The model suggests that there are universal human needs subordinate to the basic right of an individual to autonomy within society through critical participation in that chosen society. Inasmuch as profound hearing impairment negates this right, once survival is assured, every effort should be made to give each child the chance to achieve a position in which these universal needs can be met. Some might argue for an interpretation of this whereby the services for the profoundly hearing impaired dominate service provision in the developed world, due to the availability of the enabling technology of early identification and multichannel cochlear implants. All other services become 'wants', and come below meeting the basic need of the profoundly hearing impaired. In a system in which particular specialities such as otolaryngology or audiology are often cash-limited, difficult decisions would then have to be made (should, for instance, routine fitting of grommets be axed in favour of better early identification programmes; should neuro-otology clinics be axed in favour of more multichannel implants?).

Age of identification of congenitally hearing-impaired children

The age at which children are screened for hearing impairment, or at which they are suspected to have a hearing disability by a surveillance programme, has been the focus of much concern. The EC study (Martin et al., 1979; Martin, 1982) showed that almost 50% of the children included in that study (≥ 50 dB HL) had their hearing impairment confirmed by 36 months of age. The UK average was slightly better than this but was still well below the JCIH recommendation that hearing-impaired children should be enrolled in rehabilitation programmes by the age of 12 months.

More recent studies have shown evidence of some improvement in the UK (Davis and Wood, 1992; Davis et al., 1993) and in Denmark (Parving, 1993). Davis and co-workers show that over the three areas studied in the UK (which are, admittedly, well provided for in terms of audiological services), there was little difference in median age of referral to the audiology assessment services between areas. Overall the median age was 12 months, with an interquartile range of 8–21 months. The upper quartile was most variable, and depended on the severity of hearing impairment and history of NICU treatment. For children with congenital average hearing impairments in the range 40–69 dB HL, 25% were referred after 29 months of age. So, although the median age of confirmation of hearing impairment may be vastly improved, there is no room for complacency.

The inference is that a large proportion of children with moderate impairments were not found by the surveillance procedures (screening and priming of parents at routine checks) during the first 2–3 years of life for the 1980s in these areas. Some districts in the UK might have better upper quartiles, but many with less well developed audiology and community services may be much worse. However, the data are not routinely available, either in the public domain or in a form accessible to individual districts/regions. Even if the data were available through using a database such as the IHR Paediatric Audiology Record System (PARS) (Marshall et al., 1992; Marshall et al., 1993) or other means, it is not entirely clear what aspects of the data need most attention due to the low and variable nature of the numbers involved in any district and the long wait to find some of those missed.

Age of identification as an indicator of service performance

At district level (2000–10 000 births each year), a statistically useful performance indicator for the age of identification of children with a defined degree of bilateral impairment (e.g. ≥ 50 dB HL) might be an unweighted running average over a 5-year period of the median and upper quartiles of the ages of referrals, confirmation and aid fitting (where appropriate). The start and end dates of the five cohorts would have to be arranged for 6–10 years previously, i.e. in 1994 performance over the years 1985–89 would be considered. This should be one of the final indicators of how the systems worked, but does not necessarily give much information about the service performance in 1994. To compensate for this, other more process-oriented indicators should be used such as the degree of coverage and the positive predictive value for screening (i.e. the proportion of correct referrals).

Although this does not give the full picture, a review of the yield of current services and the component incremental yield on a more closely informative time-scale would be sensible. An example of this would be to take children detected before t years of age over the preceding t to 5 $+t$ years, and examine the trend in proportion of children identified before 6 or 12 months or after 2 years. Tracking this sort of performance over a period of time is more of an art in quality assurance than a science, and critical examination of each case not confirmed by 15 months by a multidisciplinary audit team may help adjust current practice to give a better quality service. Once the system has started the services as a whole could be reviewed every 3–5 years in the light of the quantitative data.

Figure 1.2 indicates that appropriately designed screening programmes might facilitate management and rehabilitation of congenitally hearing-impaired children, but poor information systems hamper management. Some of the drawbacks in the performance indicators caused by lack of numbers may be overcome by combining (against the current trend) the services and information bases over districts with a homogenous service. Thus, if three adjacent districts had a common policy on neonatal screening, checklists for parents, training health visitors to go over checklists with parents and to perform 'distraction testing' and training GPs how to utilize parental concern, combination of that data over districts would be much more informative.

Another problem of the performance indicators discussed here is that they give equal weight to all hearing impairments detected. Should a potentially profound hearing disability detected earlier count as ten times more important than a severe disability, which is rated as ten times more important than a moderate disability (and so on)?

Earlier the better?

There is a large body of opinion that early detection and intervention is best for all aspects of ability that need a hearing component. However, as always, there is sparse literature on the exact effects on abilities due to differing delays of detection. Ramkalawan and Davis (1992) have shown that children detected earlier have some better language scores than those detected late for mild–severe impairment. There is some evidence from White and White (1987) and Levitt, McGarr and Geffner (1987) that a similar state of affairs may exist in the USA. They showed a substantial depression in language and communication scores from mild through to severe hearing impairments, as did Ramkalawan and Davis (1992). Even those children detected very early with mild impairments appear to have lower scores on these variables. Markides (1986) has looked at teacher ratings of hearing-impaired children's intelligibility and these also vary with age of identification. But very few of the children in these studies were detected at birth: it has been suggested that if they had been detected at birth the discrepancy would be much smaller between these hearing-impaired children and their 'normal-hearing' peers, but no one has yet published a substantial paper on this.

Apart from scientific evidence of the benefits of early detection, it can be argued that the potential for an individual to develop adequate communication ability to participate in society is a basic human right. Thus, regardless of the individual outcome, the duty of a high-risk register, neonatal screen, or child surveillance is to safeguard that potential.

That potential has several characteristics, some of which were summarized in a recent consensus meeting on early identification, and the arguments reviewed as to the impact of early identification on each (NIH, 1993). Some of these characteristics are:

- auditory and balance development such as lateralization, development of binaural hearing and (in the longer term) ability to co-ordinate precisely in the auditory and visual domain;
- development of all types of communication skills such as turn-taking, shared meaning, preverbal and verbal communication;
- language development and acquisition, such as progressive use of an English vocabulary, ability to recognize words and use them appropriately;
- speech development, such as a progressive sophistication in use of English phonology in communication with parents and peers;
- social and emotional development, such as bonding and appropriate social behaviour (less impulsivity, aggression, constant need for parental approval);
- academic development, such as the ability to progress in a 'normal' nursery, primary or secondary school.

Despite the claims that early identification can benefit all these, there are no studies that show that detection at birth benefits the child (and family) more than detection at 6–7 months for any degree of hearing impairment. The further questions as to whether all degrees of hearing impairment would be of equal benefit (and by how much) have not been addressed. It is taken as axiomatic that detecting a child with a severe hearing impairment at 1 year of age is better than at 3 years, but to what extent does this apply to children in the mild impairment category? Should as much effort be put into finding and confirming such impairment in the first few months of life as for those with impairments ≥ 50 dB HL?

It is premature to judge this issue, as the benefits from early detection, in terms of increased quality of life for the child and its family, and in terms of the development of characteristics outlined above, have not been demonstrated. A high priority for audiological health service research should be to investigate systematically the benefits of early identification and rehabilitation of children with different degrees of hearing disability. A cautionary word on the benefits of early identification may be necessary following the work of Ruben et al. (1982) and Ramkalawan and Davis (1992). We found that, although early detection benefited language scores, the gain expected from identification at birth would still leave 80% of the mild–severely hearing-impaired children in the bottom 5% of children on some basic descriptors of language in communication. Thus, early identification should not be seen as the 'Holy Grail' but a first step towards the enablement of the child's potential through an effective intervention programme.

Further data concerning the issue of early identification and the stress that late identification places on parents are available from the study by Ramkalawan and Davis (1992). As well as measuring indices of communicative ability, they included a structured interview with the mother concerning her communication with the child, her perceptions of the quality of service that they had been given, and her views on early identification. No mother thought that identification should be delayed, and 19 of 20 thought that birth was the best time to test, despite some fears that this might be psychologically inappropriate for early bonding. Eight of the mothers said that they had been very shocked or angry when they had been told of the impairment and only eight remembered that they had been counselled about the diagnosis. There was some evidence that, taking into account the age of the child at the time of testing, the mean length of utterance (m.l.u.) was influenced by the response of the parents to the diagnosis. If the parents said they were shocked or angry the m.l.u. was lower by about 0.75 units (partial correlation −0.51, d.f. = 12, P = 0.048). The mother's own language also showed a relationship to this in terms of the rate of interaction, with the number of words per minute decreasing by 22 ($\pm$ 11) for those mothers who were shocked or angry.

If this is a real effect then early procedures such as neonatal screening should minimize not only the shock and anger that often faces parents with an unwanted diagnosis, but also the number of parents who will be false-positives in a screening programme, so that there are no barriers to essential bonding of the child within the family.

Infant screening: the major issues

In the first edition of this book the major questions that ought to be answered about infant screening were suggested, and they have been further discussed by Haggard and Hughes (1991). For the main part they appear to remain the same now as then:

1. What severities and types of hearing impairment should be detected, and by what age?
2. When should hearing screens be conducted?
3. Who should be screened?
4. Which screening methods should be used?
5. Who should do the screening, what training is necessary and what responsibilities assumed?
6. How much should be spent on screening, and who should pay?
7. What are the targets and associated indicators for screening systems?

There is no need to update the arguments that surround these questions. As yet there is no consensus on the first of these questions. There is no doubt that the answer depends on the overall system, as well as the ability to diagnose mild hearing impairments in the first year of life and to implement any meaningful rehabilitation. As an operational definition I propose a three-stage screening strategy in the first 5 years of life in which targeted neonatal screening should concern itself with detecting bilateral ≥ 50 dB HL impairments, further surveillance or screening in the first year of life should try to detect bilateral ≥ 40 dB HL impairments and school screens should try to detect unilateral and bilateral ≥ 30 dB HL impairments and other children with a suspected hearing disability. Opportunistic case finding should be concerned with any hearing problem that is contributing or potentially contributing to hearing disability and/or delayed development of skills depending on auditory input.

The final paragraph that we agreed in the previous edition of this book is worth repeating, while bearing these targets in mind (my brackets [ ]):

...A combination of several methods may prove the optimal [neonatal] screening package, though it remains to be shown whether the gain from any combination is worth the extra complexity. In the meantime, the infra-structure (personnel, equipment, liaison [database]) for a screening pro-gramme can be set up, with particular emphasis being placed on the ability to evaluate the system once it is up and running. Initially resources will have to be highly focused ... then gradually increasing the coverage of the pro-gramme and investing in new equipment [and techniques] when it has been adequately evaluated. The effort involved in the initial emphasis will not be lost when the coverage is widened ...(p. 14)

At present, as detailed elsewhere in this book, the technology exists to implement neonatal screening. The logical first step in substantially reducing the age of identification of hearing impairments is through targeted neonatal screening for children with history of NICU treatment, family history of congenital hearing impairments and children with craniofacial abnormalities. The method and protocol are still under debate for this population. The most sensitive method would be to use otoacoustic emissions and screening ABR, but if time is of the essence either otoacoustic emissions with conditional screening ABR for the emission failures or screening ABR alone would be reasonable first steps in organizing such a service.

The NIH consensus meeting (NIH, 1993) recommended that :

- '... *all* [my emphasis] hearing impaired infants should be identified and treatment initiated by 6 months of age. In order to achieve this objective, the panel recommends universal screening for hearing impairment prior to 3 months of age.'
- '... *all* new-borns, both high and low risk, should be screened for hearing impairment prior to hospital discharge.'
- '... Because 20–30% of hearing impaired infants will acquire their hearing loss during early childhood, universal neonatal screening is not a replacement for ongoing surveillance throughout infancy and early childhood.'
- '... School entry screening will continue to provide a final opportunity for universal identification of children with significant hearing loss.'

It is clear that the consensus meeting had the same problems identified in this chapter of defining which children need to be found (i.e. could benefit from detection). The median age of identification in the USA was guessed to be about 3 years of age (NIH, 1993), and the public health organization in that country is different from that in the UK. Nevertheless, there is no doubt that this consensus will add to the voice for universal neonatal screening in the UK. The results of the planned trial of universal neonatal screening in the Wessex region (1993–96) should attempt to examine the benefits that universal neonatal screening might have in the UK public health system. In addition there are various professional and ad-hoc groups working on quality standards for early identification in England, Scotland and Wales that should provide a focus for individual districts in the next year or so.

As part of such standards, uniform collection of data is a necessity. A *minimum* data set as part of a screening programme is shown in

Appendix 1. This is compatible with the data collected in the Paediatric Audiology Record System (PARS) (Davis et al. 1988; Marshall et al., 1992, 1993) and may be used as a stand-alone paper and pencil system or for incorporation in other standard hospital data bases. It is a minimum set for audit and local epidemiological purposes, and of course can and should perhaps be elaborated to include other aspects of interest, provided the aims in collecting the data are well defined.

Summary

I have tried to present a public health perspective to hearing impairments, emphasizing the need to integrate the approaches to minimizing the incidence of hearing impairment and the prevalence of hearing and other disability due to hearing impairment.

Screening for congenital hearing impairments and the development of good, well-defined information at all levels of the service are seen as playing an integral role in these approaches. A key element that would help this development would be the implementation of the recommendation that 'one person should take on the responsibilities for co-ordinating the programme of hearing screening' (Hall, 1991).

The prevalence of hearing impairment, at the age of about 3 years, appeared to be consistent in the UK over a number of years for bilateral impairments of 80 dB HL or greater, at about 1 in 2000 births. However, for impairments of lesser degrees of severity the data are not as uniform.

The major risk groupings of history of NICU treatment, family history of congenital hearing problem and craniofacial abnormality account for about two-thirds of hearing-impaired children in three areas of the UK. This does not generalize to Copenhagen, and it may not do so to other districts of the UK.

The median age of identification in three areas of the UK, for cohorts between 1983 and 1988, was about 12 months, with an upper quartile of 21 months.

Substantial inroads need to be made, as a matter of very high priority, into the benefits (including economic) of early detection of congenital hearing impairments at different degrees of severity and from the above three risk groups.

The pressure to implement universal neonatal screening may increase in the UK, because of the NIH consensus in the USA. However, such change should be preceded by proper evaluation in the UK context and a development of the paediatric audiology infrastructure.

The priorities of the audiological health systems in the UK should take account not only of availability of future new technology (e.g. smaller implants, automated otoacoustic emission systems) but also of the public health context into which it is proposed these developments are placed.

Acknowledgements

Thanks are due to Agnete Parving, Sandra Rowe, Tina Ramkalawan, Jane Sancho, Hilary Webb and Sally Wood for extensive help with the provision of some of the data analysed, re-analysed and discussed in this chapter, to Heather Fortnum in helping formulate Appendix 1 (page 40) and to Kathryn Southworth for comments on a previous draft of the chapter.

Glossary

Public health perspective

The key elements of a public health perspective are the efforts of society to protect, promote and restore individual health, e.g. The Health of the Nation programme contains many of these elements with a goal of preventing disease and reducing disability to increase the quality of life for all people in the UK (unfortunately, the key issue here of auditory health promotion was not a high priority in this programme but as the appropriate needs assessment emerges in the UK through the epidemiology of childhood hearing impairment and disability that priority may change).

Epidemiology

The study of the distribution and determinants of hearing disorders in populations, and the application of this knowledge to prioritise the different types of hearing disorders.

Prevalence (PR)

The proportion (or number) of individuals with a defined level and type of hearing impairment in a specified population cohort (e.g. 3–5 year olds).

Incidence

The number of new instances of a defined level and type of hearing impairment occurring during a given period in a specified population.

Health promotion

The process of enabling people to have more control over and to increase their health. This is achieved through health education, disease prevention and health protection.

Child health surveillance

This is synonymous with secondary prevention, i.e. reduction of prevalence of disease and disability. It involves early detection and intervention through a variety of means, including opportunistic case finding, screening and incorporation of concern about hearing into systematic reviews of a child's development.

Screening

A rapid process that identifies, in a defined population, a subgroup with a high probability of having a hearing impairment or disability. This subgroup is then referred for further assessment.

Target group

The subgroup of the population with a defined level (e.g. 50 dB HL) and type (e.g. congenital sensorineural/mixed) of hearing impairment (or disability) that is the subject of a screening programme.

Sensitivity

The percentage (or proportion S) of all those in a pre-defined target group who are detected by the screening process.

Coverage

The proportion of the defined population who are tested. Coverage has two elements:

- the actual proportion of the defined population tested (C_t); and
- the proportion of tested children with a definitive test result (C_r).

Most protocols would treat the second element as a test fail and hence the *programme sensitivity* would be:

$$C_t \times s$$

Programme sensitivity has to be calculated over a long enough period, and with a long enough delay, to make the results meaningful – usually a 5-year period with a 5-year delay for a typical district.

Specificity

The proportion (P) of all individuals defined as unimpaired who correctly pass the screening process.

Positive predictive value (PPV)

The proportion of those failing a screening test who are actually hearing impaired. The additional diagnostic cost of screening programme is directly related to the PPV and the prevalence:

$$\text{Cost } \alpha \text{ PR} \times \text{PPV.}$$

Yield

The proportion of the defined population who are in the target group that have been detected by the screening programme.

Actual incremental yield

The marginal yield of individual parts of the surveillance programme, e.g. neonatal screening, parental concern, health visitor screening, school screening.

Quality standards in early identification

A shared protocol that sets targets for different process and outcome components of a hearing surveillance programme. The elements of the programme might be wide ranging, e.g. coverage, training of personnel, methods used for screening. Such targets might include:

- appointment of individual responsible for hearing screening (at district level);
- appointment of a hearing screening audit team (at a regional level);
- an annual level of coverage (e.g. 95%) of the defined population by the screen; the annual false alarm rate (e.g. less than 7%) of the screen;
- average (e.g. over 5 years for a district) yield of the programme;
- average upper quartile of the age of confirmation of hearing impairment (e.g. below 15 months, over a 5-year period for a district);
- cost per screen attempted;
- average time from referral to confirmation of diagnosis;
- average annual proportion of congenitally hearing-impaired children and their families who accept genetic counselling;
- average annual proportion of congenitally hearing-impaired children with 'unknown' aetiology.

Audit

The routine use of process and outcome indicators to evaluate the effectiveness of a programme and the efficiency with which that degree of effectiveness is achieved, taking into account both clinical and public health objectives and the need to acquire an appropriate local epidemiology of childhood hearing impairments.

Pathology

A disease state or structural disorder of the hearing organ, which can in principle be observed, e.g. damage to cochlea, damage to auditory nerve, abnormality of the middle ear or outer ear.

Impairment

An abnormal function of the auditory system, e.g. decreased auditory sensitivity, binaural integration, ability to resolve different sound frequencies with respect to population norms. The most commonly used measure is threshold of hearing measured in dB HL, by an approved method of pure tone audiometry. However, in very young children the threshold is derived from an electrical response to a click stimulus and is measured in dBn HL. (See Chapters 6 and 7 for a discussion of these techniques.)

Disability

The reduced ability of an individual in tasks that require an auditory input (e.g. correct orientation to sounds, perception of speech in quiet, perception of speech in competition with other noise, ability to communicate effectively with other people). Auditory disability in very young (under 1 year) and young children is difficult to define and more difficult to measure. It is suggested that the definition of disability is enlarged to include the effect of hearing impairment on developmental processes necessary for the acquisition of language, speech and communicative competence, that normally require some form of auditory input.

Handicap

The adverse effect of hearing disability on the quality of life of an individual or family unit. This would include such aspects as lack of educational opportunity, additional societal and individual effort needed to support 'normal' educational activities and targets, the lack of social and emotional development, constraints on leisure activities, the interaction of hearing disability with other specific handicaps and the 'constraints' on future employment and financial security.

References

Brookhouser, P.E. (1993). Incidence/Prevalence. In: *NIH Consensus Development Conference on Early Identification of Hearing Impairment in Infants and Young Children*. Bethesda, MD: National Institute of Health, pp.27–36.

Butler, N.R. and Golding, J. (1986). *From Birth to Five*. Oxford: Pergamon Press.

Cochrane, A. (1964). *Effectiveness and Efficiency: Random Reflections on Health Services*. Nuffield Provincial Hospitals Trust.

Cochrane, A. and Holland, W.W. (1969). Validation of screening procedures. *British Medical Bulletin* 27, 3–8.

Das, V.K. (1988). Aetiology of bilateral sensori-neural deafness in children. In: Barajas, J.J. and Borg, E. (Eds), *Overview and evaluation of the hearing-impaired child: Imaging and audiology. Scandinavian Audiology Supplementum* 30.

Davidson, J., Hyde, M.L. and Alberti, P.W. (1989). Epidemiologic patterns in childhood hearing loss: a review. *International Journal of Pediatric Otorhinolaryngology* 17, 239–266.

Davis, A.C. (1983). Hearing disorders in the population: first phase findings of the MRC National Study of Hearing. In: Lutman, M.E. and Haggard, M.P. (Eds), *Hearing Science and Hearing Disorders*. London: Academic Press, pp. 35–60.

Davis, A.C. (1987). Epidemiology of hearing disorders. In: Stephens, S.D.G. (ed.), *Scott-Brown's Otolaryngology* 5th edn, Vol. 2, *Adult Audiology*. London: Butterworth, pp. 90–126.

Davis, A.C. (1989). The prevalence of hearing impairment and reported hearing disability among adults in Great Britain. *International Journal of Epidemiology* 18, 911–917.

Davis, A.C. (1993). The prevalence of deafness. In: Ballantyne, J., Martin, J.A. and Martin, A. (Eds), *Deafness*. London: Whurr, pp. 1–11.

Davis, A.C. and Wood, S. (1992). The epidemiology of childhood hearing impairment: factors relevant to planning of services. *British Journal of Audiology* 26, 77–91.

Davis, A.C., Wood, S., Webb, H. and Rowe, S. (1993). Risk factors for childhood hearing disorders. *Journal of the American Audiological Association* (in press).

Davis, A.C., Haggard, M.P., Sancho, J., Marshall, D., Hughes, E. and Wood, S. (1988). Standardised paediatric audiology records. IHR internal report Series A No 6.

Dias, O. (1990). Surdez Infantil: Estudo Clinico e Epidemiologico. Lisboa University MD thesis.

Doyal, L. and Gough, I.(1991). *A Theory of Human Need*. London: Macmillan.

Feinmesser, M., Tell, L. and Levi, H. (1986). Etiology of childhood deafness with reference to the group of unknown cause. *Audiology* 25, 65–69.

Fortnum, H. (1992). Hearing impairment after bacterial meningitis: a review. *Archives of Disease in Childhood* 67, 1128–1133.

Fortnum, H. and Davis, A.C. (1993a). Epidemiology of bacterial meningitis. *Archives of Disease in Childhood* 68, 763–767.

Fortnum, H. and Davis, A.C. (1993b). Hearing impairment in children after bacterial meningitis: incidence and resource implications. *British Journal of Audiology* 27(1), 43–52.

Fraser, G. (1987). The genetics of deafness. In: Evans, J.N.G. (Ed), *Scott-Brown's Otolaryngology* 5th edn, Vol. 6, *Paediatric Otolaryngology*, pp. 26–34. London: Butterworth

Gerber, S. (1990). *Prevention: The Etiology of Communicative Disorders in Children*. New Jersey: Prentice Hall.

Haggard, M.P. (1992). Screening children's hearing. *British Journal of Audiology* **26**, 209–215.

Haggard, M.P. and Hughes, E. (1991). *Screening Children's Hearing*. London: HMSO.

Hall, D.M.B. (1991). *Health for All Children*, 2nd edn. Oxford: OUP.

Health of the Nation (1992). London: HMSO.

Johnson, A. and Ashurst, H. (1990). Screening for sensorineural hearing loss by health visitors. *Archives of Disease in Childhood* **65**, 841–845.

Joint Committee on Infant Hearing (JCIH) (1991). 1990 Position Statement. *ASHA* **33**, 3–6.

Kankkunen, A. (1982). Preschool children with impaired hearing. *Acta Otolaryngologica Supplementum* **391**, 1–124.

Lalande, N.M., Hetu, R. and Lambert, J. (1986). Is occupational noise exposure during pregnancy a risk factor of damage to the auditory system of the fetus? *American Journal of Industrial Medicine* **10**, 427–435.

Levitt, H., McGarr, N. and Geffner, D. (1987). Development of language and communication in hearing-impaired children. *ASHA Monographs* **26**, 9–24.

Majumder, P.P., Ramesh, A. and Chinnapan, D. (1989). On the genetics of prelingual deafness. *American Journal of Human Genetics* **44**, 86–99.

Markides, A. (1986). Age at fitting hearing aids and speech intelligibility. *British Journal of Audiology* **20**, 165–168.

Marshall, D.H., Fortnum, H., Davis, A.C. and Haggard, M. (1992). *The IHR Paediatric Audiology Record System (PARS)*. Gravesend, Kent: Public Sector Software.

Marshall, D., Fortnum, H., Davis, A.C. and Haggard, M. (1993). *Paediatric Audiology Records System (PARS) Manual*. IHR Internal report Series A No 12

Martin, J.A.M. (1982). Aetiological factors relating to childhood deafness in the European Community. *Audiology* **21**, 149–158.

Martin, J.A.M., Hennebert, D., Bentzen, O., Morgon, A., Holm, C., McCullen, O., Iurato, S., Meyer, L. de Jonge, G.A., Colley, J.R.T. and Moore, W.J. (1979). *Childhood Deafness in the European Community*. Brussels: Commission of the European Communities.

Mauk, G.W. and Behrens, T.R. (1993). Historical, political, and technological context associated with early identification of hearing loss. *Seminars in Hearing* **14**, 1–17.

Mauk, G.W., White, K.R., Mortensen, L.B. and Behrens, T.R. (1991). The effectiveness of screening programmes based on high-risk characteristics in early identification of hearing impairment. *Ear and Hearing* **12**, 312–319.

Miller, E. (1991). Rubella in the United Kingdom. *Epidemiology and Infection* **107**, 31–42.

Morton, N.M. (1991). Genetic epidemiology of hearing impairment. *Annals of the New York Academy of Science* **630**, 16–31.

National Health Service and Community Care Act 1990. London: HMSO.

Newton, V.E. (1985). Aetiology of bilateral sensori-neural hearing loss in young children. *Journal of Laryngology and Otology* Supplement 10.

NIH (1993). *Early Identification of Hearing Impairment in Infants and Young Children*. Bethesda: National Institutes of Health.

Parving, A. (1983). Epidemiology of hearing loss and aetiological diagnosis of hearing impairment in children. *International Journal of Pediatric*

Otorhinolaryngology **5**, 151–165.

Parving, A. (1988). Hearing disabled children: epidemiology and identification. *Scandinavian Audiology* **30**, 21–23.

Parving, A. (1993). Congenital hearing disability – epidemiology and identification. *International Journal of Pediatric Otorhinolaryngology* (in press).

Peckham, C. (1986). Hearing impairments in childhood. *British Medical Bulletin* **42**, 145–149.

Pujol, R., Lavigne Rebillard, M. and Uziel, A. (1991). The development of the human cochlea. *Acta Otolaryngologica Supplementum* **482**, 7–13.

Ramkalawan, T. and Davis, A.C. (1992). The effects of hearing loss and age of intervention on some language metrics in a population of young hearing-impaired children. *British Journal of Audiology* **26**, 97–107.

Ruben, R.J., Levine, R., Fishman, G., Baldinger, E., Feldman W. et al. (1982). Moderate to severe sensorineural hearing-impaired child: analysis of etiology, intervention and outcome. *Laryngoscope* **92**, 38–48.

Sancho, J., Hughes, E., Davis, A. and Haggard, M. (1988). Epidemiological basis for screening hearing. In: McCormick, B. (Ed.), *Paediatric Audiology 0–5 years*. London: Taylor and Francis.

Schein, J. and Delk, M.T. (1974). *The Deaf Population of the United States*. Maryland: National Association of the Deaf.

Sheridan, M. (1972). Reported incidence of hearing loss in children of seven years. *Development Medicine and Child Neurology* **14**, 296–303.

Stevens, A. (1991). *Assessing Health Care Needs*. London: NHS Management Executive.

Taylor, I. (1980). The prevention of sensorineural deafness. *Journal of Laryngology and Otology* **94**, 1327–1343.

Upfold, L. and Isepy, J. (1982). Childhood deafness in Australia: incidence and maternal rubella 1949–1980. *Medical Journal of Australia* **2**, 323–326.

Watkin, P.M., Baldwin, M. and Laoide, S. (1991). Parental suspicion and identification of hearing impairment. *Archives of Disease in Childhood* **65**, 846–850.

Watkin, P.M., Baldwin, M. and McEnery, G. (1991). Neonatal at-risk screening and the identification of deafness. *Archives of Disease in Childhood* **66**, 1130–1135.

Welsh Office (1991). *Report of the working party for a protocol for the investigation of hearing loss in children in Wales*. Cardiff: Welsh Office.

White, S. and White, R. (1987). The effects of hearing status of the family and the age of intervention on receptive and expressive oral language skills in hearing impaired infants. In: Levitt, H., McGarr, N. and Geffner, D. (Eds), *Development of Language and Communication in Hearing-impaired Children, ASHA monographs* **26**, 9–24.

Williamson, I. and Steel, K. (1990). The aetiology of hearing impairment. *Hereditary Deafness Newsletter* **5**, 7–15.

Wilson, J.M.G. and Jungner, G. (1968). *Principles and Practice of Screening for Disease*. Public Health Papers No 34. Geneva: WHO.

Appendix 1 NEONATAL HEARING SCREENING DATA RECORD

Biographical data

Name _____ DOB _____ Sex _____

Serial number _____ Hospital / Körner number _____

Consultant code_____ GP code_____ HV code_____

District code _____ Region code _____ NICU history _____

Family history _____ Birthweight _____ gms_____ lbs oz Gestation _____wks

High risk factors _____ _____ _____ Syndrome _____

Test details   Test 1 - Date _____   Test 2 - Date _____

Reason/Tester   _____ / _____   _____ / _____

Left ear result   _____   _____

Right ear result   _____   _____

Method   _____   _____

Time taken   _____   _____

Screening level and scale   _____   _____

Onward referral to: Diagnostic ABR _____ Audiological scientist __ Genetic counsellor ____

                     Social worker _____ ENT _____ GP _____

                     Paediatrician_____ (S)CMO _____ Ophthalmologist_____

                     Other _____

Follow up (to be completed for all children with abnormal diagnostic ABR results)

Date of confirmation of hearing impairment: _____

Severity of hearing impairment   Left ear _____   Right ear _____

Type of hearing impairment   Left ear _____   Right ear _____

Hearing aid fitted_____

FIELD CHOICES

High risk factors:

1	None
2	Rubella
3	Meningitis
4	CMV
5	Jaundice
6	Respiratory problems
7	Asphyxia
8	Transfusion
9	Ototoxic drugs
10	Abnormal cranial scan
11	Cleft palate
12	Ear deformity
13	Cerebral palsy
14	Syndrome
15	Consanguinity
16	Other

Syndrome:

1	Wildervants syndrome
2	Downs syndrome
3	Mandibulo Facial Dysostosis [MFO]
4	Pierre-Robin syndrome [PRS]
5	Deafness Earpits syndrome [DES]
6	Alports syndrome [deafness with neuritis DNS]
7	Deafness with optic atrophy [DOA]
8	Pendreds syndrome
9	Jervell and Lange-Neilson syndrome
10	Usher syndrome
11	X-linked
12	Wardenbergs syndrome
13	CHARGE
14	Other

Reason for test:

1	Not done
2	Universal
3	SCBU
4	HR screen
5	Concern

Result:

1	No result
2	Refer
3	Doubtful
4	Pass

Method:

1	ARC6
2	ARC6 (E)
3	ARC8
4	POEMS
5	Other EOAE
6	ALGO
7	ABR (SM)
8	ABR
9	Other

Scale:

1	dBA
2	dBSPL
3	dBHL
4	dBnHL

Severity:

0	<20 dB HL
1	20-40 dB HL
2	41-70 dB HL
[2a	41-49 dB HL]
[2b	50-70 dB HL]
3	71-95 dB HL
4	96-120 dB HL
5	>120 dB HL

Type:

1	No conductive element
2	Conductive element (abnormal tympanogram)

Chapter 2
Otological considerations in the first 5 years of life

KEVIN P. GIBBIN

Introduction

Paediatric otology covers a wide field, requiring understanding of basic embryology and in particular organogenesis of the ear, post-natal anatomical development, otophysiology and, of course, a knowledge of developmental paediatrics. Similarly it is important to be aware that diseases of the ears need to be considered in relation to upper respiratory tract diseases and other abnormalities.

Although there are many parallels with and similarities to adult otological practice there are important differences; a simple but important example is the anatomy of the neonatal ear and facial nerve. The importance of a knowledge of otopathology, aetiology and pathogenesis of ear disorders cannot be too highly stressed although it needs to be realized that there are many opposing views in management, particularly for example in the case of secretory otitis, the single most common cause of deafness in children.

Although the otologist is clearly concerned with the medical management of deafness, many other facets of otology may also be of concern, including problems of vertigo, facial nerve pathology and cosmetic deformities of the outer ear. These topics will not be discussed in this chapter except where they may be of relevance to the problems of the child with a hearing loss: they form an important part of the knowledge required by the paediatric otologist none the less. Discussion of these topics may be found in a more generalized textbook of otology.

Embryological considerations

Paediatric otological interest starts in the early stages of fetal development, there being a number of factors that may adversely influence the development of the human ear.

The human ear develops from three separate sources: the *inner ear* is a neuro-ectodermal derivative developing from the otic placode, forming the auditory vesicle or otocyst. This subsequently develops into the membranous labyrinth, the semicircular canals being well developed by the sixth week. The cochlea begins to develop at this stage and at 4 months is almost in its adult form. The primitive otocyst carries with it a layer of mesoderm which subsequently differentiates into the otic capsule, initially cartilage and subsequently a bony capsule.

The *auricle* develops from the first visceral cleft, an ectodermal furrow between the first and second bronchial arches, the ear canal developing as an invagination from the same cleft. This ectodermal development takes place mainly between the sixth and fourteenth week of intrauterine development.

The *middle ear cleft*, comprising the eustachian tube, middle ear and mastoid antrum, develops from the tubotympanic recess, an outpouching of the first pharyngeal pouch. By the end of the second fetal month the eustachian tube may be identified; the ossicles may also be defined at this stage, developing from first and second branchial arch mesoderm. The mastoid antrum is present by the seventh month but the mastoid air cells do not develop until the end of fetal life.

Pre- and perinatal causes of deafness

From the above brief description of the embryology of the ear it may be seen that any interference with its development between approximately the sixth and fourteenth weeks may produce severe abnormalities of outer, middle or inner ears or all three components. Notable examples of such defects are caused, for example, by rubella and by teratogenic drugs, Thalidomide being the most notorious example, although quinine has also been reported as causing deafness when taken in pregnancy (Taylor, 1934; Schuknecht, 1974), as has chloroquine (Hart and Naunton, 1964). In addition to induced otological defects, abnormalities may be caused by hereditary developmental disorders, a prime example being Treacher Collins syndrome, an example of which is shown in Figure 2.1.

These developmental abnormalities may be placed in four separate groups:

- abnormalities of the pinna varying from minor degrees of malformation to total absence, the latter often associated with
- abnormal development/absence (aplasia) of the external auditory canal;
- abnormalities of the middle ear cleft, including ossicular abnormalities;
- inner ear defects.

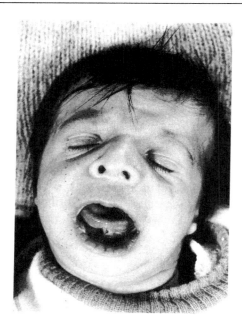

Figure 2.1 Treacher Collins syndrome.

Atresia or aplasia of the external or middle ear may be unilateral or bilateral and it is debatable whether surgery should be attempted in either case. If surgery is contemplated full radiological investigation is necessary, although there is a broad measure of agreement that the most severe forms of aural atresia should not be operated upon.

Intrauterine insult may result not only in abnormality of the external or middle ear but also in inner ear abnormalities and sensorineural hearing loss. However, over the past 10 years or so aetiological factors in these cases of congenital sensorineural deafness have changed. Before rubella immunization programmes, rubella was a relatively common cause of deafness (coupled with other manifestations of the rubella syndrome), with a reported incidence of 16% in 1969 in European countries (Minoli and Moro, 1985). In a recent survey carried out in Nottingham (Pabla, McCormick and Gibbin, 1991) of a total of 19 cases of both pre- and postnatally acquired sensorineural deafness, only one was deemed to be caused by rubella infection.

Other causes of prenatally acquired sensorineural deafness include infection with cytomegalovirus, a herpes virus. It causes characteristic large intranuclear inclusions in infected cells, evidence of the virus having been found in various inner ear structures including Reissner's membrane, stria vascularis, cells of the organ of Corti and neurons of the spiral ganglion (Stagno et al., 1977). Minoli and Moro (1985), in discussing the incidence of cytomegalovirus deafness, quote a 13% incidence of sensorineural deafness, often bilateral and severe, among the children with asymptomatic infection who constitute 95% of those with congenital cytomegalovirus infection; of those with clinical signs of cytomegalovirus 30% develop hearing loss.

Drug exposure in pregnancy has already been discussed but many drugs other than those mentioned above (including the aminoglucosides) may be toxic to the developing ear. In one case in the Nottingham series (Pabla et al., 1991) the deafness was considered to be due to maternal use of anticonvulsants during the pregnancy. Uziel (1985) has hypothesized that the last trimester of pregnancy and the neonatal period may represent a period of increased sensitivity to ototoxic antibiotics.

With increasing skill in resuscitating very small preterm babies, more of these children are found with severe sensorineural deafness; 11 of the 19 children with acquired sensorineural deafness in the Nottingham series had deafness thought to be caused by prematurity (four), hypoxia (four), jaundice (one) and fetal distress (two).

It may be that the sensorineural deafness develops as a result of a combination of factors in these cases; low birth weight may be associated with other factors such as traumatic delivery, neonatal asphyxia and hypoxia, and respiratory distress syndrome. Cochlear damage may also occur during acidosis (Despland and Galambos, 1980), and neonatal intracranial haemorrhage may also play a role. In addition to these factors it has been suggested that incubator noise may play a part in the development of sensorineural deafness in premature and low birth weight infants; it has been demonstrated in young animals that there are critical periods during which the cochlea is most vulnerable to acoustic trauma (Bock and Saunders, 1977); however, the evidence is somewhat equivocal.

Rhesus haemolytic disease is a rare cause for sensorineural deafness, following the introduction within the last 20 years of a programme of anti-D inoculation in cases of maternal–fetal rhesus incompatibility. The part played by hyperbilirubinaemia in full term healthy infants remains in doubt; however, hyperbilirubinaemia may coexist with hypoxia and neonatal sepsis in low birth weight infants and these babies are more at risk from the toxic effects of raised serum bilirubin.

This is no exhaustive reference list, and the reader is referred to Newton (1985) for details from a recent study of 111 cases in the Manchester area.

Table 2.1 summarizes and classifies the main pre- and perinatal causes of deafness, but can only be a superficial view of a wide-ranging subject. Fraser (1976) has discussed the various causes of profound deafness in childhood. There are many ways of sub-classifying aetiological factors in deafness and Fraser subdivides the causes as:

• deafness determined by mendelian inheritance;
• deafness as part of malformation syndrome not demonstrably

Table 2.1 Prenatal and perinatal causes of deafness

Genetic causes	Deafness without other defects Deafness associated with other abnormalities, such as Waardenburg's, Pendred's, Usher's, Klippel–Feil, Treacher Collins (conductive) Chromosomal abnormalities
Non-genetic causes	Prenatal: rubella, ototoxic/teratogenic drugs, pre-eclampsia/toxaemia, cytomegalovirus infection, chromosomal abnormalities Perinatal: prematurity, hypoxia/fetal distress, jaundice

    determined by simple mendelian inheritance;
* acquired deafness – pre-, peri- and postnatally acquired;
* 'unknown' causes.

Genetically determined deafness

Although deafness syndromes provide a convenient means of grouping defects, with the deafness either as a main feature of the syndrome or as an optional inclusion within the syndrome, it should be noted that many such syndromes have a genetic or chromosomal basis.

Developments in molecular biology and genetics have widened perspectives on childhood deafness and in a number of instances the gene locus for a particular deafness syndrome can now be identified.

Although all effort will be directed towards the habilitation or rehabilitation of a deaf child, the cause of the hearing loss needs to be identified. Single gene defects account for half of all childhood deafness and genetic investigation may therefore be an important part of the diagnostic protocol.

Autosomal dominant causes of deafness include Waardenburg's syndrome, osteogenesis imperfecta and Treacher Collins syndrome. *Autosomal recessive* causes include Usher's syndrome, Hurler's syndrome, osteopetrosis and Cockayne syndrome. *X-linked* causes include Alport's syndrome, albinism and deafness, Hunter's syndrome, Norries' syndrome, oto-palato-digital syndrome and mixed deafness syndrome.

Using techniques of gene localization by genetic linkage analysis, it is possible to identify the locus on the individual chromosomes of a specific gene; such techniques have dramatically improved the efficiency of linkage studies (Farrer, 1992).

With these developments, it is important that children with suspected genetic deafness should be referred to a clinical geneticist for assessment and for genetic counselling of the parents. Advice will need to be given to the child when he or she reaches reproductive age.

Genetic counselling of a family is not to be seen solely as a means of preventing the birth of further children to those parents but as a means of explaining the cause of the deafness, alleviating guilt feelings and helping parents develop positive avenues for beginning to cope with and live with deafness in the family.

Deafness syndromes

Many of the deafness–malformation syndromes have a genetic basis, but not all do so and any method of classifying the syndromes should recognize these. A convenient method of grouping the syndromes is by association with defects in other systems or parts of the body, such as:

- deafness associated with skeletal/craniofacial abnormalities;
- deafness associated with neurological disorders;
- deafness associated with ectodermal/pigmentary abnormalities;
- deafness associated with ophthalmological disorders;
- chromosomal abnormalities;
- deafness associated with metabolic/endocrine/renal disorders;
- deafness associated with other miscellaneous anomalies.

The following section lists many of the more commonly seen deafness syndromes, but is not exhaustive and the reader is referred to one of the major texts on the subject such as Gorlin and Pindborg (1964), Fraser (1976), Northern and Downs (1978) and Bluestone and Stool (1983).

Deafness associated with skeletal/craniofacial abnormalities

Absence of tibia

This is a recessive, severe sensorineural deafness associated with absence of one or both tibias.

Achondroplasia

Achondroplasia is a dominant/fresh mutation causing a conductive or sensorineural loss. The syndrome typically is associated with a skeletal abnormality with poor growth of cartilaginous bone but normal periosteal bone. Hydrocephalus may occur and deafness may be present. Many cases are due to fresh mutation.

Acrocephalosyndactyly (Apert's syndrome)

Defects include craniofacial dysostosis, syndactyly, brachycephaly, hypertelorism, proptosis, saddle-nose and spina bifida. The facial appearances are characteristic.

Crouzon's syndrome

This is a dominant syndrome, causing mixed hearing loss. Typically there is central prominence of the forehead with abnormal fusion of skull sutures. Ears may be low set and there may be many middle ear anomalies.

Cervico-oculo-acoustic dysplasia (Klippel–Feil syndrome)

This condition involves fusion of some or all of the cervical vertebrae, producing a very short neck (as seen in Figure 2.2). Both inner and middle ear anomalies may be present and recurrent meningitis has been described in association with this (Richards and Gibbin, 1977).

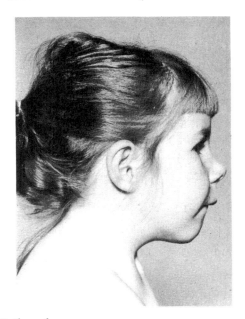

Figure 2.2 Klippel–Feil syndrome.

Cleft palate and lip (conductive deafness)

This is one of the most common of the deafness syndromes and results in secretary otitis secondary to the myopalatal anomalies.

Moebius' syndrome

This is a recessive sensorineural or conductive deafness. The most common feature of this syndrome is the bilateral facial palsy but there may be other abnormalities.

Osteogenesis imperfecta

An autosomal dominant condition, typically a conductive loss. Deafness is thought to be due to otosclerotic changes in the stapedial footplate and there is a high incidence of infant death associated with the syndrome due to recurrent bone fractures.

Goldenhar's syndrome (oculo-auriculo-vertebral dysplasia)

The aetiology of this syndrome is unknown. It is a conductive hearing loss associated with microtia/atresia of the external auditory canal. There is unilateral facial hypoplasia, extraocular muscle defects and musculoskeletal abnormalities may be present (Figure 2.3).

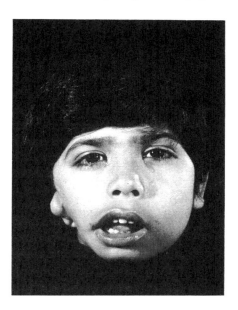

Figure 2.3 Goldenhar's syndrome.

Osteopetrosis (Albers–Schoenberg disease)

This recessive syndrome is characterized by a progressive sensorineural or conductive hearing loss. Classically these children have very thickened cortices to the long bones with growth retardation. Despite their thickness, the bones are paradoxically rather brittle.

Pierre Robin syndrome

A dominant, congenital, conductive and also sensorineural hearing loss. The typical findings of Pierre Robin syndrome include cleft palate, recessed lower jaw and chin. Other abnormalities have been reported in association with this condition.

Treacher Collins syndrome (mandibular dysostosis or first arch syndrome)

This is an autosomal dominant condition (Figure 2.1). The features classically include hypoplastic malae, anti-mongoloid palpebral fissures, notching of the lower eyelids, abnormal pinnae (often low set and with steeply sloping external auditory meati), receding chin. Deafness is usually conductive and may be associated with total aplasia of the external ear and ear canal.

Deafness associated with neurological disorders

Cerebral palsy

This accounts for the largest group of neurological conditions associated with deafness, usually a mild to moderate sensorineural loss. The syndrome is characterized by spasticity, abnormal limb movements and mental handicap. It is caused by brain damage occurring during fetal or early infant life.

Cockayne syndrome

A recessive autosomal condition causing progressive deafness and growth and mental handicap in early childhood.

Severe infantile muscular dystrophy

Another autosomal recessive condition in which mild to moderate high tone is associated with typical muscle wasting.

Deafness associated with ectodermal or pigmentary anomalies

Ectodermal dysplasia

This condition is inherited by dominant transmission with poor penetrance and variable expressivity. It is characterized by progressive sensorineural or conductive hearing loss, lobster claw deformity of hands and feet, cleft lip/palate and sometimes microcephaly.

Pili torti

A recessive condition in which severe sensorineural loss accompanies the typical picture of dry, brittle, twisted hair.

Piebaldedness

Piebaldedness may be recessive, dominant or X-linked, and is associated with sensorineural deafness.

Waardenburg's syndrome

This dominantly inherited condition is perhaps the best known of disorders of this group and involves mild to severe sensorineural deafness which may be unilateral or bilateral and may be progressive. Typical white forelock, white areas on eyebrows and eyelashes, heterochromia iridis are seen (Figure 2.4).

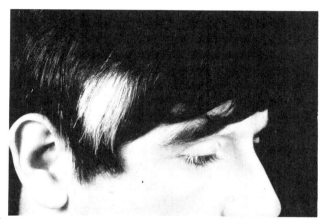

Figure 2.4 Waardenburg's syndrome.

Deafness associated with ophthalmological disorders

Duane's syndrome

A recessive severe sensorineural and/or conductive loss associated with the typical bilateral sixth cranial nerve (abducens) palsy. Other ear anomalies have been described.

Laurence–Moon–Biedl syndrome

This is a recessive progressive sensorineural loss associated with retinitis pigmentosa, mental handicap, hypogonadism and spastic paraplegia.

Refsum's syndrome

Recessive sensorineural deafness with delayed-onset blindness, ataxia, obesity, ichthyosis and polyneuritis.

Usher's syndrome

Recessive moderate-to-severe sensorineural loss. Blindness of delayed onset due to retinitis pigmentosa. There may be mental handicap, vertigo and epilepsy.

Chromosomal abnormalities

Down's syndrome (trisomy 21)

This is the most common of the chromosomal abnormalities causing deafness. Typical facial features with hyponasality and frequent or persistent upper respiratory tract disorders. Mental handicap is present but may appear worse than it is because of the associated hearing loss. Typical otological features include a very high incidence of secretory otitis, narrow hairy ear canals with dry scaling skin.

Long arm 18 deletion syndrome

This condition involves growth and mental impairment, microcephaly, malformation of pinnae and ear canals. It is typically associated with a conductive loss.

Trisomy 13–15

Microphthalmia, cleft lip and palate, often with mental handicap, microcephaly and seizures are associated with this condition. Both conductive and sensorineural loss may be found with abnormalities of ear canals, ossicles and inner ear.

Trisomy 18

This condition involves microcephaly and mental handicap; deformities of the ear may be present. Typically the hearing loss is profound.

Turner's syndrome

Turner's syndrome is associated with a sensorineural or conductive loss. The readily recognizable defects include webbed neck, webbing of digits, high arched palate, micrognathia.

Deafness associated with metabolic/endocrine/renal disorders

Alport's syndrome

An autosomal dominant condition, affecting men more severely than women. Progressive hereditary nephritis associated with progressive sensorineural deafness, starting in pre-adolescence.

Nephrosis and urinary tract malformations

Sex linked or recessive disorder comprising renal anomalies and conductive deafness.

Pendred's syndrome

A recessive profound deafness associated with goitre which in some cases may be noted at birth.

Renal genital syndrome

Recessive; renal and genital abnormalities, low set ears, aplastic external auditory canals and conductive deafness.

Miscellaneous

CHARGE syndrome

Congenital, non-hereditary defects – syndrome comprising *c*oloboma, *h*eart disease, *a*tretic nasal choanae, *r*etarded development, *g*enital hypoplasia and (external) *e*ar anomalies. Usually associated with sensorineural deafness.

Jervell and Lange–Nielsen syndrome

Recessive. Profound sensorineural deafness associated with electrocardiographic abnormalities. Death usually occurs in childhood.

Preauricular abnormalities

Dominant; conductive loss with preauricular pits, tags and sinuses.

Postnatal causes of sensorineural deafness

Table 2.2 lists the possible causes of post-natal sensorineural deafness; however, meningitis and mumps both remain prominent as important factors. It is very important that a detailed history is taken and that the child born with sensorineural deafness is thoroughly investigated; similarly an understanding of the development of the ear is needed.

Management of sensorineural deafness

The otologist is concerned not only with the diagnosis of the hearing loss but also with its management. It is essential that, in the case of the

Table 2.2 Postnatal causes of sensorineural deafness

Genetic causes	Familial sensorineural deafness Genetic deafness syndromes with delayed onset of hearing loss
Non-genetic causes	Meningitis Mumps (usually unilateral) Trauma Measles Ototoxic agents

severely deaf child, the management involves a closely knit team comprising otologist, paediatric audiological scientist, physiological measurement technician (audiology) and teacher of the deaf. If other defects are known or suspected early referral to a developmental paediatrician is indicated. If a genetic cause is known or suspected then the otologist should liaise with a clinical geneticist. Most important of all is close involvement of the parents in the management team. Hearing aid provision is a fundamental part of the management and is discussed in Chapters 10, 11 and 12.

The otologist plays an important role in diagnosis and treatment of sensorineural deafness, and in detecting and treating any conductive hearing loss found in these children. Children with sensorineural deafness have the same risk of developing secretory otitis, the most common cause of childhood deafness, as their otherwise normally hearing peers. The effect of a superimposed conductive hearing loss on a child with sensorineural deafness may reduce the benefit of even the most powerful hearing aid. It remains an individual decision when to take action to treat such a superimposed conductive hearing loss, but it is the author's view that such action should be taken promptly once the conductive component is diagnosed; a conductive loss of 30 dB in addition to, say, a sensorineural deafness of 90–100 dB is likely to cause very adverse effects.

In the UK the prevalence of severe or profound sensorineural deafness is 1–2 per 1000 (Davis and Wood, 1992); in a small number of children with profound sensorineural deafness, conventional amplification will be neither adequate nor appropriate and cochlear implantation may now be considered for these children. The detailed audiological criteria for cochlear implantation may vary from one centre to another but broad consensus agrees that the child should have had an adequate trial of suitable conventional amplification coupled with appropriate other support. In Nottingham the criteria for implantation include (hearing) aided responses to sound-field warble tones in excess of 70 dB(A) across the frequency range 500 Hz to 4 kHz.

In the UK children with congenital losses were not initially considered suitable for cochlear implantation but experience now suggests that this group of children may benefit greatly from an implant.

Benefits of cochlear implantation may be both primary and secondary (Mecklenburg, Demorest and Staller, 1991), including improved speech perception, enhanced lipreading skills, improved voice quality, improved speech production and increased phonological repertoire with improved single word receptive vocabulary. There may also be tertiary effects, with benefit to education and intellectual development and longer term employment prospects (Gibbin, 1992).

Middle ear pathology and conductive hearing loss

In numerical terms children with middle ear disorders present a larger problem from infancy through the early school years than that associated with sensorineural deafness, even though any associated hearing loss may be minor or fluctuant. The problem of middle ear disorders may be considered in two broad groups:

1. Non-suppurative otitis media (includes otitis media with effusion (OME), tympanosclerosis, atelectasis and adhesive otitis media).
2. Suppurative otitis media, which encompasses acute otitis media and chronic suppurative otitis media (CSOM), the latter usually being considered in two broad groups: tubotympanic disease, a 'benign' or safe mucosal disease and attico-antral disease, often associated with cholesteatoma and considered to be 'unsafe'.

Acute suppurative otitis media

In the UK acute suppurative otitis media (ASOM) is rarely seen in hospital practice unless complications supervene or the condition fails to resolve. Even so, it presents a considerable workload in general practice, with an overall episode rate of 27.6 per 1000 (Royal College of General Practitioners, 1986). The highest incidence is at 6–12 months of age with a second peak around the time of school entry (Brook and Burke, 1992). The majority of children (84%) have an acute otitis media at some time in early life (Brownlee, de Loach and Jackson, 1969).

ASOM typically occurs behind an intact tympanic membrane but can recur in children with a persistent perforation of the membrana tensa. The condition is characterized by an acute febrile illness with severe ear pain, frequently followed by an aural discharge. Treatment is usually by antibiotics, preferably a penicillin or erythromycin. Recent discussion has questioned whether antibiotics should be used at all (Mygind et al.,

1981; Van Buchem et al., 1981; Bain, 1990; Browning, 1990; Burke et al., 1991; Claessen et al., 1992). Some authors suggest that use of antibiotics in ASOM may predispose to chronic middle ear effusions.

The relationship between ASOM and otitis media with effusion will be discussed later. It is important to note that ASOM may occur in children of all ages including infants, when its diagnosis may be more difficult as it often presents in a more non-specific manner with pyrexia, malaise and vomiting. In these cases the diagnosis is made on otoscopy, the typical red bulging drum being easily visible.

Chronic suppurative otitis media

Chronic suppurative otitis media (CSOM) may be categorized as tubotympanic disease or attico-antral disease.

Tubotympanic disease

This is a condition in which the underlying pathology is a chronic mucositis of the middle ear, either ascending via the eustachian tube from upper respiratory tract sepsis producing a tubotympanitis, or associated with chronic mastoid infection or tympanomastoiditis. Examination of the child with a persistent mucoid or mucopurulent aural discharge will reveal a central tympanic perforation of variable size: classically, in tubotympanitis the perforation will be anterior in the membrana tensa and posterior in cases of tympanomastoiditis. Figure 2.5 shows the tympanic membrane and related middle ear structures.

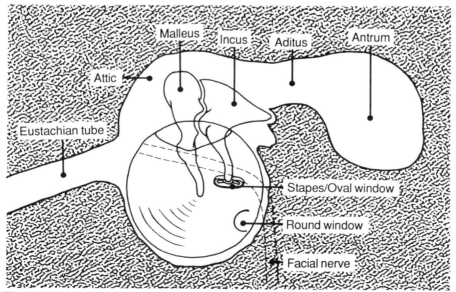

Figure 2.5 Diagrammatic representation of the anatomy of the middle ear.

Examination of the upper respiratory tract may show evidence of infective rhinitis, sinusitis or adenoiditis; tonsillitis is not considered to be a cause of acute or chronic suppurative otitis media.

Attico-antral disease

Attico-antral disease is associated with an attic defect, a perforation or retraction pocket in the membrana flaccida. It is usually associated with a scanty but offensive discharge from the ear from which can be cultured coliform bacteria and other Gram-negative organisms such as *Proteus* and *Pseudomonas spp.* Assessment of these children requires examination of the ear using an operating microscope and it is often necessary to undertake this under general anaesthesia in order to carry out adequate suction toilet. Essentially, the management of this condition is surgical, requiring formal exploration of the ear with the main aim of the operation being to secure a safe dry ear, conservation of hearing being of secondary importance.

The definitive operation in cases of established cholesteatoma, a collection of actively desquamating squamous epithelium within the middle ear cleft, is modified radical mastoidectomy in which the mastoid antrum and air cell system are exteriorized via the ear canal, the integrity of the middle ear space being maintained where necessary by use of temporalis fascial autograft to repair the defect in the tympanic membrane. Although in the adult cholesteatoma usually occurs in a sclerotic mastoid, paediatric cholesteatoma often presents in a well pneumatized temporal bone with consequent widespread bony involvement.

Both tubotympanic and attico-antral disease may produce a conductive hearing loss; in the event of a labyrinthine fistula, a more likely occurrence in attico-antral disease, sensorineural deafness may occur, coupled with a history of vertigo.

Management of the hearing loss in either form of CSOM is determined by the nature of the underlying disease process. Conductive deafness secondary to tubotympanic disease can be treated surgically, carrying out a tympanoplastic procedure, grafting the perforation and performing ossiculoplasty. However, the indications for this type of surgery in young children are debatable, those opposing such surgery in children under a certain age maintaining that surgical success rate and the likelihood of further ASOM with resultant re-perforation render it inappropriate. Recently, however, evidence has been presented showing that surgical reconstruction of ears in children is not contra-indicated on these grounds and that myringoplasty has a good chance of success irrespective of the patient's age.

It is fortunately uncommon for cholesteatoma to affect both ears in children, the other ear usually being normal; the child can therefore usually manage well both socially and developmentally without surgery or without the need for a hearing aid.

Otitis media with effusion

Incidence

OME is the single most common cause of deafness in childhood, occurring in children of all ages. Estimates of the prevalence of conductive deafness due to this vary widely with age and the method of diagnosis: OME may be seen in children under the age of 12 months. Tos et al. (1986) have carried out a study on the epidemiology and natural history of OME in three cohorts of Danish children using tympanometry as a basis for initial assessment. In their first cohort of children 60% of the 150 children tested at 12 months demonstrated abnormal tympanograms, 13% with flat, type B, traces (Jerger, 1972). At ages 2 and 3 years the prevalence varied from 7% to 19% and at ages 4 and 5 years from 11% to 18%. This study also confirmed the seasonal variation of the point prevalence of type B tympanograms, which was approximately 15% for the first year and 30% for the second, third, fourth and fifth years, spontaneous remission of type B being common in all age groups. Giebink, Le and Paparella (1982) have shown mucoid otitis media to be most prevalent in the 0–1 year age group. In a cross-sectional study Birch and Elbrond (1984) showed that of children aged 9 months to 7 years in day care centres the maximum proportion of bilateral type B tympanograms was found in 1 year olds. Van Cauwenberge (1986) has shown that 16% of apparently healthy preschool children aged 2;6–6 years had fluid in their ears (this figure possibly being higher because different diagnostic tools gave conflicting results). The highest percentage of OME was seen at the age of 2–3 years, with a gradual decrease with increasing age. This compares with Sade's (1979) view that a completely random sample would show the predominant age of occurrence to be 3–6 years.

Pestallozza has reported (Pestallozza, G., 1987, personal communication) that incidence of type B tympanometry decreases from 65% at 2 years to 25% or below at 5 years, stating also that attacks of ASOM are directly related to the frequency of OME and decrease from 36% at 2 years to 7% at 5 years. In the same presentation Pestallozza quoted an incidence of OME and ASOM of 30–67% in children under 12 months based on otoscopy, and 14–61% based on tympanometry.

Rach, Zielhuis and van den Broek (1986) have demonstrated that 39% of 1099 children examined were shown to have a middle ear effusion in at least one ear by tympanometry; 21% of the children had bilateral effusions. They also showed a marked seasonal effect, 39% of ears having a flat type B curve in winter which dropped to 24 % in summer, with a steady state in the number of C1 and C2 tympanograms.

It is very difficult to estimate the figures for prevalence and incidence of OME in different age groups because of seasonal, and possibly geographical and other, variations. However, there is compelling evidence that OME is widespread in children under the age of 5 years. Even if only a small percentage of the total numbers of children with OME need treatment there is still a major medical problem to be dealt with.

The question of whether OME is a modern phenomenon has been raised by Black (1984b). He stated that by the late 1970s glue ear had become the most common reason for childhood surgery in England and Wales, with similar changes occurring in the USA where it has been estimated that 1000 000 children are treated each year. Although OME has been recognised since the early 19th century (and possibly even before the seventeenth century), Black is unable to find references with details of incidence or prevalence of the condition. It is not possible to answer the question of whether the incidence of OME has increased in recent years or even whether there is a true increase in the condition. Fiellau-Nikolajsen et al. (1979) questioned whether, despite reports supporting an increased prevalence, there had been a *genuine* increase in the prevalence of the condition. Haggard et al. (1992) have shown that improved screening yields a large increase in the numbers of children failing the (7–9 months) screen who have abnormal hearing. They showed that screening and assessment can find a number of children in their first year having referable (to an otolaryngologist) middle ear disease corresponding to about 1.5% of the age cohort.

Aetiology and pathogenesis

It has been stated (Gibb, 1979) that malfunction of the eustachian tube is universally agreed to be the essential underlying cause. Undoubtedly eustachian dysfunction plays a role in the aetiology of this condition, but it is also undoubtedly true that the above statement is a major oversimplification of what is probably a multifactorial condition, the following possibly playing a part in the development of OME.

Eustachian dysfunction

This may reflect organic obstruction evidenced by the occurrence of serous otitis media in cases of nasopharyngeal carcinoma where direct invasion of the nasopharyngeal portion of the tube is likely. Although nasopharyngeal carcinoma is more commonly a disease of adults, cases are seen in childhood, some of these demonstrating unilateral middle ear effusions as in adults. Evidence for other purely mechanical causes may be found in the high incidence of OME in children with cleft palate, where there is limitation of the action of tensor palati muscle (Holborrow, 1962). Paradise, Bluestone and Felder (1969) found that virtually all infants under 20 months with cleft palate suffer from otitis media, frequently in its secretory form.

Bluestone and Beery (1976) discussed at length the pathogenesis of OME and suggested that there are two types of eustachian tube obstruction: mechanical and functional. They felt that nasal obstruction may also be involved in the pathogenesis of middle ear effusions; swallowing in the presence of nasal obstruction results in an initial positive phase and then a negative nasopharyngeal air pressure.

Another factor which may be relevant to the aetiology of OME in children is the relatively wider lumen and more horizontal course of the eustachian tube in infants and young children.

Adenoids

The vexed question of adenoid mass, tonsil mass, adenoiditis and tonsillitis in relation to OME continues to cause discussion. Many studies have been carried out in order to answer the many questions raised: for example, in a review of the literature Hibbert and Stell (1982) quoted 26 authors who blamed large adenoids for the presence of OME, but they found no difference between the size of the adenoids in a group of children admitted for adenoidectomy as part of the management of OME compared with an age and sex matched group, thus raising doubts as to the role of the adenoids as an aetiological factor of OME (Hibbert and Stell, 1982). This supported the view of Fiellau-Nikolajsen, Falbe-Hansen and Knudstrup (1980), who found no difference at 6 months between two groups in a controlled trial of adenoidectomy and myringotomy versus myringotomy alone in 3-year-old children. Sade (1979) came to a similar conclusion to Fiellau-Nikajsen, and in a 2-year controlled prospective study Widemar et al. (1985) drew the same conclusion. However, Maw (1983) has shown that adenoidectomy confers benefit in the management of such children, implying that the adenoids may have an aetiological role in the development of OME. This study showed clearly that no benefit was gained from tonsillectomy. Nieto, Calvo and Garcia (1983) came to a similar conclusion about the role of the adenoids, stating that increased prevalence of purulent rhinorrhoea in children with OME suggests an infective cause for this condition and it may well be that this is related to the size of the adenoid.

Elverland et al. (1981) reported on a series of 166 children followed up for 5 years; adenoidectomy was carried out in connection with the first insertion of grommets on the basis of recurrent symptoms of nasal obstruction and resulted in a significant reduction in the need for repeated insertion of tympanostomy tubes in patients younger than 8 years old. They suggest that, rather than the adenoids obstructing the nasopharyngeal lumen of the eustachian tube, effusions occur due to eustachian malfunction secondary to poor nasopharyngeal ventilation. Sniffing and swallowing in the presence of adenoidal enlargement may result in an involuntary Toynbee manoeuvre (Lamp, 1973). Elverland et al.'s suggestion may be relevant to children with Down's syndrome who have several possible factors predisposing them to OME, muscular hypotonia and upper airway sepsis possibly both contributing as aetiological and pathogenetic factors.

Other views on the part played by the adenoids are contained in a paper by Tuohimaa and Palva (1987), albeit in a slightly older age group. They showed that the size of the adenoids had an effect on preoperative intra-tympanic pressure. In children with large adenoids, the difference was highly significant. Tonsillectomy had no effect on intratympanic pressure. Collins et al. (1985) have suggested that the histamine content of adenoids is the important factor; children with bilateral OME were found to have increased amounts of histamine in their adenoid tissue compared to a group with no signs or symptoms of OME.

Another consideration is that the adenoids may act as a reservoir of infection; Ruokonen, Sandelin and Makinen (1979) showed significantly more positive cultures of *Haemophilus influenzae* and virus isolates in adenoid tissue removed from patients with middle ear effusions than in adenoids from patients with simple hypertrophy and no ear disease. This conflicts with the results of Maw and Speller's (1985) investigation which found no such differences in *Streptococcus pneumoniae* and *H. influenzae*. Osborne et al. (1987) have reported on a group of 69 children who underwent adenoidectomy, analysing the adenoid tissue bacteriologically for both type and amount of organism per gram of adenoid tissue: there was no significant difference between the four subgroups with symptoms of nasal obstruction, glue ear, recurrent probable otitis media and recurrent sore throats with probable tonsillitis.

Mills, Uttley and McIntyre (1985) drew a similar conclusion; they found no difference in the incidence of either *S. pneumoniae* or *H. influenzae* in the postnasal spaces of children who had had their adenoids removed and those who had not. They did, however, report positive middle ear cultures in chronic secretory otitis media, again *S. pneumoniae* and *H. influenzae* being the predominant pathogens, the *H. influenzae* serotype most commonly isolated being type e rather than type b.

Maxillary sinusitis was considered by Grote and Kuijpers (1980) as a possible factor in the aetiology and pathogenesis of OME in a combined retrospective and prospective study; they concluded that middle ear effusion is often associated with infective disease of the maxillary sinuses.

The discussion on the role of the adenoids becomes even more problematical in considering the aetiology and pathogenesis of OME in very young children when the adenoids are rarely enlarged, the adenoids reaching a peak size at about the age of 4 years.

Other factors

Numerous other aetiological factors have been postulated for OME:

- Allergic diatheses have been proposed and rejected by various authors, and Black (1985b) concluded that by 1981 most of the published research suggested that allergy was not usually responsible for glue ear; more recent work challenges that view.
- Overuse, abuse or misuse of antibiotics has also been held to be responsible, a view countered by an MRC report in 1957; it has been suggested that OME is a sequel to inadequately treated ASOM, resulting in persistent low grade mucosal disease (Gibb, 1979).
- Black (1985b) has provided a review of the causes of glue ear and includes hereditary factors in his list of causes. More recently, Rockley and Rhys Evans (1986) reported on a study of 73 children with persistent OME; in 66% of these children one or both parents had abnormalities of the tympanic membrane compared with 26% of non-affected cohorts, and they were able to exclude environmental influences in the study. Although findings point to a hereditary predisposing factor to middle ear disease, Rockley and Rhys-Evans could find no indications as to what that factor may be.
- Other factors that Black considered include social conditions, air pollution, socioeconomic status and family size and child care: Brooks (1969) was unable to find a difference in incidence of OME between children in an urban environment and a clean seaside resort; Harvey (1975) noted a high incidence of OME in areas of higher population density than areas of lower population density. Again, on the question of family size, Black quoted references with conflicting conclusions.
- Discussion has also centred on the role of smoking in OME: Kraemer et al. (1983) found that parental smoking increased the risk of OME fourfold; Pukander (1982) found no effect; Pukander et al. (1985) found a slight but not significant increase in risk for *acute* otitis media attributable to maternal smoking; in a study of salivary cotinine concentrations and OME in 7-year-old children, Strachan, Jarvis and Feyerabend (1989) noted that one-third of the cases studied were statistically attributable to exposure to tobacco smoke. However, Barr and Coatesworth (1991) felt that smoking was unlikely to be a risk factor for OME although it *may* have an association with the disorder.
- Mills and Brain (1985) confirmed a relationship between ASOM and OME (and also supported the conventional image of the child with OME as a mouth breather with nasal symptoms). Patients may be predisposed to develop ASOM by the possession of a chronic effusion; alternatively, incomplete resolution of ASOM may lead to the

development of OME. Teele, Klein and Rosner (1980) have shown that an effusion may persist for weeks to months following an episode of acute otitis media.

Summary

It seems probable that OME is a truly multifactorial condition, with eustachian tube function and anatomy as perhaps one of the more important factors; sepsis with related mucosal oedema may also be important. It seems probable that allergy may play only a minor role, if any.

Effects and clinical presentation of secretory otitis

The effects of OME may be usefully considered under two main headings:

1. Hearing loss.
2. Other otological sequelae.

Hearing loss

Sade (1979) has termed OME 'the silent syndrome'; the hearing threshold in cases of OME may vary from normal to about 50 dB, the average loss being about 28 dB (Cohen and Sade, 1982) (Figure 2.6). One of the major difficulties in assessing the hearing of any child with OME is the possibility of fluctuating auditory thresholds. Despite both otoscopic and tympanometric confirmation of persistence of the effusion it is unclear why the hearing varies with continuing presence of fluid in the middle ear. OME is the most common hearing disorder in children, the hearing loss being demonstrable in children of all ages using the appropriate testing techniques.

Deafness may present in a number of ways, in some instances determined by the age of the child. In infants, hearing loss may be suspected when the child fails the health visitor screening test, normally carried out between the ages of 6 and 9 months; the hearing loss is subsequently confirmed by further testing under properly controlled conditions.

At any age parental concern or doubt about a child's hearing should result in careful assessment. The parent may give a very clear history of the child not responding to sound, but there may be many instances of merely a lingering uncertainty as to the child's responsiveness to sound. The history may be more clear-cut for older children, as comparisons may be made within the family. The deafness may, however, present with a secondary symptom, again depending on the age of the

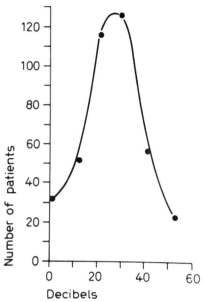

Figure 2.6 Distribution of degree of hearing impairment in SEM (from Sade, 1979).

child. Delay in speech and language development may be an important pointer to a hearing loss and such a history should lead to careful assessment. It is the author's view that before corrective speech therapy is undertaken with children with speech and language delay, hearing assessment should be carried out; it is important to note that, due to the evanescent nature of OME and to its variable effects on hearing, a child may pass a health visitor test despite the presence of fluid in their ears. Bamford and Saunders (1985) have discussed other reasons why children with OME may pass a hearing screening test, recording that as many as 60% of children with OME may not be detected by pure tone audiometry.

The effects of a conductive loss on speech and language development are documented in Chapter 3 and will not be repeated here, but in the author's experience many children with speech delay with a hearing loss due to secretory otitis show dramatic improvement once the loss is corrected by surgical treatment. The possible pitfalls and problems of failure to diagnose an early hearing loss are documented by a parent (Morton, 1987) in a letter to *The Guardian*. Another possible secondary effect of a fluctuating conductive loss is on the development of the necessary auditory strategies for speech perception, an effect that may be irreversible (Downs, 1977).

Hall and Hill (1986) postulate that five variables must be considered in assessing why OME can have a devastating effect on some children yet be of trivial importance to others:

1. the age at which the disorder occurs;
2. the duration of the episodes;
3. the severity of the loss;
4. intrinsic qualities in the child;
5. the child's environment.

Behavioural disturbances may indicate an underlying hearing difficulty, particularly if the hearing had been normal. Such disorders may include disobedience, apparent because the child does not hear an instruction or real because the child ignores the instruction (possibly as an attention-seeking device). Previously dry children may become enuretic; the child may become withdrawn or may show tantrums. Not *all* children with behavioural disturbances have a hearing loss, but deafness should be considered in the differential diagnosis of these children.

Other otological sequelae

Children with OME may have a history of other features which may point to the diagnosis as well as presenting with hearing loss.

Frequent attacks of ASOM

This relationship has already been discussed.

Earache

Children with OME experience bouts of mild earache quite frequently. These episodes may cause the child to become miserable, but the child is not unwell, not pyrexial and mild analgesia is usually sufficient to dispel the symptoms. These bouts are not to be confused with the severe pain of acute suppurative otitis media.

Vertigo

Sade (1979) has stated that he has never seen this in children, but Blayney and Colman (1984) reported a series of 27 children with vertigo, OME being a cause in five. In the author's experience a very small number of children with OME are late in walking but show immediate improvement once the effusions resolve or are drained. Jones et al. (1990) have shown that middle ear effusion has a significant effect on balance – ventilating the ear restored the balance to normal.

In addition to the conditions mentioned above, OME may produce other *otological* changes which can be assessed only by careful examination of the ear.

Atelectasis

This term signifies collapse of the tympanic membrane which may be localized to a particular area of the drum, or may be generalized and may vary from slight retraction of the tympanic membrane to its total collapse onto the promontory.

Adhesive otitis

This term is applied to the condition in which fibrous adhesions are present in the middle ear as a result of previous inflammation. It may be associated with atelectasis, but instead of being thinned the tympanic membrane is commonly thickened, dull in appearance and immobile.

Tympanosclerosis

Tympanosclerosis is a hyaline degeneration occurring within the submucosa of the middle ear and, although it is most easily seen in the drum itself, it may occur elsewhere in the middle ear. Calcification commonly occurs, producing 'chalk deposits'. The typical appearance is of an antero-inferior crescentic white appearance in the tympanic membrane; there may, however, be plaques elsewhere in the drum head. The net result may be a conductive hearing loss due either to loss of mobility of the drum or to fixation of the ossicular chain.

Cholesterol granuloma

In some instances the tympanic membrane may appear dark blue, the so-called idiopathic haemotympanum. The effusion in these cases is dark brown, often pearlescent. Idiopathic haemotympanum is often associated with cholesterol granuloma. Histologically, cholesterol crystals are deposited in the submucosa with a surrounding foreign body giant cell reaction.

Cholesteatoma

Deguine (1986) has concluded that as OME and cholesteatoma have essentially the same aetiological basis (eustachian tube dysfunction) they constitute evolutionary stages of the same disease, a view compatible with that of Tumarkin (1961). However, there are many other theories of the aetiology and pathogenesis of cholesteatoma. Tos (1981) has discussed the relationship between OME in childhood and chronic otitis in adults and has proposed that chronic middle ear disease results directly from OME in childhood.

Examination for OME

The following is a brief summary of the otologist's examination: full otological examination includes examination of the nose nasopharynx and oropharynx as well as an assessment of the child's general development; the presence of other abnormalities must be noted.

Examination of the ears of a young child is not always easy, but it is important to persevere because aural examination is an essential part of the assessment of the child. Abnormalities of the pinna and ear canal, the presence of accessory auricles and preauricular pits or sinuses should be noted. Visualization of the eardrum may show no abnormality in cases of sensorineural deafness but a sensorineural hearing loss does not preclude other otological abnormalities (and vice versa).

Otoscopy may be carried out using the electric auroscope or by using a head mirror. In both cases pneumatic otoscopy should be performed. When using the head mirror this is easily carried out using the Siegle speculum; in the case of the electric hand-held auroscope a separate rubber bulb may then be attached to a nipple on the auroscope itself. An important point often overlooked is the need to avoid hurting or frightening the child; holding the auroscope correctly will help reduce the risk. The auroscope should be held rather like a pen, using the right hand for the right ear and allowing the ulnar border of the hand to rest lightly against the side of the child's head. This ensures that in the event of the child moving suddenly the auroscope will also move and the speculum will not be driven into the child's ear. At the same time the free hand can be used to retract the pinna – posteriorly in the case of older children but inferiorly in the case of an infant – in order to help visualize the tympanic membrane.

The tympanic membrane should be inspected methodically, both the pars tensa and the attic part being carefully examined. If a perforation is present its site and size should be carefully detailed. The appearance in cases of secretory otitis may vary widely from almost normal to quite severe degrees of atelectasis and retraction, with or without the presence of tympanosclerosis. There is usually loss, or a breaking up, of the normal light reflex; the drum may be retracted, the handle of the malleus lying more horizontally than normal and the lateral process of the malleus being more prominent. The colour of the drum in this condition may vary from an almost normal pale pink/grey to yellow or even blue. It may occasionally be more pink in colour, which may lead the unsuspecting to diagnose acute suppurative otitis media. Air bubbles or fluid may be seen, although this is less common than widely supposed. Perhaps the most common appearance of the drum in secretory otitis media is of a dull, featureless, slightly retracted pars tensa. In these cases use of the pneumatic otoscope will be at its most advantageous, demonstrating reduced or absent mobility of the drum.

Assessment of the child with middle ear pathology includes full examination of the upper respiratory tract; although the adenoids reach a peak size typically at the age of 4 years adenoid hypertrophy may be seen in children of any age, even in infants of less than 1 year old.

After clinical examination the child's hearing is assessed and tympanometry carried out; although this is the more accepted method of operation it is not axiomatic and in the author's weekly clinic in the Nottingham Children's Hearing Assessment Centre the children have usually undergone audiological assessment before the medical consultation.

Treatment of OME

Three important topics need to be considered under this heading: 'Why?', 'When?' and 'How?'. It may perhaps be appropriate to consider the third question first as, although the heading 'Treatment of OME' implies surgical measures, this is not necessarily so and treatment can be considered in the non-surgical as well as the surgical domain.

Perhaps the single most important measure in the treatment of any child with a hearing loss is advice and counselling of the parents; in cases where a hearing loss is diagnosed, even where the parents were not previously aware of the child not hearing properly, the first step must be to appraise them of the condition and explain its possible effects. (This will often be the case where screening results in the onward referral of the child and subsequent diagnosis of hearing loss.) This then can be coupled with advice on what steps the parents can take. In the case of the child detected at 6–9 months old, he or she may be 12 months or older before being seen by an otologist. The parents should be reminded to speak very clearly when talking to their child, facing him or her, and to devote perhaps rather more time to the child than might have been the case with a normally hearing child. The parents can also be given an advice sheet as a more lasting reminder of the measures they should implement. In the case of a slightly older child at nursery school, it is important that the care assistants or teachers are aware of the child's deafness in order to take appropriate measures; again this should be coupled with provision of an advice sheet. It may be helpful for the parents to enquire regularly as to whether the hearing loss is causing any difficulties, such an inquiry being a tactful reminder of the child's hearing loss to those at the nursery.

In discussing other modalities of treatment of OME two considerations apply:

1. Treatment of the hearing loss.
2. Treatment of other sequelae or aspects of OME, such as atelectasis, earache.

Audiological assessment is important in establishing the child's level of hearing, but no two children will experience the same degree of disability or handicap from a given audiometric pure tone threshold – therefore other factors need to be considered. Parental questioning needs to be relevant to the age of the child, for example, a child of 2 years who has no more than a few words of vocabulary with poor pronunciation may be considered in need of active management. Other features already indicated when discussing clinical presentation may point towards a need for medical intervention – for example, disobedience or behavioural disturbance as well as very obvious communication difficulties. In the assessment, a guide to the ability of the slightly older child to discriminate may be seen in the results of the McCormick Toy Discrimination Test, which is also a useful means of demonstrating to the parents an aspect of the child's disability.

In answering the question 'When?' perhaps the single most important point is to note the need of avoiding early surgical treatment in view of the high spontaneous resolution rate (Buckley and Hinton, 1991; Shah, 1991; Effective Health Care Bulletin, 1992; De Melker, 1993).

Non-surgical treatment may include oral or nasal decongestants, mucolytics and antibiotics. A survey by Cherry (1986) showed that 80% of a group of otolaryngologists surveyed used some form of conservative medical treatment; of these over 80% used oral decongestants, two-thirds used topical nasal decongestants and just over half used mucolytics. Antibacterial treatment was used by 40%.

Published work suggests that for established effusions decongestant therapy has little benefit (Fraser, Mehta and Fraser, 1977). Conflicting efficacy of mucolytics may be seen in several published studies quoted by Cherry. Marks, Mills and Shaheen (1981) found cotrimoxazole to be effective in 64% of children with OME, although the relapse rate was high with a net cure rate of 28% after 1 year (Marks, Mills and Shaheen, 1983). Rosenfeld and Post (1992) have concluded in a meta-analysis that antibiotics have a clinically and statistically significant impact on resolution of OME. In the light of the present evidence it seems reasonable and logical to undertake a trial of antibacterial therapy using cotrimoxazole in children with a history of OME of relatively recent onset, perhaps using oral decongestant therapy for those children who experience deafness and other symptoms of OME only with coryzal infections.

Choice of surgical treatment is a minefield and is the subject of much individual bias (Smith and Maw, 1991); an attempt at meta-analysis proved impossible due to the heterogeneity of the trials reviewed (Bodner et al., 1991). Stephenson and Haggard (1992) have discussed the design of surgical trials for OME. An increased rate of surgery since 1974 (Black, 1984a) has been shown and Black (1985a) has also demonstrated geographical variation in the use of surgery within the UK and between England and Wales and the USA. Most trials of surgical treatment for OME have centred around children of early school age, none specifically addressing the question of the very young child. Surgery is most often performed in children of 5–8 years, when ear effusions tend to improve anyway (Drug and Therapeutics Bulletin, 1986a).

In Nottingham a total of 494 children under the age of 5 years received surgery for middle ear effusions in 1985, a surgical rate of 10.26 per 100 otolaryngological catchment population. This is less than in other major departments within the Trent Region, Trent having lower surgical treatment rates for otitis media and mastoidectomy than the average for England and Wales (University of Leeds, 1992). The Nottingham rate has increased from 1.75 in 1979, reflecting increasing diagnosis of the condition; the Nottingham Children's Hearing Assessment Centre (CHAC) opened in 1981. In an early series of 2000 children from CHAC (McCormick et al., 1984), 322 (16%) were referred for an otological opinion and of these 130 (6.5% of the whole group) were listed for surgery; 24 of these were under the age of 2 years.

Surgical treatment includes myringotomy (in which the eardrum is incised and the fluid aspirated by suction, with or without insertion of a ventilation tube) and adenoidectomy (either alone or combined with one or other of the above procedures).

The role of the adenoids in the aetiology and pathogenesis of OME has already been discussed. The role of adenoidectomy has been discussed in *Drug and Therapeutics Bulletin* (1986b). Four trials (Rynnel-Dagoo, Ahlbom and Schiratzki, 1978; Fiellau-Nikolajsen, Falbe-Hansen and Knudstrup, 1980; Roydhouse, 1980; Widemar et al., 1985) have shown adenoidectomy to be of no value in the treatment of OME. However, Maw (1983) and Bulman, Brook and Berry (1984) have both shown adenoidectomy to be of benefit, albeit in children of 2–11 and 4–9 years respectively, the mean age being 5;3 years: Fiellau-Nikolajsen's group studied 3-year-old children. Black et al. (1986) have reported on a controlled trial of adenoidectomy in the treatment of glue ear; they found an additional short-term benefit of adenoidectomy over ear operation, but by 6 months this benefit was no longer statistically significant. The mean age of the children in their group was 6;4 years with a range of 4–9 years. More recently Black, Crowther and Freeland (1990) have concluded that if the principal aim of surgery is to restore hearing then insertion of a grommet is the treatment of choice; the addition of adenoidectomy will increase the likelihood of restoration of normal middle ear function.

In analysing these results it seems that adenoidectomy may be of value in the school-age child, typically the age where adenoids reach peak size, but not necessarily in younger children. However, adenoidectomy may be indicated for reasons other than OME even in very young children and should be assessed separately from the management of OME.

The question of whether to carry out insertion of a ventilation tube as well as myringotomy remains largely unresolved. There is no doubt that insertion of grommets carries the risk of long-term damage to the tympanic membrane and of cholesteatoma formation (Shah, 1971; Kilby, Richards and Hart, 1972; Brown, Richards and Ambegaokar, 1978; Ben Ami et al., 1983; Curley, 1986; Skinner, Lesser and Richards, unpublished results). Nevertheless, there is an immediate audiometric benefit to be gained from insertion of a grommet, although the benefit tends to be lost after 6–12 months (Brown, Richards and Ambegaokar, 1978; To, Pahor and Robin, 1984). Curley (1986) has found that the 3–4 year age group had the greatest mean number of admissions for insertion of grommets (2), compared with 1.69 for those under 3 years. The decision to insert a grommet should be based on preoperative otoscopic, audiometric and tympanometric assessment. Administration of nitrous oxide anaesthesia causes a rise of intratympanic pressure (Singh and Kirk, 1979; Rees and Freeland, 1992) and this can result in clearance of an effusion from the ear.

This author proposes, therefore, that in long-established cases with clear criteria of audiological disability, older children should receive adenoidectomy and myringotomy, reserving insertion of grommets for those with recurrent effusions following this. In the younger child the immediate hearing gain to be expected following myringotomy with insertion of grommets may outweigh the potential disadvantages, and it is the author's practice to insert Shephard's grommets in these children.

Typically Shephard-type grommets remain in place for an average of 6–9 months (Gibb and MacKenzie, 1985) before spontaneous extrusion. Long-term ventilation may be achieved by Goode T-tubes or Per Lee grommets, the latter being the author's choice. East (1986) has reported on the persistence of the Per Lee grommet for several years, supporting Gibb and MacKenzie (Figure 2.7).

The two groups most likely to suffer long-term OME are children with cleft palate (where a Per Lee grommet may be used), and children with Down's syndrome. This latter group presents special problems and several reasons, including the narrow lumen of the external auditory canals, preclude the routine use of grommets in their management.

The presence of a small-lumen ventilating tube such as the Shephard type, need not prevent the child swimming, as discussed by Marks and Mills (1983), Smelt and Monkhouse (1983), Marks, Mills and Shaheen (1985) and Pringle (1992). It seems prudent to advise against immersing the head when swimming and to insert a simple plug using fine cotton wool rubbed in petroleum jelly, even though there may be no evidence to support the need for either of these measures.

Finally, if other measures fail or are inappropriate, a conductive loss

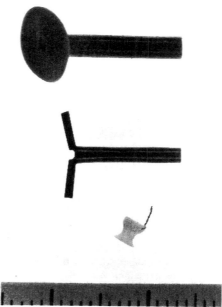

Figure 2.7 Aural grommets: Per Lee tube (top); Goode T-tube (middle); Shephard (bottom).

may be helped by the use of a hearing aid: this may be particularly appropriate in children with Down's syndrome.

Conclusion

The otologist plays a central role in the management of children with hearing loss in relating the wide aspects of the child's development to the specifically audiological problem associated with the deafness. While retaining an objective view of the management, the otologist needs a sympathetic approach to the child and to the parents. Close liaison with audiologists and education authorities, as well as with other relevant medical personnel, is essential.

References

Bain, J. (1990). Childhood otalgia; acute otitis media. *British Medical Journal* 300, 1006–1007.

Bamford, J. and Saunders, E. (1985). *Hearing Impairment, Auditory Perception and Language Disability.* London: Edward Arnold.

Barr, G.S. and Coatesworth, A.P. (1991). Passive smoking and otitis media with effusion. *British Medical Journal* 303, 1032–1033.

Ben Ami, M., Rosen, G., Schlezinger, T., Konack, S. and Ben Ami, N. (1983). Otitis media with effusion, complications after treatment. *Journal of Laryngology and Otology* 97, 1091–1094.

Birch, L. and Elbrond, O. (1984). Prospective epidemiological investigation of secretory otitis media in children attending day-care centres. *ORL* 46, 229–234.

Black, N. (1984a). Surgery for glue ear – a modern epidemic. *Lancet* i, 835–837.

Black, N.A. (1984b). Is glue ear a modern phenomenon? A historical review of the medical literature. *Clinical Otolaryngology* 9, 155–164.

Black, N.A. (1985a). Geographical variations in the use of surgery for glue ear. *Journal of the Royal Society of Medicine* 78, 641–648.

Black, N. (1985b). Causes of glue ear. *Journal of Laryngology and Otology* 99, 953–966.

Black, N., Crowther, J. and Freeland, A.P. (1986). The effectiveness of adenoidectomy in the treatment of glue ear; a randomised controlled trial. *Clinical Otolaryngology* 11, 149–156.

Black, N.A., Sanderson, C.F.B., Freeland, A.P. and Vessey, M.P. (1990). A randomised control trial of surgery for glue ear. *British Medical Journal* 300, 1551–1556.

Blayney, A.W. and Colman, B.H. (1984). Dizziness in childhood. *Clinical Otolaryngology* 9, 77–86.

Bluestone, C.D. and Beery, Q.C. (1976). Concepts on the pathogenesis of middle ear effusions. *Annals of Otology, Rhinology and Laryngology* 85 (suppl. 25).

Bluestone, C.D. and Stool, S.E. (1983). *Pediatric Otolaryngology*. Philadelphia: W.B. Saunders.

Bock, G.R. and Saunders, J.C. (1977). A critical period of acoustic trauma in the hamster and its relation to cochlear development. *Science* 197, 396–398.

Bodner, E.E., Browning, G.G., Chalmers, F.T. and Chalmers, T.C. (1991). Can meta-analysis help uncertainty in surgery for otitis media in children? *Journal of Laryngology and Otology* 105, 812–819.

Brook, I. and Burke, P. (1992). The management of acute, serous and chronic otitis: the role of anaerobic bacteria. *Journal of Hospital Infection* 22 (suppl. A), 75–87.

Brooks, D.N. (1969). The use of the electro-acoustic impedance bridge in the assessment of middle ear function. *International Audiology* 8, 563–569.

Brown, M.J.K.M., Richards, S.H. and Ambegaokar, A.G. (1978). Grommets and glue ear; a five year follow-up of a controlled trial. *Journal of the Royal Society of Medicine* 71, 353–356.

Browning, G.G. (1990). Childhood otalgia; acute otitis media. *British Medical Journal* 300, 1005–1006.

Brownlee, R.D., de Loach, W.R. and Jackson, H.P. (1969). Otitis media in children. Incidence, treatment and prognosis in pediatric practice. *Journal of Pediatrics* 75, 636–642.

Buckley, G. and Hinton, A. (1991). Otitis media with effusion shows a progressive resolution with time. *Clinical Otolaryngology* 16, 354–357.

Bulman, C.H., Brook, S.J. and Berry, M.G. (1984). A prospective randomised controlled trial of adenoidectomy vs. grommet insertion in the treatment of glue ear. *Clinical Otolaryngology* 9, 647–76.

Burke, P., Bain, J., Robinson, D. and Dunleavey, J. (1991). Acute red ear in children: controlled trial of non-antibiotic treatment in general practice. *British Medical Journal* 303, 558–562.

Cherry, J.R. (1986). Current conservative treatment of childhood secretory otitis media. *Journal of Laryngology and Otology* 100, 1019–1026.

Claessen, J.Q.P.J., Appelman, C.L.M., Touw-Otten, F.W.M.M., de Melker, R.A. and Hordijk, G.J. (1992). A review of clinical trials regarding treatment of acute otitis media. *Clinical Otolaryngology* 17, 251–257.

Cohen, D. and Sade, J. (1972). Hearing in secretory otitis media. *Canadian Journal of Otolaryngology* 11, 27–29.

Collins, M.P., Church, M.K., Bakhshi, K. and Osborne, J. (1985). Adenoid histamine and its possible relationship to secretory otitis media. *Journal of Laryngology and Otology* 99, 685–691.

Curley, J.W.A. (1986). Grommet insertion: some basic questions answered. *Clinical Otolaryngology* 11, 1–4.

Davis, A. and Wood, S. (1992). The epidemiology of childhood hearing impairment: factors relevant to planning of services. *British Journal of Audiology* 26, 77–90.

Deguine, C. (1986). The relationship between secretory otitis and cholesteatoma. In: Sade, J. (Ed.) *Acute and Secretory Otitis Media*, pp. 111–116. Amsterdam: Kugler.

De Melker, R.A. (1993). Treating persistent glue ear in children. *British Medical Journal* 306, 5–6.

Despland, P. and Galambos, R. (1980). The auditory brainstem response (ABR) is a useful diagnostic tool in the infant intensive care unit. *Pediatric Research* 14, 154–158.

Downs, M.P. (1977). The expanding imperatives of early identification. In: Bess F. (Ed.), *Childhood Deafness: Causation, Assessment and Management*, New York: Grune and Stratton.

Drug and Therapeutics Bulletin (1986a). Glue ear in children, medical management. *Drug and Therapeutics Bulletin* 24, 22–24.

Drug and Therapeutics Bulletin (1986b). The surgical management of glue ear. *Drug and Therapeutics Bulletin* 24, 49–51.

East, D. (1986). The use of Per Lee ventilation tubes in the management of refractory secretory otitis media. *Journal of Laryngology and Otology* 100, 509–513.

Elverland, H.H., Mair, I.W.S., Haugeto, O.K. and Schroder, K.E. (1981). Influence of adenoid hypertrophy on secretory otitis media. *Annals of Otolaryngology* 90, 7–11.

Farrer, L.A. (1992). Gene localization by linkage analysis. *Otolaryngology Clinics of North America* 25, 907–922.

Fiellau-Nikolajsen, M., Lous, J., Vang-Pedersen, S. and Schousboe, H.H. (1979). Tympanometry in three year old children. *Archives of Otolaryngology* 105, 461–466.

Fiellau-Nikolajsen, M., Falbe-Hansen, J. and Knudstrup, P. (1980). Adenoidectomy for middle ear disorders; a randomised controlled trial. *Clinical Otolaryngology* 5, 323–328.

Fraser, G.R. (1976). *The Causes of Profound Deafness in Childhood*. London: Baillière Tindall.

Fraser, J.G., Mehta, M. and Fraser, P.M. (1977). The medical treatment of secretory otitis media. *Journal of Laryngology and Otology* 91, 757–765.

Gibb, A.G. (1979). Non-suppurative otitis media. In: Ballantyne, J. and Groves, J. (Eds), *Scott-Brown's Diseases of the Ear, Nose and Throat*, 4th edn, pp. 193–236. London: Butterworths.

Gibb, A.G. and MacKenzie, I.J. (1985). The extrusion rate of grommets. *Otolaryngology, Head and Neck Surgery* 93, 695–699.

Gibbin, K.P. (1992). Paediatric cochlear implantation. *Archives of Disease in Childhood* 67, 669 -671.

Giebink, G.S., Le, C.T. and Paparella, M.M. (1982). Epidemiology of otitis media with effusion in children. *Archives of Otolaryngology* 108, 563–566.

Gorlin, R.J. and Pindborg, J.J. (1964). *Syndromes of the Head and Neck*. New York: McGraw-Hill.

Grote, J.J. and Kuijpers, W. (1980). Middle ear effusion and sinusitis. *Journal of Laryngology and Otology* **94**, 177–184.

Haggard, M.P., McCormick, B., Gannon, M.M. and Spencer, H. (1992). The paediatric otological case load resulting from improved screening in the first year of life. *Clinical Otolaryngology* **17**, 34–43.

Hall, D.M.B. and Hill, P. (1986). When does secretory otitis media affect language development? *Archives of Disease in Childhood* **61**, 42–47.

Hart, C. and Naunton, R. (1964). The ototoxicity of chloroquine phosphate. *Archives of Otolaryngology* **80**, 407–412.

Harvey, R.M. (1975). Environmental factors in glue ear. *Journal of Laryngology and Otology* **89**, 73–77.

Hibbert, J. and Stell, P.M. (1982). The role of enlarged adenoids in the aetiology of secretory otitis media. *Clinical Otolaryngology* **7**, 253–256.

Holborrow, C.A. (1962). Deafness associated with cleft palate. *Journal of Laryngology and Otology* **76**, 762–768.

Jerger, J. (1972). Studies in impedance audiometry. *Acta Otolaryngologica* **96**, 513–523.

Jones, N.S., Radomskij, P., Prichard, J.N. and Snashall, S.E. (1990). Imbalance and chronic secretory otitis media in children; effect of myringotomy and insertion of ventilation tubes on body sway. *Annals of Otology, Rhinology and Laryngology* **99**, 477–481.

Kilby, D., Richards, S.H. and Hart, G. (1972). Grommets and glue ears: two year results. *Journal of Laryngology and Otology* **86**, 881–888.

Kraemer, M.J., Richardson, M.A., Weiss, N.S., Furukawa, C.T., Shaapiro, G.G., Pierson, W.E. and Bierman, C.W. (1983). Risk factors for persistent middle ear effusions. Otitis media, catarrh, cigarette smoke exposure and atopy. *Journal of the American Medical Association* **249**, 1022–1025.

Lamp, C.B. (1973). Chronic secretory otitis media: aetiological factors and pathological mechanisms. *Laryngoscope* **83**, 276–291.

McCormick, B., Wood, S.A., Cope, Y. and Spavins, F.M. (1984). Analysis of records from an open access audiology device. *British Journal of Audiology* **18**, 127–132.

Marks, N.J. (1985). Secretory otitis media: grommets and swimming (Editorial). *Clinical Otolaryngology* **10**, 1–2.

Marks, N.J., Mills, R.P. and Shaheen, O.H.A. (1981). A controlled trial of co-trimoxazole therapy in serous otitis media. *Journal of Laryngology and Otology* **95**, 1003–1010.

Marks, N.J., Mills, R.P. and Shaheen, O.H.A. (1983). Co-trimoxazole in the treatment of serous otitis: a follow-up report. *Journal of Laryngology and Otology* **97**, 213–216.

Maw, A.R. (1983). Chronic otitis media with effusion (glue ear) and adenotonsillectomy; prospective randomised controlled study. *British Medical Journal* **287**, 1586–1588.

Maw, A.R. and Speller, D.C.E. (1985). Are the tonsils and adenoids a reservoir of infection in otitis media with effusion(glue ear)? *Clinical Otolaryngology* **10**, 265–270.

Mecklenburg, D.J., Demorest, M.E. and Staller, J.S. (1991). Scope and design of clinical trial of the Nucleus multichannel cochlear implant in children. *Ear and Hearing* **12** (suppl.), 10s–14s.

Mills, R. and Brain, C. (1985). A history of acute suppurative otitis media and allergic symptomatology in children with secretory otitis media and controls. *Clinical Otolaryngology* 10, 303–306.

Mills, R.P., Uttley, A.H.C. and McIntyre, M.F. (1985). A bacteriological study of the middle ear and upper respiratory tract in children with chronic secretory otitis media. *Clinical Otolaryngology* 10, 335-342.

Minoli I. and Moro, G. (1985). Constraints of intensive care units and follow-up studies in prematures. *Acta Otolaryngologica Supplementum* 421, 62-67.

Morton, A. (1987). *The Guardian* 3 February.

MRC Working Party for Research in General Practice (1957). Acute otitis media in general practice. *The Lancet* ii, 510-514.

Mygind, N., Neistrup-Larsen, K.-I., Thomsen, J., Thomsen V.F., Josefsson, K. and Sorensen, H. (1981). Penicillin in acute otitis media; a double blind placebo controlled trial. *Clinical Otolaryngology* 6, 5-14.

Newton, V.E. (1985). Aetiology of bilateral sensorineural hearing loss in young children. *Journal of Laryngology and Otology* (suppl. 10).

Nieto, C.S., Calvo, R.M. and Garcia, P.B. (1983). Aetiological factors in chronic secretory otitis in relation to age. *Clinical Otolaryngology* 8, 171-174.

Northern, J.L. and Downs, M.P. (1978). *Hearing in Children*. Baltimore: Williams and Wilkins.

Osborne, J.E., Telford D., Barr, G. and Roberts, C. (1987). Adenoid infection; its relationship to otitis media, glue ear and tonsillitis. *Clinical Otolaryngology* 12, 261-264.

Pabla, H.S., McCormick, B. and Gibbin, K.P. (1991). Retrospective study of the prevalence of bilateral sensorineural deafness in childhood. *International Journal of Paediatric Otolaryngology* 22, 161–165.

Paradise, J.L., Bluestone, C.D. and Felder, H. (1969). The universality of otitis media in 50 infants with cleft palate. *Pediatrics* 44, 35–42.

Pringle, M.B. (1992). Swimming and grommets. *British Medical Journal* 304, 198.

Pukander J. (1982). Acute otitis media among rural children in Finland. *International Journal of Paediatric Otolaryngology*, 4, 325–332.

Pukander, J., Luoptonen, J., Timonen, M. and Karma, P. (1985). Risk factors affecting the occurrence of acute otitis media among 2–3 year old urban children. *Acta Oto-Laryngologica* 100, 260–265.

Rach, G.H., Zielhuis, G.A. and van den Broek, P. (1986). The prevalence of otitis media with effusion in two year old children in the Netherlands. In: Sade, J. (Ed.), *Acute and Secretory Otitis Media*, pp. 135–137. Amsterdam: Kugler.

Rees, G.L. and Freeland, A.P. (1992). The effect of anaesthesia on tympanograms of children undergoing grommet insertion. *Clinical Otolaryngology* 17, 200–202.

Richards, S.H. and Gibbin, K.P. (1977). Recurrent meningitis due to congenital fistula of the stapedial footplate. *Journal of Laryngology and Otology* 91, 1063–1071.

Rockley, T.J. and Rhys Evans, P.H. (1986). Secretory otitis media. *Journal of Laryngology and Otology* 100, 389–394.

Rosenfeld, R.M. and Post, J.C. (1992). Meta-analysis of antibiotics for the treatment of otitis media with effusion. *Otolaryngology, Head and Neck Surgery* 106, 378–386.

Royal College of General Practitioners (1986). *Morbidity Statistics from General Practice: Third National Study 1981–1982*. London: HMSO.

Roydhouse, N. (1980). Adenoidectomy for otitis media with mucoid effusion. *Annals of Otology, Rhinology and Laryngology* 68 (suppl.), 312–315.

Ruokonen, J., Sandelin, K. and Makinen, J. (1979). Adenoids and otitis media with effusion. *Annals of Otology, Rhinology and Laryngology* **88**, 166–171.

Rynnel-Dagoo, B., Ahlbom, A. and Schiratzki, H. (1978). Effects of adenoidectomy: a controlled two year follow-up. *Annals of Otology, Rhinology and Laryngology* **87**, 272–278.

Sade, J. (1979). *Secretory Otitis Media and its Sequelae.* New York: Churchill Livingstone.

Schuknecht, H.F. (1974). *Pathology of the Ear.* Cambridge, MA: Harvard University Press.

Shah, N. (1971). Use of grommets in glue ear. *Journal of Laryngology and Otology* **85**, 283–287.

Shah, N. (1991). Otitis media and its sequelae. *Journal of the Royal Society of Medicine* **84**, 581–586.

Singh, C.B. and Kirk, R. (1979). The effect of nitrous oxide on middle ear pressure in children during anaesthesia. *Journal of Laryngology and Otology* **93**, 349–356.

Smelt, G.J.C. and Monkhouse, W.S. (1985). The effect of bathwater, seawater and swimming on the guinea pig middle ear. *Journal of Laryngology and Otology* **99**, 1209–1216.

Smith, I.M. and Maw, A.R. (1991). Secretory otitis media: a review of management by consultant otolaryngologists. *Clinical Otolaryngology* **16**, 266–270.

Stagno, S., Reynolds, D.W., Amos, C.W., Dahle, A.J., McCollister, F.P., Mohindra, I., Ermocilla, R. and Alford, A.A. (1977). Auditory and visual defects resulting from symptomatic and subclinical congenital cytomegalovirus and toxoplasma infection. *Pediatrics* **59**, 659–667.

Stephenson, H. and Haggard, M.P. (1992). Rationale and design of surgical trials for otitis media with effusion. *Clinical Otolaryngology* **17**, 67–78.

Strachan, D.P., Jarvis, M.J. and Feyerabend, C. (1989). Passive smoking, salivary cotinine concentrations and middle ear effusion in 7 year old children. *British Medical Journal* **298**, 1549 -1552.

Taylor, H. (1934). Prenatal medication as a possible aetiologic factor of deafness in the new born. *Archives of Otolaryngology* **20**, 790–793.

Teele, D.W., Klein, J.O. and Rosner, B.A. (1980). Epidemiology of otitis media in children. *Annals of Otology, Rhinology and Laryngology* **89**, 5–6.

To, S.S., Pahor, A.H. and Robon, P.E. (1984). A prospective trial of unilateral grommets for bilateral secretory otitis media in children. *Clinical Otolaryngology* **9**, 115–118.

Tos, M. (1981) Upon the relationship between secretory otitis in childhood and chronic otitis and its sequelae in adults. *Journal of Laryngology and Otology* **95**, 1011–1022.

Tos, M., Stangerup, S.E., Hvid, G., Andreassen, U.K. and Thomsen, J. (1986). Epidemiology and natural history of secretory otitis. In: Sade, J. (Ed.), *Acute and Secretory Otitis*, pp. 95–106. Amsterdam: Kugler.

Tumarkin, A. (1961). Pre-epidermosis. *Journal of Laryngology and Otology* **75**, 487–500.

Tuohimaa, P. and Palva, T. (1987). The effect of tonsillectomy and adenoidectomy on intratympanic pressure. *Journal of Laryngology and Otology* **101**, 892–896.

University of Leeds (1992). *Effective Health Care Bulletin* **4**.

Uziel, A. (1985). Non genetic factors affecting hearing development. *Acta Oto-Laryngologica Supplementum* **421**, 57–61.

Van Buchem, F.L., Dunk, J.H.M. and Van'T Hof, M.A. (1981). Therapy of acute otitis media: myringotomy, antibiotics or neither? A double blind study in children. *The Lancet* **ii**, 883–887.

Van Cauwenberge, P.B. (1986). The character of acute and secretory otitis media. In: Sade, J. (Ed.), *Acute and Secretory Otitis*, pp. 3–11. Amsterdam, Kugler.

Widemar, L., Svenson, C., Rynnel-Dagoo, B. and Schiratzki, H. (1985). The effect of adenoidectomy on secretory otitis media; a 2 year controlled prospective study. *Clinical Otolaryngology* **10**, 345–350.

Chapter 3
Consequences of otitis media for speech and language

M.P. HAGGARD, J.A. BIRKIN and D.P. PRINGLE

In this chapter we examine language delay as a consequence (sequela) of ear disease in early childhood. We do so, not because we believe that the language domain necessarily contains the most important or the most reliable (i.e. statistically significant) sequelae, but rather because this is the aspect of behavioural deficit traditionally most widely cited as related to ear disease in childhood. We use the term 'ear disease' by intent, because it is even more cautious as to specific 'diagnosis' than the term otitis media with effusion (OME). This has become a more favoured term than secretory otitis media (SOM), because acute otitis media (AOM) commonly occurs in the same children and an effusion and a hearing loss can be present in both conditions; OME does not preclude AOM. Both AOM and OME may be sequentially related and have many risk factors in common. At the risk of acronym fatigue, we use the term MEH (middle ear history), as a history will usually include both AOM and SOM in a way that is difficult to separate. On the basis of the epidemiological literature on prevalence, duration and natural history we assume that in most affected children the vast majority of days of auditory deprivation within a MEH will involve SOM.

Haggard and Hughes (1991) review the epidemiological literature which there is not space to review fully here. In brief, SOM (or OME) is extremely common from the latter half of the first year of life through to about 6 years (cumulative incidence of at least one episode over 80%). However, only about 5% of children have long-persisting histories. After about 6 years of age the rate of final remission is high, although a small percentage continue to have otopathological sequelae. Between these, the point prevalence (i.e. the percentage of children at any one time with fluid in both ears) ranges from under 10% in summer to over 20% in winter. The seasonal variation in otitis media is connected with infections of the respiratory tract and there is some evidence that attacks are precipitated by viral action, to which the secretory immune reaction enables bacteria to take hold. Risk factors for OME include:

- small head size;
- certain anatomical predispositions in the head (particularly in pathological forms such as Down's syndrome or cleft palate that lead to poor eustachian tube function);
- passive smoking (as a pollutant exacerbating the effusions);
- lack of breast feeding in the early months.

There are numerous others, but no risk factor is overwhelmingly strong. The causal status of some types of risk factor, such as socioeconomic group is unclear; these may simply mark the co-occurrence of several weak and obscure but causal risk factors. It seems that one group of factors relates to susceptibility to infection, another to clearance of fluid and the ability or otherwise to maintain a ventilated middle ear, and a third to the production of particularly viscous and colloid effusions. This brief epidemiological caricature generates four questions that pose potential problems for the study of sequelae:

1. Where is the line to be drawn, in respect of severity and persistence, so as to define those cases that are of genuine concern?
2. What is the impact of the fluctuating nature of the condition in many children – extra confusion through changeableness – or restriction of the long-term cumulative deprivation?
3. How does the time course of individual natural histories relate to periods of maximum vulnerability for sequelae?
4. What other characteristics of a child, in his or her constitution or environment, predispose a child suffering from OME to severity and persistence towards greater adverse effects (synergism for sequelae), and are these factors also correlated with the risk factors for occurrence, or for severity and persistence?

The literature on sequelae holds a partial answer to (3), but the other issues remain a source of confusion and disagreement about the likely impact of OME.

Analysis of the problem of language sequelae

Most writings, original or derivative, on OME sequelae refer to language deficits. The historical emphasis on language delay as the main sequela appears to have grown up for three reasons.

First, there happens to exist a profession (speech and language therapy or speech pathology), providing assessment and rehabilitation for a range of language problems to which OME, as well as sensorineural hearing loss, may contribute. This profession's statement of its interests, and services offered, plus its availability as a referral channel for cases viewed medically as problematic and resistant to simple medical solutions, helps to determine awareness of language problems.

Secondly, and partly as a result, there are tests, norms and a body of theory and experiment concerning language structure and language processing. The study of language has always had a strong developmental emphasis; the means whereby children acquire the apparently distinctive human faculty of language has exercised philosophers for centuries.

Thirdly, whereas spatial and mechanical skills can rely on other sense modalities, the intimate association between the auditory input and language hardly requires evidence to assert. In short, we call this explanation for OME sequelae the hearing/language hypothesis.

These historical factors overemphasizing language in OME are reasons not to doubt the evidence on language sequelae, but to take a broader view of sequelae. Much of the earlier clinical research was performed on a 'logically retrospective' basis, i.e. with clinical samples of children having language delay, looking 'backwards' for OME as a precipitating factor. If we were taking samples from the population we would choose them to qualify *only* on the same focal defining attribute under scrutiny (e.g. MEH), or ensure that other possibly compounding factors were equally present in the MEH and control groups. Because referral criteria are based more upon impact than on presence of a precisely defined causal attribute, clinical samples tend to have slightly raised prevalences of other pathologies (for example, intrinsic language backwardness); these co-present pathologies in clinic-based samples are often not factored out or even recorded. Where there is reason to believe that such factors are synergistic (a pair of factors producing more effect than expected from summing their separate contributions) the typical logically retrospective clinical studies will tend to exaggerate the magnitude of the causal influence of the one factor focused on. (For a more exhaustive treatment of this and other problems in the study of sequelae of MEH, see Haggard and Hughes, 1991.)

A major difficulty in designing and interpreting language sequelae studies has been lack of a theoretical expectation of what aspect of language MEH should most influence: syntax, lexicon, semantics, pragmatics or phonology? receptive or expressive functions? quality or quantity? These are important issues for two reasons: first, if tests of all functions were included in a study but only one showed the expected deficit with MEH, we might not be able to show whether this was a specific and interesting influence or a chance finding (this uncertainty arises because so many opportunities would have been created by performing statistical tests on so many variables); secondly, the appropriate level of concern about impact might differ according to who is asked – should we care about mispronunciations (minor articulation disorder) for almost cosmetic reasons of social conformity even if there is no measurable barrier to effective communication? Do we wish to emphasize syntax and lexicon, so as to favour cognition and educational progress, or is overall communication in a social environment, depending on pragmatics – i.e. the appropriate use of language as a medium – more important? Objective and firm answers to these questions cannot be given. The research evidence points to minor deficits in most aspects of language and speech in whatever aspect they have been sought.

Where deficits in aspects of language have been attributed to MEH, there has rarely been adequate control for two relevant effects, which can be thought of almost as artefacts:

1. Organically based variables other than the effective hearing level, such as general illness having its effect through mood and days absent from school.
2. Possible synergistic factors, as suggested above, that would need to be co-present with MEH to produce any appreciable level of deficit, through gross deprivation of language inputs.

Although evidence is scarce, a plausible list of these synergistic factors would include the verbal stimulation level in preschool education, the cultural level of the home, eyesight, family position, number of siblings, sleeping patterns and perinatal history.

Reported 'language delay' is, in the extreme, one key sign according to which parents and professionals suspect and identify cases of hearing loss, especially where there is no effective universal early screening system of high coverage and high sensitivity. However, the level of concern about language expressed by parents of children with OME is not especially high. If language does play a key role in other aspects of development, then some idea of how it might come to do so is necessary. Figure 3.1, from Haggard and Hughes (1991), indicates where language may fit into the complex of related sequelae of MEH. By the standards of likely complexity of real adaptive processes in development, this diagram is not complex, although it is more complex than the simple causal associations conjectured in most paediatric and audiological writings about MEH. This minimum necessary complexity is required by the nature of the evidence on variability. In particular, two of the best large studies of sequelae, the Dunedin Study (Chalmers et al., 1989) and the Boston Study (Teele et al., 1990), show MEH deficits for tests of motor skill and non-verbal IQ respectively that are as large as those shown on verbal/language tests. The former are tests which one would *not* expect to be directly affected by auditory deprivation. From the point of view of the obvious hearing/language hypothesis, this is a little worrying. We do not yet know whether the non-specific but extensive (environmentally mediated) factors suggested by 'illness effects' are sufficient to explain such non-verbal effects, or whether an *intrinsic* underlying factor, such as a deficiency of the immune system, should be invoked to explain both otitis media and its sequelae as joint

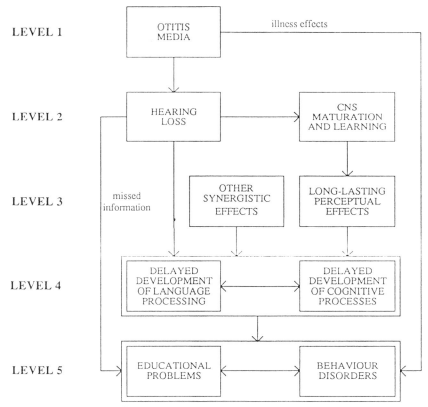

Figure 3.1 Sequelae of otitis media and routes linking them.

products of a common cause. A third possibility is that early cognitive function is so heavily dependent upon language that no such thing as a completely 'non-verbal test' for control purposes actually exists. From the point of view of treatment, the role of intrinsic non-environmental risk factors may have been under-emphasized in the past, because these were wrongly thought to be not as susceptible to, and hence to undermine the case for, (environmental) intervention. That does not necessarily follow: rather, a complex mixture of intrinsic and extrinsic influences is usual for disease and for disability. Therefore the argument for an intervention such as surgery depends crucially upon the evidence as to whether intervention lessens impact of disease. It does not depend on the intrinsic/extrinsic balance within the mix of cause factors, or on presence of a specific relationship between the domain of intervention and the causal factor. (In other words, we should not necessarily advocate behavioural intervention exclusively for behavioural deficits, nor surgical intervention exclusively for organic outcomes.)

Before proceeding to review controlled studies of whether MEH does affect language, we report some preliminary evidence from a

Table 3.1 Percentage of parents (*n* = 107) of children diagnosed as having OME expressing their degree of concern over six aspects of language and speech

	None, not sure, doesn't apply	A little concern	A lot of concern
Late speech	62.3	8.9	27.8
Mispronunciations	47.2	24.7	28.1
Unclear speech to parents	64.0	10.5	25.6
Unclear speech to adults	63.2	14.9	21.8
Unclear speech to other children	69.7	10.5	19.8
Immature speech	67.4	5.6	27.0

study of parental concern over the various types of sign or symptom held to be part of, or possibly included in the clinical presentation of MEH. Table 3.1 shows parental expressions of concern over various aspects of speech and language in a sample of children with OME diagnosed by otolaryngologists. Concern over language was no higher than the average concern over illness, behaviour, balance and other sign/symptom areas. Within language, the concern levels and reporting frequencies are relatively homogenous, with the exception of mispronunciation, which is reported more frequently. It is interesting that parents appear more concerned about the social deviance aspect of the phonetic form of language than about failure to achieve its purpose, namely communication. Clearly this is an aspect of language that can be detected easily by the ear in the absence of the clear reference values usually required (as in a normed test). Not shown in Table 3.1, but reported elsewhere (Haggard et al., 1993), was a slight trend for professionals (otolaryngologists and general practitioners) to place language high among their areas of concern, but for parents to place it slightly lower than, for example, minor behaviour disorders occurring during periods of reduced hearing.

The preceding discussion of historical concentration on language serves to explain how such a misalignment between the concerns of parents and those of professionals could arise. These data are a subjective aspect of health beliefs and do not reflect either objective prevalences or objective measures of disability or health need. However, they are useful in documenting what matters to parents and hence what combinations of signs and symptoms they are likely to mention when pressing forward, for referral or treatment.

Evidence

There are a restricted number of ways of determining whether the health beliefs about impact of MEH are grounded in reality. Small controlled studies of well-defined clinical groups can contribute valuable insight and are briefly reviewed later. However, for the purpose of knowing whether a deficit really occurs in some aspect of language, in which aspect, and how large the deficit is, large studies are the only useful source. Table 3.2 summarizes 15 reports of 13 studies, each having over 50 subjects. It includes some large population cohort studies in which the actual numbers in the affected group, or the numbers in particular subgroups, were smaller than 50, but population studies have particular value in showing the relationship of a defined group justifying clinical concern to the normal population. Although sheer size is not a substitute for control, larger studies are more able to attest the reality of effects that are of probably small magnitude, and to quantify the magnitude precisely. They are also less likely to produce systematic selection biases or random findings. A large study will also involve a higher percentage of all the children in a particular district that might have been sampled as meeting definition.

A further type of bias requires brief mention. Where there is a professional reason to believe that an effect exists, certain selective processes or biases intrude. First, only *plausible* hypotheses tend to be tested and positive results submitted for publication, because editors and readers like a positive result. This point is a force for caution and, subject to the qualification about false conclusions introduced by biases, tends to lend assurance to the overall conclusion from a body of literature even if such a literature becomes repetitive. The second point is more worrying: only the *positive* trends get selected for further detailed analysis, tabulation and inclusion in an abstract, which is all that many readers will see. The process of persisting to publication and surviving editorial review discriminates highly against null findings. There is no way to precisely balance the second, more risk-prone, influence with the first, more conservative, one. Those who interpret the literature must be aware of all these selection processes and try to separate the restricted interpretation of what the data can support from broader inferences about impact of disease or treatment and the associated policy recommendations. We later provide a short prose account of the overall conclusions permitted from the literature. A fuller account of results, arguments and interpretation of the literature on language sequelae would make for interesting debate, but amid the contemporary trend to systematic reviews and summary overviews we rely mainly on a summary table. Reviews of the traditional type are available in Haggard and Hughes (1991) and Roberts et al. (1991). A brief overview of useful points made in smaller studies follows.

Small studies

It is sometimes possible to combine good matching on the major relevant factors known to influence the outcome variable(s) and to study

Table 3.2 Summary of findings from 13 large studies

Authors	Subjects	Language and speech measures
Kaplan et al. (1973)	489 Eskimo children followed from 0 to 10 years. One or more episodes of otitis media had been experienced in 76% (of whom 78% had had their first attack before 2 years); 41% had perforation and scars; 16% had hearing loss of 26 dB; 25% had hearing in normal range but had a measurable air–bone gap.	Weschler Intelligence Scale for Children (WISC), four verbal subtests. Modified for comprehension, similarities in order to be relevant for subjects (digit span not modified) Metropolitan Achievement Test (MAT) (language)
Gottlieb, Zinkus and Thompson (1979)	213 schoolchildren divided into: A (educationally handicapped with significant auditory processing deficits) and B (learning disabled with no auditory perceptual disturbances) Further subdivided: (1) those with a history of otitis media; (2) those with no such history	Speech and language pathologist analysed speech, language, articulation and auditory processing skills. Physicians Developmental Screening Test (PDST), screened for developmental delays, perceptual weaknesses, academic deficiencies. Child was considered language delayed if it could not construct simple 2–3 word phrases by 24 months
Howie et al. (1979)	Schoolchildren (144 in total) test group, with three or more attacks of OME in first 18 months. Control group no OME. Matched pairs: sex, birth date, father's occupation, school attended, year of testing (i.e. school year). All patients treated with antibiotics	Science Research Associates Test (SRAT) (academic achievement: language, arts, reading, maths)

Findings/conclusions	Comments	Non-language measures used
Number of episodes of otitis media was related to tympanic membrane abnormalities, low verbal/achievement scores. Subjects with otitis media before 2 years and/or a 26+ dB hearing loss had significantly impaired verbal ability, reading, language, maths. Similar findings were made for subjects with recovered hearing	Onset and number of bouts had a major role in impairing verbal development. Low mean verbal score for whole cohort, due to cultural/language biases of tests. Early identification of otitis media could avoid later language difficulties	WISC (four non-verbal tests), Bender–Gestalt 'draw a person' test, MAT (reading and maths)
In group A 40.8% were language delayed. In group B 17.1% were delayed. Subgroups 1 and 2 had similar numbers of delayed subjects. Study appears to show link between recurrent middle ear disease, central auditory deficits and delayed language development	Interpretation must be cautious because study was retrospective and not blinded. Development of long-term auditory processing (perceptual) deficits may be due to chronic otitis media before 3 years. Preschool period may be a 'latent period of educational jeopardy' in which identification of 'risk' signs could help avoid certain psycho-educational disorders	WISC (Revised) (IQ), also auditory, visual perception subtests. Wide Range Achievement Test (WRAT) (reading, spelling, arithmetic skills). Illinois Test of Psycholinguistic Abilities (ITPA) (auditory and visual processing abilities). Clinical interview (behaviour, personality, self-concept)
Three or more episodes of OME during the first 18 months (supposed critical period) leads to impeded academic achievement	Greater frequency and sensitivity of measures needed to avoid overlooking short bouts of OME, as even these may have implications for handicapped children. Auditory related language skills may be more accurately evaluated by an individual language test than a written one	

Table 3.2 *(contd)*

Authors	Subjects	Language and speech measures
Silva et al. (1982)	47 children with bilateral OME. 355 normal when tested at 5 years of age. No significant background differences between groups	Dunedin Articulation Screening Scale (DASS), Reynell Developmental Language Scale (RDLS) (speech articulation, verbal comprehension and expression)
Stewart et al. (1984) (continuation of study in preceding entry)	959 followed from 3 to 9 years. Split into seven groups depending on incidence and severity of OME. Most OME sequelae not statistically significant by 9 years	RDLS, ITPA, Dunedin Articulation Checklist (DAC) (verbal comprehension and expression, speech articulation, language)
Teele et al. (1984)	205 3 year olds (who had three or more bouts of OME by 2 years). Control group. All from variety of socioeconomic backgrounds	Peabody Picture Vocabulary Test (PPVT) revised; Zimmermann Pre-school Language Scale (ZPLS), verbal ability quotient/comprehension quotient; Fisher–Logemann/Gold mann–Friscoe (Woodstock) test of articulation (F–L/G–F), comprehension, vocabulary, articulation
Teele et al. (1990)	207 7 year olds, ranked according to number of days with MEE (0–2 years)	PPVT, Berko Morphology 'WUG' Test (WUG), Brunte–Lezine Test (BLT), F–L/G–F (W) (subsample) (emphasizing structural aspects of language)

Findings/conclusions	Comments	Non-language measures used
Bilateral OME group were disadvantaged in speech articulation abilities, verbal comprehension, motor development and intelligence	Reduced distorted auditory input due to OME could result in language delay. Link between OME and behaviour problems suggests need to examine 'problem' children for OME. Identification or diagnosis using hearing loss alone may allow one-third of cases of OME to be missed	McCarthy Scale of Children's Abilities (SCA) (total motor test). Stanford–Binet Intelligence Scale (S-BIS), child scale-A (motor development, IQ, behaviour)
Bilateral OME groups: (3 years) significantly disadvantaged in verbal comprehension/expression; (5 years) disadvantaged in verbal expression/IQ; (9 years) disadvantages no longer significant between groups, but most severely affected group still disadvantaged in articulation	OME associated with significant disadvantages in speech articulation, verbal comprehension and expression (and IQ) up to 7 years of age. Differences tend to disappear with age and treatment, but delayed speech is still evident at 9 years	S-BIS (IQ 5 years), WRAT (reading 7–9 years), WISC (IQ 7 years)
Prolonged bouts of MEE led to lower scores. MEE in first 6–12 months associated with lowest scores. More noticeable in children with higher socio-economic status	Study did not indicate whether low scores may persist. If they do not, it would suggest that present treatment is adequate. If they persist need to rethink present treatment	
Time with MEE before 3 years was significantly associated with lower speech/language scores, IQ, and school performance at 7 years. After 3 years OME was not a significant predictor of articulatory/morphological ability	Duration of sequelae unknown. Intervention could avoid problems. Parent–child interaction, type of day-care, critical period of vulnerability may all determine extent of sequelae	WISC-R, MAT (IQ, reading and maths ability)

Table 3.2 *(contd)*

Authors	Subjects	Language and speech measures
Menyuk (1986)	205 children with three or more or one or fewer episodes of otitis media by 2 years of age. Subjects drawn from urban and suburban areas, 80% of each were low or middle socio-economic status. Subjects were tested at 3 then 7 years	At 3 years: PPVT, ZPLS, G-F, language sample analysed for structural complexity/MLU. At 7 years: F–L/G-F (W), WUG, PPVT, BLT (speech sound articulation and discrimination, lexical comprehension and pro-duction)
Friel-Patti et al. (1987)	500 children aged 6–27 months at beginning of study. 93 subjects had language evaluation at 18 months, middle to high middle socio-economic status. 24% had evidence of OME in at least one ear	Sequenced Inventory of Communicative Development (SICD) (receptive and expres-sive), REEL, Vineland Adaptive Behaviour Scales (VABS) (revised), PPVT (revised), G–F test of articulation. Systematic Analysis of Language Transcripts (SALT) analysed lan-guage samples (receptive and expressive skills, syntax, phonology, mor-phology)
Friel-Patti and Finitzo (1990) (continuation of study in preceding entry)	483 middle-class children followed from 6 to 24 months. Hearing was measured at 6 months then at 6-monthly inter-vals. Average hearing level calculated then divided into 'better' and 'worse' hearing groups. Number of days with OME computed;73.5% of total had had bouts of OME. Note: 99 of total number were excluded from the language mea-sure	SICD (receptive and expressive) measured at 6-monthly intervals from 1 year (comprehension, production, discrimina-tion)

Findings/conclusions	Comments	Non-language measures used
3 years: performance differences seen in group from middle socio-economic status, possibly due to developmental spurt in relatively otitis media-free subjects. 7 years: time with otitis media detrimentally affected performance. Socio-economic status had less effect. Differences tended to occur in production, which suggests early persistent otitis media delays rather than distorts development	Early recurrent otitis media can have long-term effects (four or more bouts had most effect). 'Critical level' in distortion of information processing may be needed before language suffers. Predictions made about children most at risk (i.e. low socioeconomic status, multiple bouts) and about areas of language/speech affected. Discrimination/comprehension of language show effects of early persistent otitis media before production problems	
Significant relationship between ear history and language performance at 18 months – particularly for receptive language scores. Language delay is related to number of episodes of OME. OME contributory, not exclusive, factor in delay	Prediction: OM group likely to exhibit further expressive language deficit with time. High incidence of undetected otitis media renders retrospective studies of limited validity. Parental reports possibly unreliable	Auditory brainstem response (ABR) and audiometry (auditory sensitivity)
Time with OME before 12 months was negatively related to the SICD (receptive) score at 1 year. Similar correlations were seen at 18-month SICD (expressive). Group average hearing level before 12 months, was correlated with receptive language at 12, 18 and 24 months. Children with better hearing before 12 months showed higher receptive/expressive language performance at 2 years	The relationship between OME and language is mediated by hearing. Better language was associated with better hearing and fewer days of OME. Differences, not gross delays were seen	ABR (to rule out sensorineural hearing loss)

Table 3.2 *(contd)*

Authors	Subjects	Language and speech measures
Lous et al. (1988)	463 8 year olds, of whom 26 had long-lasting SOM. A control group of 26 matched for age, sex, school, grade level and controlled for classroom and social status	PPVT (revised), WISC (verbal) (receptive vocabulary, general information, comprehension, arithmetic, similarities and vocabulary)
Lous (1990)	384 7 year olds (unselected): 187 boys, 197 girls. Parents' social strata, handedness, type of child care, number of siblings, mother's occupation, otological history, place of residence etc., noted	Statens Institut Tallidende, Odense (SITO) (phonology) (requires auditory capacity together with recognition and comprehension of elements and meaning of a sentence)
Rach et al. (1991)	43 (out of population of 1439) Dutch children (4–6 years old) with bilateral OME on two separate occasions, assigned to treatment/non treatment groups. Matched controls used for 'optimal' language development reference	Reynell standardized for Dutch (measures verbal, comprehension and expression capacity). Test administered 6 months before and 6 months after children were assigned to groups
Knishkowy et al. (1991)	233 children (followed from 0–3 years). Part of community programme for promotion of growth and development. 67% had had one or more episodes of OME in last 3 years	BLT (language subscore – 2 years). Israel Ministry of Health recommended speech screening test (3 years)

Findings/conclusions	Comments	Non-language measures used
Long-term SOM did not cause mean test scores to drop significantly. Greater variability of scores was seen on PPVT (revised) and WISC for case group	Authors recommend further studies needed to explain SOM/language development relationship	Silent word reading test (OS-400)
Using ANOVA, an association between phonology score and tympanogram type in better ear was found at 7 years. For otological history and pure tone screening no association was seen. Time with OME and occurrence of myringotomy/intubation produced no significant differences in phonology score	Subjects' age may account for lack of significant differences, i.e. may have overcome linguistic difficulties. Background variables: mother's social group most closely associated to phonology score	Tympanometry, pure-tone screening
Bilateral OME of 3–6 months' duration caused significant impairment of expressive language skills. The effect on verbal comprehension was not significant. Children who received ventilating tubes did not perform significantly better	Persistence of the expressive language deficit is uncertain	
Early OME has deleterious effect on language/development up to 3 years of age. Enrichment programme possibly reduced differences between groups	Hearing deficit had more effect on language acquisition/expression than on pronunciation. Higher socio-economic status had lower incidence of OME. Ethnic bias in speech test may contribute to performance differences	BLT (postural, social and coordination subscores). Israel Ministry of Health hearing screening test. S-BIS (IQ)

Table 3.2 *(contd)*

Authors	Subjects	Language and speech measures
Roberts et al. (1991)	63 children (followed from 0 to 6 years): 30 middle class, 33 low income. Ear status monitored from 0 to 3 years (duration of OME was recorded)	At age 4–6: Miller–Yoder Language Comprehension Test, (M-Y LCT), Clinical Evaluation of Language Functions (CELF), PPVT, Bankson Language Screening Test (BLST) (Semantic section), SALT analysed language samples (comprehension, processing and production abilites, receptive vocabulary)

cases intensively enough to provide reliable measures of outcome when this is done. Small studies can economically provide insights into important variables, interactions and probable processes in developmental delay, although they are not suitable for determining the magnitude of impact. The literature on MEH sequelae was 'inaugurated' by Holm and Kunze (1969) with such a small matched study, but there is some doubt as to whether their effect may have been due to continuing mild hearing impairment present at the time of test. Wallace et al. (1988) looked at 'emerging language' in 1 year olds, with the receptive and expressive scales of the Sequenced Inventory of Communication Development, and found an OME deficit on the latter but not the former. Jerger et al. (1983) and Gravel and Wallace (1992), following up their earlier study group, have shown that children with an early (up to 1 year) MEH perform less well under conditions of competing stimulation when reporting back single sentences than do children without a MEH. The equivalent signal-to-noise ratios for 50% intelligibility in the latter study differed by 3 dB. Although 3 dB would constitute a small difference in the threshold in quiet, in noise this is a large effect, equivalent to a 20–30% difference in accuracy. Although this is perhaps as much an auditory or cognitive ability as a language ability, it illustrates one pathway in Figure 3.1 by which effective input may be impoverished beyond the point where disease remits. For such a task it is not yet known how long-lasting the difference may be in a sample of children (or adults) in which rigorous control for ear pathology or asymmetries of hearing is instituted. Interestingly, the Gravel and Wallace 1992 investigation also showed a small effect of a perinatal high-risk

Findings/conclusions	Comments	Non-language measures used
History of otitis media had no major detrimental effect on language	Suggested reasons for null result: interaction between otitis media and other risk factors; small sample. Gender differences were seen in otitis media and language but were inconsistent	

history/asphyxia or birth weight below 1500 g but only in the MEH group; numbers were too small to attest to statistical significance. Finally, we should remember that children do not develop in a vacuum. Black et al. (1988) succeeded in showing a greater number of failures in receptive language at 14 months than in expressive (as expected). They also showed that mothers who encouraged development by adopting a teaching role had children with higher development scores (as expected). Unexpectedly, the children with persistent otitis media had less sociable mothers. Here we see the common belief confirmed of how a parent can influence a child's language cognition and behaviour, and also how the child's health status may contribute to the quality of dyadic interaction with potential consequences for interpersonal behaviour. The inherited organic constitution may be determining the effective environment by failing to reward the parent. Because of this 'chicken and egg' problem, interpretations of environmental influences have to be cautious.

Summary of findings from 13 large studies

From a corpus of reports on 13 studies with 50 or more subjects, several points about the possible existence of any relationship between early recurrent otitis media and language development can be made. The various studies referred to middle ear disease in different ways. As some of these terms are used almost interchangeably, and as AOM and OME are associated, any distinction between their effects on sequelae can probably not be sustained. From the studies summarized in Table

3.2, the evidence is only moderately consistent, but the issues have not been sufficiently focused to describe the evidence as directly conflicting. One area of agreement is the probable lack of any *long-term* effects on formal aspects of language from early recurrent OME. The 13 studies can be categorized into two groups, those which find some adverse effect of OME on a language proficiency score ($n = 9$), and those which do not ($n = 3$). Several studies acknowledge the limitations in their findings in terms of confounding background variables. The particular variables that may or may not have been adequately controlled raise considerations too technical to examine here.

In the studies that did observe an effect, particular aspects of language may have been affected, but evidence is lacking for any particularly characteristic profile of OME effects. Teele et al. (1984, 1990) showed a detrimental effect on vocabulary, articulation and the structural aspects of language from early history of otitis media. Articulation effects were also shown by Silva et al. (1982) and Stewart et al. (1984). Friel-Patti et al. (1987), demonstrated an effect on receptive language and commented that expressive language effects may become apparent as the child gets older. Friel-Patti and Finitzo (1990) found similar results but concluded that differences in performance, not delays, were being shown. Conversely, developmental language delay was shown by Gottlieb, Zinkus and Thompson (1979) and Menyuk (1986). Similarly, language acquisition was shown by Kniskowy et al. (1991) to be delayed and expressive language detrimentally affected. Kaplan et al. (1973), Silva et al. (1982) and Stewart et al. (1984) showed that a detrimental effect on verbal comprehension was linked to early recurrent otitis media. Discrimination and comprehension of language differences were noted before 2 years of age by Menyuk (1986), who also recorded production differences. Knishkowy et al. (1990) and Rach et al. (1991) recorded an effect solely on expressive language.

Some studies failed to find any *specific* overall effect of early recurrent OME on language, but showed general academic achievement to be detrimentally affected (Howie et al., 1979). Others saw a dose–response effect within the MEH group alone, i.e. in terms of severity and duration of bouts. Rach et al. (1991) noted the larger effects on language from background variables such as socioeconomic status than from OME, but documented a dose–response effect for time with OME in the age range 2–4 years. Although more convincing than a simple association of categories, this dose–response relationship does not itself introduce control for possible non-auditory causal links. A stronger underlying systematic predisposition could be directly associated with language problems in another way and lead to a more persistent history. One study (Roberts et al., 1991) showed no link at all between OME and language. These authors inferred that methodological limitations of previous studies and the interaction of OME with various other risk factors for sequelae in the different studies would together serve to explain the contradictory findings about deficits in language.

From the studies that did show an effect, it appears that early age of onset, long duration and number of bouts of OME made language difficulties more likely. Several studies showing a deleterious effect on language observe both receptive and expressive language deficits, although the latter have been more commonly found. Background variables, such as socio-economic and ethnic status, also affect language performance (Lous, 1990; Kniskowy et al., 1991), requiring careful control for these variables.

There is much less certainty about longer term sequelae of persistent early recurrent OME. If effects were likely to be persistent then treatment and intervention strategies would need re-thinking in order to go some way to ameliorate any subsequent academic disadvantage. However, Stewart et al. (1984) and Lous (1990) did not envisage long-term effects as being likely, and in those articles in which this was considered the general consensus of opinion is sceptical. Only Menyuk (1986) has considered long-term effects likely.

In summary, some detrimental effects on language of early persistent or recurrent otitis media have been shown in several areas of language and the majority of large studies published have shown an effect. The dominant trend is for the largest effect to accompany early age of onset, and long duration of episodes of OME. Language sequelae for MEH cannot therefore be dismissed as a fiction: nor can they be taken as the most essential, severe or long-term part of the presentation in OME. We do not see sufficient evidence of large effects to emphasize language as hitherto defined and tested as the exclusive area of concern or a justification for treatment on its own. Equally, language should not comprise the exclusive measure of outcome in trials of treatment: aspects of cognition, interpersonal behaviour and social aspects of communication are likely to be just as important. These general cautionary remarks do not undermine the value of checking clinically for MEH in individual language-delayed children, or for language sequelae in children with MEH, as there is tentative evidence for synergism in sequelae.

Implications

Two interesting practical implications follow from this literature.

First, if delay or distortion in some aspect of language is building up to constitute a sequela, to what extent can it also be regarded as part of the presentation and hence validly used for screening, assessment and of differential planning of management? We formerly viewed such a possibility as an admission of defeat in the context of possible preventive screening, it being preferable to detect the underlying MEH or hearing loss before cumulative sequelae have had time to occur. This view is perhaps too utopian and too extreme in its logic, and we have since been convinced by the arguments of Ruben (1991). If language delay is detectable shortly after 1 year in some children then, against the background that many children are still not identified as having a hearing problem or otitis media until much later, there may well still be room for a surveillance approach, with treatment and language rehabilitation as options. The issue then arises of what instrument (e.g. parental questionnaire or language test) should be used on what sorts of population, at what age. Currently, despite various attempts at recommendation there is no universal language screen in most countries and the term 'screen' should be used cautiously in this context. However, a well standardized, culturally appropriate, short, simple and valid (i.e. predictive) language test for 1–4 year olds suspected of having MEH could be very useful. It could not determine how much of any deficit was due to MEH as opposed to other factors but it could quantify the need for intervention. Tests such as the Sequenced Inventory of Communicative Development and the Receptive Expressive Emergent Language Scale have had success in research in very young children, and questions from these could be standardized as a subset to accompany other clinically available information. If otolaryngologists and speech and language therapists are validly to base their activities on an assessment of the extent of language deficit rather than on a single chance observation or parental report, then some development work towards a clinically appropriate test is necessary, building upon the research findings reviewed here.

The second issue concerns the efficacy of language interventions. Although opinions have been expressed about what is deemed clinically appropriate (Hasenstab, 1987), there is no good controlled trial information on the effectiveness of any well-specified regime of language therapy or supplementary auditory stimulation in OME. On the assumption that levels of language performance result from an interplay of environmental factors with factors intrinsic to the child, there is some hope that stimulation could indeed be effective. Evidence from other conditions in which mild language disability does not arise chiefly from OME (or necessarily from a deprivation of auditory input) gives some grounds for hope. For example, Mineo and Goldstein (1990) showed that an intervention programme which developed one linguistic area at a time could lead to generalization of skills in developmentally delayed preschool children. Brooks-Gunn et al. (1992) using a cognitive development enhancement programme showed an improvement in the language skills of low-birth-weight children, whose mothers had undergone only relatively basic education and who were considered 'environmentally at risk' as a result.

Another type of precedent on which we can draw concerns conventionally hearing-impaired children, although in the 'treatment' hearing aids are not separated from the auditory rehabilitation. Parving (1992), using type of school as an indication of the outcome of preschool intervention, showed that intervention and early identification of hearing loss often resulted in a hearing-impaired child being able to join mainstream education (as opposed to a special unit or school for the deaf). Rittenhouse et al. (1990) looked at two groups (signing/non-signing) of severely hearing-impaired children who received 20 months' intervention and showed significant progress on all language measures. Intervention consisted of hearing aids and language stimulation. From this small group of examples there appears little doubt as to the potential value of intervention programmes for hearing-impaired children. This raises the issue of whether it would be appropriate or even ethical to separate treatment (or hearing aids) from rehabilitation. Probably with the milder effects of OME this would be acceptable. With accumulating certainty about the sequelae in language, cognition and behaviour, and about the ways of measuring these skills, we may expect to see target groups of children with OME designated. It will then be possible to suggest appropriate language interventions and subject them to evaluation. However, as far as effective behavioural intervention specific to OME goes, the research literature points to an interesting and promising possibility, rather than to any firm scientific basis as yet for remedial language interventions. Surgery therefore remains the main treatment option (see Chapter 2).

References

Black, M.M., Gerson, L.F., Freeland, C.A., Nair, P., Rubin, J.S. and Hutcheson, J.J. (1988). Language screening for infants prone to Otitis Media. *Journal of Pediatric Psychology* 13, 423–433.

Brooks-Gunn, J., Gross, R.T., Kraemer, H.C., Spiker, D. and Shapiro, S. (1992). Enhancing the cognitive outcomes of low birth weight, premature infants: for whom is the intervention most effective? *Pediatrics* 89, 1209–1215.

Chalmers, D., Stewart, I., Silva, P. and Mulvena, A. (1989). *Otitis Media with Effusion in Children – the Dunedin Study*. London: MacKeith Press.

Friel-Patti, S. and Finitzo, T. (1990). Language learning in a prospective study of otitis media with effusion in the first two years of life. *Journal of Speech and Hearing Research* 33, 188–194.

Friel-Patti, S., Finitzo, T., Formby, E. and Brown, K.C. (1987). A prospective study of early middle ear disease and speech-language development. *Texas Journal of Audiology and Speech Pathology* 13, 39–42.

Gravel, J.S. and Wallace, I.F. (1992). Listening and language at 4 years of age: effects of early otitis media. *Journal of Speech and Hearing Research* 35, 588–595.

Gottlieb, M.I., Zinkus, P.W. and Thompson, A. (1979). Chronic middle ear disease and auditory perceptual deficits. Is there a link? *Clinical Pediatrics* 18, 725–732.

Haggard, M. and Hughes, E. (1991). *Screening Children's Hearing: A Review of the Literature and the Implications of Otitis Media.* London: HMSO.

Haggard, M.P., Birkin, J.A., Browning, G.G., Gatehouse, S. and Lewis, S. (1993). Behavioral sequelae of otitis media with effusion. *Journal of Pediatric Infectious Diseases* (in press).

Hasenstab, M.S. (1987). *Language Learning and Otitis Media.* London: Taylor and Francis.

Holm, V.A. and Kunze, L.H. (1969). Effect of chronic otitis media on language and speech development. *Pediatrics* **43**, 833–889.

Howie, V.M., Jensen, N.J., Fleming, J.W., Peeler, M.B. and Meigs, S. (1979). The effect of early onset of OM on educational attainment. *International Journal of Otorhinolaryngology* **1**, 151–155.

Hutton, J.B. (1983). Effect of middle ear pathology on selected psychoeducational measures following surgical treatment. *Perceptual and Motor Skills* **57**, 1095–1100.

Jerger, S., Jerger, J., Alford, B.R. and Abrams, S. (1983). Development of speech intelligibility in children with recurrent otitis media. *Ear and Hearing* **4**, 138–145.

Kaplan, G.J, Fleshman, J.K., Bender, T.R., Baum, C. and Clark, P.S. (1973). Long term effects of otitis media: a 10 year cohort study of Alaskan Eskimo children. *Pediatrics* **52**, 577–584.

Knishkowy, B., Palti, H., Adler, B. and Tepper, D. (1991). Effect of otitis media on development: a community based study. *Early Human Development* **26**, 101–111.

Lous, J. (1990). Secretory otitis media and phonology when starting school. *Scandinavian Audiology* **19**, 215–222.

Lous, J., Fiellau-Nikolajsen, M. and Jeppesen, A.L. (1988). Secretory otitis media and language development: a six year follow up study with case control. *International Journal of Pediatric Otorhinolaryngology* **15**, 185–203.

Menyuk, P. (1986). Predicting speech and language problems with persistent otitis media. In: Kavanagh, J.F (Ed.), *Otitis Media and Child Development*, pp. 83–91. Parkton, MD: York Press.

Mineo, B.A. and Goldstein, H. (1990). Generalized learning of receptive and expressive actionobject responses by language-delayed preschoolers. *Journal of Speech and Hearing Disorders* **55**, 665–678.

Parving, A. (1992). Intervention and the hearing-impaired child – an evaluation of outcome. *International Journal of Pediatric Otorhinolaryngology* **23**, 151–159.

Rach, G.H., Zielhuis, G.A., Van Baarle, P.W. and Van Den Broek, P. (1991). The effect of treatment with ventilating tubes on language development in preschool children with otitis media with effusion. *Clinical Otolaryngology* **16**, 128–132.

Rittenhouse, R.K., White, K., Lowitzer, C. and Shisler, L. (1990). The costs and benefits of providing early intervention to very young, severely hearing-impaired children in the United States: The conceptual outline of a longitudinal research study and some preliminary findings. *British Journal of Disorders of Communication* **25**, 195–208.

Roberts, J.E., Burchinal, M.R., Davis, B.P., Collier, A.M. and Henderson, F.W. (1991). Otitis media in early childhood and later language. *Journal of Speech and Hearing Research* **34**, 1158–1168.

Ruben, R.J. (1991). Language screening as a factor in the management of the pediatric otolaryngologic patient. *Archives of Otolaryngology* **117**, 1021–1025

Silva, P.A., Kirkland, C., Simpson, A., Stewart, I.A. and Williams, S.M. (1982). Some developmental and behavioural problems associated with bilateral otitis media with effusion. *Journal of Learning Disabilities* **15**, 417–421.

Stewart, I., Kirkland, C., Simpson, A., Silva, P. and Williams, S. (1984). Some developmental characteristics associated with otitis media with effusion. In: Lim, D.J., Bluestone, C.D., Klein, J.O. and Nelson, J.D. (Eds), *Recent Advances in Otitis Media with Effusion*, pp. 329–331. Philadelphia: Marcel Decker.

Teele, D.W., Klein, J.O., Rosner, B.A. and The Greater Boston Otitis Media Study group (1984). Otitis media with effusion during the first 3 years of life and development of speech and language. *Pediatrics* **74**, 282–287.

Teele, D.W., Klein, S.O., Chase, C., Menyuk, P. and Rosner, B.A. (1990). Otitis media in infancy and intellectual ability, school achievement, speech and language at 7 years. *Journal of Infectious Diseases* **162**, 685–694.

Wallace, I.F., Gravel, J.S., McCarton, C.M., Stapells, D.R., Bernstein, R.S. and Ruben, R.J. (1988). Otitis media, auditory sensitivity and language outcomes at 1 year. *The Laryngoscope* **98**, 64–70.

Chapter 4
Behavioural hearing tests 6 months to 3;6 years

BARRY McCORMICK

Introduction

Behavioural hearing tests (BHT) are used more widely than any other tests in paediatric audiology practice and most practitioners use techniques based on the *Ewing* approach first described by Ewing and Ewing (see for example Ewing and Ewing, 1944). This chapter describes the writer's interpretation of the Ewing approach. Visual reinforcement audiometry (VRA) is an additional and very useful technique and is given full coverage in Chapter 5.

It is interesting to observe that practitioners who received initial training in the Ewing methods often tend to continue to use the techniques because they satisfy the requirements very effectively and efficiently. The tests discussed in Chapters 7, 8 and 9 should be available to provide complementary and in some cases supplementary information, but rarely will these tests completely replace behavioural methods because of time, equipment and resource constraints and also because BHT methods have the potential to provide more extensive information about the child's auditory responses including the detection and processing of, and total reaction to, auditory signals including speech. To give some sort of perspective here, from our open access audiology service which covers three health districts and a catchment population of 1 million (12 000 births per year) with its well-documented service commitment and referral system (McCormick et al., 1984) we have found that auditory brain stem response (ABR) tests are needed to back up BHT methods in 3% of the cases seen in the paediatric audiology clinic (Mason, McCormick and Wood, 1988). The BHT or VRA methods provide the foundation for the paediatric audiology service and without these the structure and comprehensiveness of the investigations would be incomplete and inadequate. It must be accepted, however, that there are many pitfalls in BHT methods and it is unfortunate that adequate coverage of the finer details of the test techniques has not been forthcoming in the literature.

The methods described in this chapter typically occupy 10–20 min of a half-hour appointment for children below the age of 3 years. The remaining time is used to obtain a history from the parents, to undertake middle ear impedance investigations and to counsel the parents.

Although BHT methods have established a respectable standing in paediatric audiology clinics they have not shared the same success in screening contexts in the community. The reasons for such failings and suggested solutions have been presented by the author elsewhere (McCormick, 1994). The main shortcomings relate to training provision, lack of guidance on standards or lack of adherence to set standards. With tighter control over such factors the BHT methods have been shown to work well in the screening context utilizing simplified versions of the tests described in this chapter. The reader is strongly advised to refer to McCormick (1994) to complement this chapter by extending BHT methods into the screening context.

Testing babies from 6 months to 18 months

The *distraction* test is the test of choice for this age group and is based on the general principles first described by Ewing and Ewing (1944) in their *distracting* test with the addition of various modifications. The test is based on the principle that the normal response observed when sound is presented to a baby is a head turn to locate the source of sound. The response is most likely to occur with the very young baby if the sound is presented in the horizontal plane of the ear.

Two testers are required to undertake the test, with one presenting the sound stimuli out of visual field and the second tester controlling the baby's attention in the forward direction. To perform this test adequately a baby must have matured to the stage of being able to sit erect and perform head turn responses in the horizontal plane. The test technique described here is normally suitable for babies from 6 months up to 18 months but in some cases, if the baby is given sufficient back and head support in, for example, a reclining seat, the technique can be applied in a modified form for babies as young as 3 or 4 months. The test is also often used in other modified forms for children older than 18 months to complement other techniques. The essential requirements for the test are:

- a quiet, tidy room (minimum area 16 m²) with an ambient noise level not exceeding 25–30 dB (A);
- a low table;
- a selection of frequency-specific sounds, for example, warble tones, narrow band noises etc.;
- a sound level meter.

The test is undertaken with the baby seated on its parent's knee facing forward and sitting erect. The parent must be instructed not to react in any way when stimulus sounds are presented, for even the slightest movement on their part could initiate a response from the baby and invalidate the test. Such inadvertent clues should be watched for carefully by the testers during the course of the test.

It is the role of the person at the front to capture and then control the baby's attention to just the right degree in preparation for the sound stimulus insertion. This is best done by attracting the baby's attention down to a low table surface situated between the tester and the baby. A useful technique here is to spin a small brightly coloured object on the table to capture the attention to a peak and then to cover the item with the hands and continue to maintain a fine attention control, by moving the fingers slightly if necessary just sufficient to prevent the baby from looking up at the tester. The sound stimulus should be presented half a second after the object has been covered. The advantage of this spinning/covering/fine control technique is that it enables the tester to observe the baby's eye and head movements without forming eye contact or eye fixation. The objective is to keep the baby's attention on the table surface rather than on the tester.

The second person's role is to remain out of the baby's visual field (assumed to extend at least 90° on each side from the baby's midline) and to present the sound stimuli at the appropriate location and time. The situation must be checked to ensure that no shadows are cast in the forward direction and no other clues are present to indicate to the baby that there is any activity behind (for example talking, creaking floorboards, perfumes, rustling clothing etc.). The sound stimuli should be presented in the horizontal plane of the baby's ears at an angle set back from the ears of not less than 30° but no more than 45°. Nothing should be allowed to enter the baby's peripheral vision including the sound source, the tester's hair, shoes etc., and great care must be taken when arranging the test situation to ensure that the lighting arrangement is such that shadows and reflections cannot be detected by the baby. Visual cueing is probably the most common invalidator of the distraction test. It is vital, of course, that the tester at the front should not glance or gesture to the tester at the back, for this may alert the baby to the presence of the second tester. The chosen stimulus sound should be presented no later than 1 s after the object has been covered on the table and it should continue for up to 10 s if the baby does not show an immediate response. During this interval the first tester should continue to maintain the fine (finger) attention control until a response in the form of a head turn is observed.

The test stimuli

It is known that sound field and earphone testing can give equally reliable and repeatable results (Byrne and Dillon, 1981; Arlinger and Jerlvall, 1987) and earphones are clearly not desirable for use with babies. A great deal has been written about babies' responsiveness to test sounds of different nature, for example, Ewing and Ewing (1944),

Mendel (1968), Hoversten and Moncur (1969), Moore, Wilson and Thompson (1977), Samples and Franklin (1978), Thompson and Folsom (1985) and McCormick (1986).

In practice, warble tone and narrow band noises are the preferred stimuli for clinical use and these can be calibrated for presentation at set distances or, alternatively, the distances can be varied and the sound levels can be recorded using a sound level meter mounted at the same distance from the instrument as the baby's ear. Manufacturer's calibrations and data relating to sound frequency content and output level should be checked independently to ensure that the instruments perform to specification.

The objective in the distraction test is to record the quietest level at which the baby responds to a range of frequency-specific sounds across the speech frequency range from 250 Hz up to 4 or 6 kHz. Responses are observed at supra-threshold levels initially and then the levels are reduced and progressively raised from quiet until the lowest level at which the baby responds on two out of three presentations is recorded for each sound. Levels as high as 100 dB(A) or more should be available when testing a child thought to be deaf. The results are recorded as the 'quietest levels needed to initiate a response' rather than as 'threshold responses'. Numerous workers have reported a progressive improvement in behavioural response sensitivity as a function of increasing age in the first years of life. For example, Kaga and Tanaka (1980) reported mean behavioural responses for 1 and 2 kHz pure tones of approximately 40 dB HL at 7 months, 25 dB HL at 2 years. Suzuki and Ogiba (1961) and Liden and Kankkunen (1969) reported the same trend but slightly different levels which they termed 'thresholds'. It is unclear as to whether babies respond at levels which can be considered to be threshold in the normal sense of the term used for pure tone audiometry and it is perhaps a mistake to think in those terms. It is, in any event, almost impossible in a sound field to test below 15 or 20 dB(A) in most clinical situations due to ambient noise problems and very few clinics claim to test below 25/30 dB(A) in practice because of such constraints. It is assumed that if a baby responds at 30 dB(A) or less at this age then it is not at risk in terms of speech and language development. Babies who respond only above 35 dB(A) are at risk and their response pattern should be tested thoroughly.

Response requirements

The normal response expected from a baby in the distraction test is a full head turn in the direction of the sound. There may be reasons, not related to hearing, which prevent the child from responding in this way. It may be that the child is not developmentally ready for the test, that the child may not be in a suitable state on the day or that there may be some mental or physical disability. A quick check of the baby's physical maturation and readiness for the test may be made by letting the child visually follow an object through a 90° arc on each side of the midline. If the baby can do this but fails to turn to sound then the response to tactile stimulation, such as a touch on the hair or ear, and to visual stimulation, such as an object deliberately brought into peripheral vision, should be checked. If quick responses are observed to the tactile and visual modalities but consistent lack of response is recorded to sounds then the indications are that a hearing problem is present. If lack of response is recorded to all three modalities there are clearly other factors present which need to be investigated. In such cases the hearing investigations must proceed using the methods described in Chapters 7, 8 and 9.

Consideration of the number of trials to be administered for each stimulus is complicated by drifts in the baby's attention and distractions such as extraneous noises. Nevertheless, some measure of consistency is needed and the author has observed that under the conditions specified here babies respond on approximately 70% of the occasions when audible sounds are presented. The rule of thumb to emerge from this is that the baby should be expected to respond on two out of three presentations of the sound and the objective of the test is to determine the quietest level at which this response pattern can be recorded.

Response reinforcement

When the baby has turned to a sound stimulus the tester should reward the response by simple means such as a smile, vocal praise, a tickle on the arm etc. She should then stay in position until the attention has been pulled back to the front by the distractor after which time he should either stay on that side or silently move to the other side in an unpredictable sequence so that the baby cannot anticipate the side of presentation of subsequent stimuli. This response reinforcement is very important and is often not performed well. Some warble tone instruments now incorporate light reinforcement systems, to supplement the human reinforcement possibilities. If a baby shows apparently no response to a particular sound it may be that the hearing sensitivity is reduced but it is also possible that the child may simply have lost interest. To check the situation further, it is often useful to incorporate the same sound in the attention-capturing activity at the front. When the sound source is covered at the front and the sound then appears (from another source) this often increases the older baby's motivation to turn. Babies above the age of 10 months or so may turn only once to each sound to satisfy their curiosity and may show little interest if the same sound is presented again. It is wise to vary the order and side of presentation to heighten the novelty factor.

No-sound trials

The child's checking or searching behaviour must be assessed during the test and this is best done by including 'control trial' or 'no-sound trial' intervals during the test. The baby's attention should be captured, controlled and phased in the normal way and the second person should move into position as if to present a sound but without actually doing so. Ideally, these observations or no-sound trials should be presented as frequently as the sound stimulus trials, but in practice this rarely happens because of time shortage. These trials must, however, be used in every test situation and at frequent intervals during the test. It is good practice to document the number of responses to no-sound trials, in addition to the sound trials.

Recording the results

The distraction test results may be measured in dB SPL, dB (A) or dB nHL. It is common clinical practice to use a sound level meter with an A weighting characteristic or, less commonly, with a linear SPL scale, and it must be remembered that these scales do not yield results which can be related directly to the audiogram. It is debatable whether conversion factors should be adopted given that the signals are not pure tones; they are of varying band widths, and the normal concept of threshold may be inappropriate if it is age-dependable in the first year or so of life. Nevertheless, on occasions it might be of interest to plot the results on an audiogram-type chart, in which case conversion factors are required. The steps needed to achieve such conversions have been discussed by Nolan (1978 and 1987), Lutman and McCormick (1987) and the resulting values from Lutman and McCormick are given in Table 4.1. Briefly, the stimulus level in dB (A) is converted to linear dB SPL by means of the A weighting correction (BS 5969, 1981; IEC 651, 1979) and compared with normal hearing at the test frequencies under binaural free-field listening conditions as given by the minimal audible field (ISO R 226, 1961). The difference between the measured threshold and normal hearing is, by definition, equivalent to the hearing threshold level in dB HL. The last column in Table 4.1 gives the composite correction factor derived according to the assumptions made above. However, until more is known about true threshold values in babies and the relationship between pure tone and complex tone thresholds, it is probably more appropriate and more precise simply to quote the measured dB (A) or dB SPL values for the stimuli used.

Table 4.1 Conversion factors from dB (A) to HL equivalent (corrections to be added)*

Frequency (Hz)	Conversion dB (A) to dB SPL	Minimum audible field (Bin) dB SPL from ISO 226	True conversion values dB (A) to dB HL equivalent
250	+9	+12	−3
500	+3	+6	−3
1000	0	+4	−4
2000	−1	+1	−2
4000	−1	−4	+3
8000	+1	+15	−14
10 000	+3	+16	−13

*From Lutman and McCormick (1987).

Test techniques 18–30 months

By the time the normal child has reached a mental age of 18 months, she should be able to understand simple verbal instructions. This broadens the horizon for the hearing test beyond the confines of auditory detection into the area of auditory discrimination of speech. This age group is, however, the most difficult and challenging to test and the typical 18-month-old child may cry a lot and show a negative tendency – often wanting to do the opposite of what adults desire or request. The child's normal negativism and short variable attention span may challenge the skills of the tester to the full. The tests described here are based on play methods, one of which was described by Ewing and Ewing (1947) under the title 'Cooperative Test'.

Testing auditory discrimination of speech

For children above the age of 3 years it is possible to undertake speech audiometry using a simplified adult-type test approach and plotting performance intensity function scores (see for example, Siegenthaler, 1969; Jerger and Jerger, 1982). This, however, is too demanding for the younger child and it is necessary to simplify both the task and the method of scoring to suit the vocabulary level and the concentration span of the child. The simplest and most widely accepted approach is to find the quietest level at which the child can discriminate between simple familiar instructions or requests. With the constraints of live presentation of speech the quietest level at which the normal child will respond correctly 80% of the time (that is to four instructions out of five) is 40 dB (A) and it is the deviation from this level that is of interest. It is not possible to define more precise target scores, such as speech reception thresholds for spondees or half peak level elevations, because of the constraints imposed by factors associated with development, attention, and co-operation. In addition, each child's spoken and receptive vocabulary will differ widely at the 18–30 month stage.

If a child has a hearing impairment of such a degree that it affects the development of speech and language, it may not be possible to undertake this part of the test. Some children with slight or moderate hearing impairments may be able to identify instructions when permitted to watch the speaker's face and/or when the instructions are presented at a very loud level and so both of these techniques should be tried. The results of the test can be reported as, for example:

He could not identify simple instructions below a raised listening level of 60 dB (A) when not permitted to watch the speaker's face.

The Four-toy Eyepointing Test (McCormick, 1994)

This test is probably the simplest available for this age group and it requires the minimum degree of co-operation from the child. Two pairs of items from the McCormick Toy Discrimination Test (described in full detail later) are used, namely cup/duck and spoon/shoe. The test is undertaken with the child seated on the parent's knee, facing the tester. The four toy items are spaced apart in an arc on a low table surface (Figure 4.1) and the child is expected to eye point to each item in response to the request 'Where is the spoon?' or 'Look at the cup', etc.

It is, of course, necessary to check that the child understands the names of the items and this is best done by asking the parent to confirm this as each item is introduced to the child at the start of the test. The tester should use a loud conversational level of voice initially and the child should be permitted to watch the tester's face during the conditioning stage of the test. Once two or three successful responses have been obtained under these conditions then the lower half of the tester's face should be covered to obliterate visual clues and the voice level should be lowered to determine the quietest level at which an 80% score can be achieved. With only four items in the display there is a 25% probability of a chance response or a learning effect if the toys are requested in a set order. To minimize the problems it will be necessary to avoid any set sequence and, on occasions, to repeatedly request the same item. If the child's attention drifts it may be helpful to swap the position of the toys to recapture the interest for a few more responses.

There are certain pitfalls which must be avoided when utilizing the eyepoint type response, the chief one being the avoidance of giving premature praise as the child's eyes glance across the toys. The response must be recorded only when the eyes have fixed on one item.

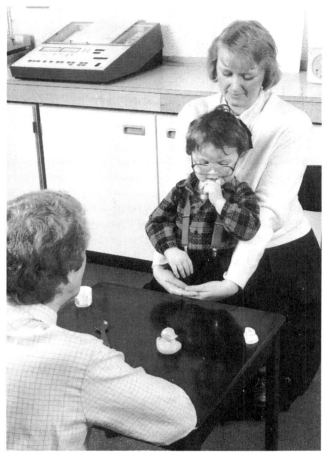

Figure 4.1 Test situation for the Four-toy Eyepointing Test.

The spacing of the toys must be sufficient to avoid ambiguity in the gaze direction if eye pointing is to be acceptable. The more mature child may co-operate by finger pointing, in which case responses can then be obtained by presenting the instructions from each side in turn rather than from directly in front of the child. Ideally, the instructions should be presented at an angle of 90° from the ear at roughly arm's length from the child so that a sound level meter can be held, or positioned on a tripod, adjacent to the child's ear. The advantage of holding the meter is that the typical head and body movements can instantly be compensated for by repositioning the meter; in effect the meter movement can be synchronzied with the head movements. The small inaccuracies in recording level resulting from sound reflections from the arm and hand are negligible compared with the rather large errors which result from changes in head position when a meter is in a fixed position. The tripod method can be used only for the mature child who will sit alone, rather than on the parent's knee, and remain still for the whole of the test; not many children will satisfy these requirements at this age.

The Cooperative Test

Compared with the Toy Discrimination Test, this test requires greater tester skill and more cooperation from the child, but it offers a useful alternative and is, in some cases, more appropriate for the active child. The objective is to develop a giving game with simple toy materials and to record the minimum listening level required for the comprehension of simple instructions, such as 'give this to teddy'. To increase the sensitivity of the test it is desirable to choose items with the same number of syllables and with acoustic similarities. Allowing for the limited vocabulary at this age, the writer's preferred items are teddy, baby (or dolly), and mummy and/or daddy. The first stage of the test is to check that the names of the items are known and then the game is established by demonstrating the giving activity in response to instructions presented initially at a loud level and with visual clues. After a few demonstrations of this nature the child should be invited to take part and it may be helpful to place the item in the child's hand and to restrain the child's hand until the instruction has been given. This enables the tester to gauge whether the child is attempting to respond impulsively and, if so, to suppress such behaviour.

The technique for recording the results, after removing visual clues and varying the presentation level and order of presentation, is the same as for the Four-toy Eyepointing Test, the only difference being that the giving action replaces the eye pointing response.

Testing responses to frequency-specific sounds

The second part of the audiological assessment for this age group is really a repeat of the distraction method used for the younger child but with slight modification. The 18-month-old child is more mature and is much more likely to show patterns of inhibition and habituation. It appears that the response is governed more by voluntary control rather than by primitive reflex, for the child may turn only once to each sound to satisfy its curiosity. There is, therefore, a need to vary the order of presentation and to take special care to ensure that the child is not aware of the side of presentation until the stimulus appears. It is helpful to have two noisemakers held symmetrically on each side in the 45° position, if checking behaviour is observed, and to include many control trials with no sound stimulus. If the child does not respond even at raised levels, it is sometimes useful to incorporate the same sound in the attention-gaining activity at the front; the temptation and motivation to turn is then heightened when the stimulus sound appears from a different location. Sometimes the verbal prompt 'Where is the noise?' may initiate a turn, but if this technique is used it is vital to include control (no sound) trials with the same prompting. The visual reinforcement audiometry discussed in Chapter 5 may be very useful at this stage.

Test techniques 2;6–3;6 years

Children with mental ages of 2;6 years and above should be capable of undertaking a simple pre-audiometry conditioning procedure known as a *performance* test and this method is used to replace the distraction test for recording responses to frequency-specific sounds.

The second part of the audiological assessment utilizes toy materials to test auditory discrimination of speech for a wider range of items than could be utilized for the younger child.

The Performance Test

In this test the child is conditioned to wait for an auditory stimulus and then to respond in a play activity such as placing a ball on a stick, a peg in a board, stacking cubes or beakers or knocking a skittle off the table. The tester must develop child-handling and timing skills and be able to make effective use of simple play materials (Figure 4.2) to maintain the child's interest and co-operation. A great merit of this test technique is

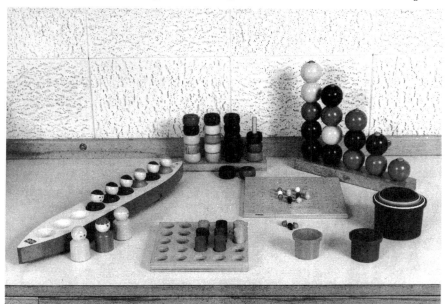

Figure 4.2 Play materials for the Performance Test.

that it can be used without the need for verbal instruction and is particularly useful when testing children with language difficulties. At this age the child should be seated in a low chair adjacent to the parent and the test materials should be placed on a low table.

The conditioning is established by demonstrating with visual and auditory prompting initially, and subsequently with the auditory stimulus alone. The conditioning sequence starts with a demonstration in which the tester holds the response item poised ready to respond and then promptly inserts it in the boat (for example) when the sound stimulus is presented. After a few demonstrations of this nature the child should be offered the toy and the tester should guide a few responses. The responses should be rewarded with a hand clap gesture and vocal praise and the stimulus level must be fairly high at first. If no signs of restraint are detected, the stimulus level should be increased and/or visual prompting should be employed (for example, a head nod when the stimulus is inserted) until a pattern of conditioning is established. One of the common pitfalls observed when this test is being used is that of inappropriate timing and specifically not leaving a sufficient pause before inserting the sound. If the child is conditioned correctly he should be prepared to wait poised ready to respond (Figure 4.3) for up to 10 s. In fact, the tester should vary the pause interval from 1–10 s quite unpredictably during the test to reduce the possibility of anticipatory responses and to identify and control any impulsive response tendency. If a child is developmentally ready for the test, reliable conditioning can normally be established after four or five demonstration responses and a further four or give guided responses. If this cannot be achieved, it will be necessary to resort to distraction methods (or visual reinforcement methods) to test the child's responses to frequency-specific stimuli.

The basic principles of the Performance Test have been described above and it is now necessary to discuss some of the finer details. It is, of course, vital that there should be no visual clues when the sound stimulus is presented, other than during the conditioning phase. If portable sound-field noise generators are used they should be held out of the child's visual field so that she cannot see movement of the tester's finger, hand, or arm, when the interrupter switch is operated. The normal position for holding the device is at an angle of 45° set back from the child's ear (Figure 4.3). Whenever the stimulus frequency is changed, the tester should be ready to re-condition the child for the new stimulus if there is any hesitation in the response. It is good practice to present each new sound at a comfortable level above the assumed threshold and then to lower the level quickly if positive responses are obtained. It must not be assumed that the conditioning will carry through to different sounds for the very young child.

If a child accepts the test situation and shows a good level of

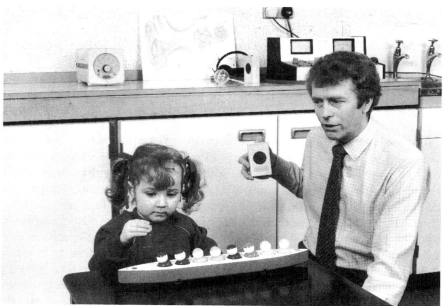

Figure 4.3 Child poised ready to respond in a Performance Test.

maturity, it might be possible to introduce the bone vibrator and later the earphones to obtain pure tone audiometric thresholds at a few frequencies. The golden rule, however, is to obtain the sound-field thresholds for two or three frequencies first because the point at which the child's co-operation might cease is often quite unpredictable. It is wise to obtain the essential information first before attempting something more ambitious, because with the mature child it will take only a short time to obtain a few sound-field thresholds, whereas the limit of the immature or uncooperative child's concentration may be exhausted by the same task. At the onset of the test it is not always possible to be sure which category the child will fall into at this age and all testers, however experienced, will admit to having misjudged certain children's abilities. The good tester will be very economical with time and this is why it is recommended that bone conduction testing should follow sound-field tests. This avoids duplicating air conduction information and, in addition, the child is often more likely to accept the physical intrusion of the smaller apparatus. Once having obtained a few bone conduction thresholds the tester may then be successful with earphones with some children. The procedure for audiometry is discussed in detail in Chapter 6 and it will be appreciated that once the child is mature enough to accept the earphones the task becomes much more straightforward.

The term *threshold* has been used in this section in a rather loose sense. The objective is to attempt to apply a standard threshold tracing method using the 'down 10 dB, up 5 dB' procedure described in Chapter 6 but it will be appreciated that this may not always be possible. With the very young child it might be necessary to use larger increments and decrements to speed up the procedure. A useful technique which can be employed with hand-held devices is to vary the distance of presentation, sweeping in smoothly from 1 m to within 10 cm of the ear, knowing that each halving of distance corresponds to a 6 dB increase in level. The sound level can then be deduced either from a pre-determined calculation or it can be measured directly with a sound level meter simply by duplicating the distance. The errors in distance estimates of this nature are acceptably low given that audiometry uses rather gross 5 dB steps and 6 dB corresponds to a doubling or halving of distance. The experienced tester can easily gauge distances which duplicate the sound levels within 5 dB.

With the availability of affordable computers the possibility of using computer games for conditioning and response reinforcement is worth considering. Children can be conditioned to press a mouse or simple joystick to elicit a reward in response to a stimulus from about the age of 3 years and early experience with the use of such methods has been encouraging. Their main application has been for prolonged testing such as cochlear implant tuning where new activities are needed. For normal clinical use the conventional play techniques can be quicker and more convenient. The pleasure children derive from the physical handling and manipulation of toy equipment should not be overlooked when considering computer game alternatives. There is a place for both methods.

If computers are to be used the following requirements must be satisfied to ensure maximum efficient use of the technique:

1. The stimulus/response/reward cycle should be fairly rapid so that a new stimulus can be presented within 5 s.
2. The stimuli should be discrete and the timing of their presentation should be variable and under the control of the tester to accommodate drifts in the child's attention.
3. False responses should be correctable or not rewarded.
4. There should be the facility to change the game rapidly if the child becomes bored.

Speech discrimination tests

Although the 2;6-year-old child has usually developed a much wider receptive and expressive vocabulary than his 18-month-old counterpart, she is often still not mature enough for full speech audiometry to be undertaken under conditions of earphone use and with a series of word lists. Consequently, it is necessary to simplify the task and to play safe initially by using live voice in a sound-field setting. Numerous tests are available in the UK (for example, Kendall Toy Test, Kendall, 1954; RNID Picture Screening Test, Reed, 1969; Dodds Insert Board, Dodds, 1972; Toy Discrimination Test, McCormick, 1977) and they have mostly been developed for use in a screening context. The Toy Discrimination Test was developed by the writer for use as a simple screening test in the community health setting but this, like some of the other tests cited, has often been adapted for use in audiology clinics. This is now the most widely used test in the UK and it is the only British test developed specifically for use with children from a mental age of 2 years.

The Toy Discrimination Test (McCormick 1977)

This test is based on the popular idea of using a single set of toys in a finger pointing task. In this case, the toys were chosen from vocabulary lists followed by field trials in clinical practice, bearing in mind the following criteria:

1. The items should be known to a normal child with a mental age of 2 years.
2. There should be paired items of monosyllables with the maximum possible degree of acoustic similarity within the constraints imposed by:
   (a) the child's limited vocabulary at this age; and
   (b) the ease with which toy representation and identification could be achieved.

The test consists of 14 toys (Figure 4.4) in seven pairs, that is:

cup/duck
spoon/shoe
man/lamb
plate/plane
horse/fork
key/tree
house/cow

The test is administered by setting out a display containing only those paired items known to the child and the child is conditioned to point to the toys on request. Children with normal hearing can identify the items at a minimum listening level of 40 dB (A) and the objective is to determine the quietest level at which the child can identify the items with 80% success (that is, four correct items located from five requests) and to measure any deviation from the 40 dB (A) normal level. The finer details of the test administration will now be discussed and these

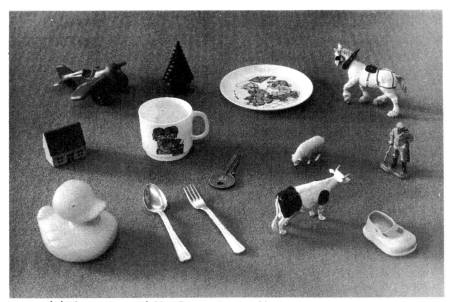

Figure 4.4 The McCormick Toy Discrimination Test.

should be noted particularly when testing the very young child. It is worth emphasizing again that maximum child co-operation at this age might be maintained only for a brief spell and it is necessary for the tester to develop timing and child-handling skills to maximize the amount of information that can be obtained from unpredictable children.

It is recommended that the child should be seated in a low chair adjacent to his or her parent, or on the parent's lap if shy or withdrawn. With the tester kneeling, or seated, across a low table positioned in front of the child, the toy items should be brought out individually and a check made to determine which ones are well known to the child. The child should be encouraged to name each item, thus enabling the tester to assess the presence and quality of the speech sounds, particularly those in the high-frequency region. If the child will not, or can not, name the toys then the parent should be asked which items they would expect the child to recognise. The final display should contain only those pairs of items which are well known to the child and the tester then demonstrates to the child that he should point to each toy in response to the request 'Show me the ...' or 'Where is the ...'. A good conversational level of voice must be used initially, with the child able to watch the tester's face for visual speech clues. Having established the conditioning, the tester should cover her mouth to obliterate visual clues and the voice level should be lowered to determine the quietest level at which the child correctly identifies four items from five requests (80% score). The test is normally undertaken with the tester in front of the child initially, but once a measure of the level required, using a sound level meter, is obtained, it may be possible to obtain further responses from each side. Ideally, the instructions should be presented at right angles to each ear at arm's length from the child, with the level being monitored with a sound level meter held just behind the child's head, level with the ear, and at the same distance from the tester. It may be possible to mount the instrument on a tripod if the child will stay in a reasonably fixed position. With the very young or immature child it may only be possible to obtain a few responses from the front before the child's attention drifts. Occasional repositioning of the toys in the display may help to recapture the attention sufficiently for a few extra responses to be obtained. If a child attempts to manipulate or play with the toys it might be helpful to use a drum stick as a pointing stick, to occupy the child's hand(s).

In the case of the very shy or withdrawn child or the child with motor difficulties, the eye pointing technique can be used with a limited range of the toys spaced well apart on the table. The pitfalls discussed earlier in this chapter must be avoided if eye pointing is used but it is well worth devoting time in an attempt to establish a response pattern of this nature with the very damaged child for she sometimes surprises not only the tester but also her parents.

One of the great merits of a sound-field test of this nature is that the child's parent(s) can observe directly the nature of the child's hearing problem. The difference between sound detection and speech discrimination can be demonstrated together with the word confusions at quiet listening levels. Children with slight or moderate hearing problems will often say 'what', or 'pardon', at the quiet listening levels and the more severely affected child might attempt to watch the face intently for speech reading clues. These signs all offer valuable indicators of the presence of the child's hearing problems and they should be discussed with the parents.

The results of the Toy Discrimination Test should be reported as for the Four-toy Eyepointing Test, that is:

A raised level of ... dB (A) was required before the child could achieve an 80% score.

This assumes, of course, that the child does not have a degree of loss of such severity as to prevent the development of speech and language. It is unlikely that the late-diagnosed child with a severe or profound hearing loss will be able to undertake this test, although it might be worth attempting the test with the child able to watch the speaker's face and using only a few easily lipreadable items such as shoe, spoon, fork and horse. The reporting of negative results if the child is unable to undertake the task, or the reporting of success with and without visual and auditory clues, can still be very informative.

The Automated McCormick/IHR Toy Discrimination Test

There are advantages and limitations in the live presentation of speech test materials to very young children.

Advantages

1. The material is presented in a very natural communication situation.
2. Visual (speech reading) clues can be used.
3. The test is non-intrusive to the child because it requires the minimum of equipment (headphones can sometimes have a disturbing and inhibiting effect on children below the age of 3 years).

Limitations

1. Inter- and intra-subject variability in voice level and intelligibility can influence the results.
2. The accurate monitoring of voice level can be problematic.
3. It may be difficult to score responses accurately while maintaining the necessary level of close interaction with the child.
4. It is not possible to test below a minimal voice level of 35/40 dB (A) in a live setting.

The Automated McCormick/IHR (Institute of Hearing Research) Toy Discrimination Test (Ousey et al., 1989; Palmer, Sheppard and Marshall, 1991) provides an innovative solution to many of the problems and it offers a highly refined and accurate method for obtaining stable, reliable, and repeatable audiometric speech test results from very young children of 2 years of age and above.

The test uses a speaker presentation of digitally stored speech waveforms of the 14 words in the Toy Discrimination Test and incorporates an adaptive scoring algorithm under microprocessor control. Conventional recording techniques cannot be used for the very young because the combination of word pairs known to each child differs. Digital recordings enable instant random access to any word combinations. The components of the test are shown in Figure 4.5 and consist of a handset linked to the control unit housed in the speaker stand.

The tester programmes the test by means of the handset control which includes a display (for the tester) indicating the output word for the current trial and the estimate of the threshold. The handset contains the following selection options:

1. Word pair selection (one select button for each word pair).
2. Stimulus presentation control (timing under tester control).
3. Score correct and incorrect buttons.

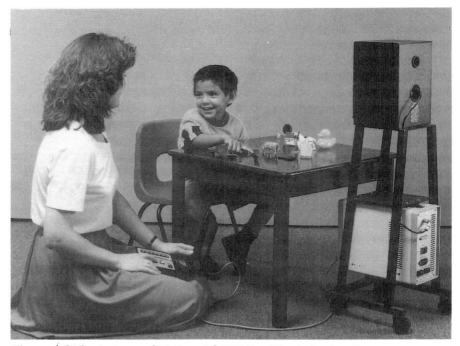

Figure 4.5 The Automated McCormick/IHR Toy Discrimination Test

4. Repeat responses at the same level (score included) or at a higher level (not scored). The latter option is used to alert a child whose attention has drifted.
5. Test in quiet or in 60 dB pink noise.
6. Warble tone selection option with frequency selection and level control in 10, 5, 2 or 1 dB steps.
7. Speaker selection (two speakers available and the stimulus words, masker noise and warble tones can be routed to either at will).
8. Optional Visual Reinforcement Audiometry Facility with one or two speakers.

Calibration signals for the words, masker noise and warble tones in dB(A) or dB SPL are also selected by the handset control.

The Automated Toy Test takes approximately 2–3 min to administer to the typical 2–5-year-old child and shows an excellent test–retest correlation of 0.93 for such children (Ousey et al., 1989). For children in this age group the normal score in quiet (typical clinical ambient noise level of less than 30 dB (A)) for the 71% correct criterion is 30/35 dB (A). For adults in the same acoustic surroundings it is approximately 20 dB (A) (18.6 dBA). These levels are much lower than can be obtained with live presentation of speech.

Testing starts with the test word presented at 72 dB(A) and consists of a running-in phase 'Point to the …' followed by the stimulus word. Initially the level is reduced by 12 dB following each correct response until the child makes an error when the level is increased by 12 dB. After the next correct response an adaptive procedure is used to control the stimulus level and to estimate the level giving the 71% correct response. The level is reduced by 6 dB following two correct responses and increased by 6 dB following an error. The transition from increasing to decreasing level, or vice versa, constitutes a reversal. The threshold is then estimated as the mean of the stimulus levels at six reversals at which time the testing automatically stops.

The correlation between speech in quiet and pure tone thresholds (average of 0.5, 1 and 4 kHz) is high with a 95% confidence interval of 11 dB (Palmer, Sheppard and Marshall, 1991) and by utilizing the speech in noise facility it is possible to investigate aspects of hearing disability in a way that hitherto had not been possible with very young children. The test is finding application in hearing aid evaluation (aided/unaided speech in noise and warble tone testing) and in the investigation of binaural hearing performance (Summerfield, 1993, personal communication) in addition to normal clinical testing. It is an excellent example of the harnessing of new technology to satisfy clinical demands. Acknowledgement for the idea of using digital recordings for this purpose goes to Professor Mark Haggard (Director of the Medical Research Council Institute of Hearing Research), who raised the idea with the author.

Summary

The testing of children below 3 years of age by behavioural methods poses many problems, which can be overcome by the skilled tester. The development of appropriate skills in child handling, in timing and in clinical decision-making constitutes an important training requirement for the paediatric audiologist. Only when such skills have been acquired and practised will the practitioner be in a good position to evaluate the values and virtues of other test developments. It is unlikely that future methods will completely replace the need for the behavioural methods because of the richness of information they provide about the child's actual use of hearing.

References

Arlinger, S.D. and Jerlvall, L.B. (1987). Reliability in warble-tone sound field audiometry. *Scandinavian Audiology* 16, 21–27.

Byrne, D. and Dillon, H. (1981). Comparative reliability of warble tone thresholds under earphones and in sound field. *Australian Journal of Audiology* 3, 12–14.

Dodds, J. (1972). An object puzzle as an indicator of hearing acuity. *Sound* 6, 49–55.

Ewing, I.R. and Ewing, A.W.G. (1944). The ascertainment of deafness in infancy and early childhood. *Journal of Laryngology and Otology* 59, 309–338.

Ewing, I.R. and Ewing, A.W.G. (1947). *Opportunities and the Deaf Child*. London: University of London Press.

Hoversten, G.H. and Moncur, J.P. (1969). Stimuli and intensity factors in testing infants. *Journal of Speech and Hearing Research* **12**, 689–702.

Jerger, S. and Jerger, J. (1982). Pediatric speech intelligibility test: Performance intensity characteristics. *Ear and Hearing* **3**, 325–334.

Kaga, K. and Tanaka, Y. (1980). Auditory brainstem response and behavioral audiometry. *Archives of Otolaryngology* **106**, 564–566.

Kendall, D.C. (1954). Audiometry for young children. *Teacher of the Deaf* **307**, 18–23.

Liden, G. and Kankkunen, A. (1969). Visual reinforcement audiometry in the management of young deaf children. *International Audiology* **8**, 99.

Lutman, M.E. and McCormick, B. (1987). Converting free-field A-weighted sound levels to hearing levels. *Journal of the British Association of Teachers of the Deaf* **11**, 127.

McCormick, B. (1977). The Toy Discrimination Test: An aid for screening the hearing of children above a mental age of two years. *Public Health* **91**, 67–73.

McCormick, B. (1986). Evaluation of a warbler in hearing screening tests. *Health Visitor* **59**, 143–144.

McCormick, B. (1994). *Screening for Hearing-Impairment in Young Children*. London: Whurr.

McCormick, B., Wood, S.A., Cope, Y. and Spavins, F.M. (1984). Analysis of records from an open access audiology service. *British Journal of Audiology* **18**, 127–132.

Mason, S., McCormick, B. and Wood, S. (1988). The Auditory Brainstem Response (ABR). *Archives of Disease in Childhood* **63**, 465–467.

Mendel, M.I. (1968). Infant responses to recorded sounds. *Journal of Speech and Hearing Research* **11**, 811–816.

Moore, J.M., Wilson, W.R. and Thompson, G. (1977). Visual reinforcement of head-turn responses in infants under 12 months of age. *Journal of Speech and Hearing Disorders* **42**, 328–334.

Nolan, M. (1978). Guidance on the interpretation of information from a sound level meter. *Journal of the British Association of Teachers of the Deaf* **2**, 169–173.

Nolan, M. (1987). Letter to the Editor. *Journal of the British Association of Teachers of the Deaf* **11**, 128–129.

Ousey, J., Sheppard, S., Twomey, T. and Palmer, A.R. (1989). The IHR–McCormick Automated Toy Discrimination Test – description and initial evaluation. *British Journal of Audiology* **23**, 245–249.

Palmer, A.R., Sheppard, S. and Marshall, D.M. (1991). Prediction of hearing thresholds in children using an automated toy discrimination test. *British Journal of Audiology* **25**, 351–356.

Reed, M. (1969). *RNID Picture Screening Test of Hearing*. London: Royal National Institute for the Deaf.

Samples, J.M. and Franklin, B. (1978). Behavioural responses in 7 to 9 month old infants to speech and non-speech stimuli. *Journal of Auditory Research* **18**, 115–123.

Siegenthaler, B. (1969). Maturation of auditory abilities in children. *Audiology* **8**, 59–71.

Suzuki, T. and Ogiba, Y. (1961). Conditioned orientation reflex audiometry. *Archives of Otolaryngology* 74, 192–198.

Thompson, G. and Folsom, R.C. (1985). Reinforced and non-reinforced head-turn responses of infants as a function of stimulus bandwidth. *Ear and Hearing* 6, 125–129.

Chapter 5
Visual reinforcement audiometry

JOHN BAMFORD and EILEEN McSPORRAN

Introduction

Although the assessment of accurate hearing thresholds is by no means the only task of the paediatric audiologist, it is nevertheless an essential requirement without which appropriate diagnosis and habilitation cannot take place. In a small number of cases (e.g. very severely handicapped infants) assessment of auditory sensitivity may only be possible using the so-called 'objective' test methods such as auditory brain stem responses and sensitivity prediction from acoustic reflex thresholds (see Chapters 7 and 9). For most children, however, it is possible to obtain an accurate estimate of sensitivity thresholds across the whole frequency range using behavioural testing techniques (sometimes referred to as 'subjective' methods). If the child is able to cooperate actively in the test procedures – generally from the age of about 3 years, pure tone audiometry may be possible. As always in paediatric audiology, flexibility of procedure is essential and modifications of the task given to the child and to the instructions and social reinforcement given by the audiologist may be needed, but the procedure remains essentially that of standard pure tone (headphone) audiometry.

For children below the age of 3 years, or those with developmental delay or particular handicaps, other behavioural testing methods must be used to assess hearing sensitivity. These other methods overlap and are to some extent alternatives. Although clear protocols are essential for *screening* tests it can be misleading to define exact protocols for the further assessment procedures because the impression may be given of rigid methodology; it is essential that aspects of calibration and equipment are defined rigorously but within that rigour it is just as important to stress the necessity for a flexible approach to the child and for the audiologist to take into account the *whole* child. In what follows, reference will frequently be made to particular age ranges for which particular techniques are appropriate. The caveat will be made here, but applies throughout, that the determinant of the approach best used is not chronological age but developmental age – and in particular the status of the child's auditory attention. Cooper, Moodley and Reynell (1978) provide a useful summary of the development of attention, which passes through extreme distractibility in the first year of life, fairly inflexible attention to concrete aspects of the environment in the second year, a more flexible and shifting attention control in the third year of life, to the stage in the fourth year at which the child can choose to control its own attention. It is at this stage that the child may be able to undertake the cooperative requirements of formal pure tone audiometry.

From birth to about 6 months behavioural responses to sound will not clearly reflect auditory thresholds and the audiologist may have to rely on qualitative observation of the child's responses in order to draw conclusions about auditory sensitivity. Such methods have been subsumed under the title Behavioural Observation Audiometry (BOA, see Wilson and Thompson, 1984 for a review). From about 6 to 18 months of age, distraction testing is widely used in the UK, followed by the so-called cooperative (18–30 months) and performance methods (30–36 months). Play audiometry is another term used for performance testing; it refers to that stage at which a child, although not yet able to wear headphones and cooperate with pure tone audiometry, is nevertheless able to join in a task that requires it actively to direct its attention to sounds – to listen – and respond by placing a brick in a box, a peg in a board etc. This may be possible at 30 months or earlier in some cases. These techniques are reviewed in Chapter 4.

A further behavioural technique which is usable, bearing in mind the general development, from about 6 or 7 months through to 3 years of age is visual reinforcement audiometry (VRA). This is a powerful and simple technique, well suited to the kind of authoritative audiological assessments required at the referral levels of assessment.

Historical background

It is not the aim of this chapter to review in detail the early literature on VRA. Such reviews are available elsewhere (see, for example, Kankkunen, 1982; Wilson and Thompson, 1984). Nevertheless, some historical perspective may be useful.

VRA is occasionally suggested to be a descendant of the 'peep-show' technique described by Dix and Hallpike (1947) and used by, for example, Barr (1955) for pure tone audiometry in young children. This technique was, however, more akin to play audiometry or performance testing in which the child cooperates in the task to the extent that it actively listens for sound signals to which it responds appropriately. VRA is more properly associated with the younger pre-active listening methods in which a response (such as head turning) is elicited by gaining the child's attention.

Suzuki and Ogiba (1961) first described the technique of conditioning orientation reflex (COR) audiometry. In COR the infant sits on a parent's knee in front of apparatus that contains two small loudspeakers at about 30° on either side of the midline and 70 cm apart. Above each speaker is a doll which could be illuminated to make it visible. The tester sits behind the apparatus and observes the child over the top. A pure tone at an intensity estimated to be about 40 dB above threshold is presented for 3 or 4 s from one of the loudspeakers and at the same time the doll above that loudspeaker is illuminated. The sound (or sound and light) elicit a turning response, the orientation reflex, towards the source. After an interval of 2 or 3 s, the same tone–light stimulation is presented from the other side. This conditioning procedure, in which sound and light are associated, is repeated three or four times from different sides in order that the child makes the association between sound and (pleasurable or rewarding) light. Once this association has been made the sound is presented alone, and only if the child turns appropriately is the response rewarded or reinforced with the visual stimulus. Successive trials use signals of lower intensity levels until thresholds are reached and the child's responses cease.

Although the COR technique as described by Suzuki and Ogiba is no longer used, and the rather cumbersome apparatus has been superseded by much simpler methods, it was the precursor of today's VRA procedures and used many of the essential principles to be found in VRA. In particular, the use of visual reinforcement of the sound stimulus elicits responses that are more frequent and more stable, allowing the audiologist the time to assess responses for a variety of signals down to near-threshold levels. While the sound on its own will elicit a clear orientation reflex, that response is quickly extinguished if no reward (or meaning) is associated with the sound. Some broad-band sounds such as voice or rattle will elicit turning responses for several trials without an additional visual reinforcer, but even these will extinguish too quickly for the purposes of threshold assessment (the broad-band nature of such stimuli makes children more responsive to them than to pure tones, rather than any alleged 'familiarity' effect – see Bench and Mentz, 1975; Thompson and Folsom, 1985). The use of a visual reinforcer not only allows more test time (because more responses are elicited), but also allows the use of very frequency-specific signals such as warble tones. In effect, the visual reinforcer makes the rather meaningless warble tones more interesting to the child. The use of specific sounds, which are now given more interest, in turn makes the precise control of the child's attention less crucial to the success of the test, although the child's state of attention will always remain an important factor. Suzuki and Ogiba correctly pointed out that their COR procedure is a mixture of classical (pavlovian) and operant (instrumental) conditioning. In initial trials the procedure is more akin to classical conditioning in that a conditioned association is established between the contiguous sound and light. After the initial conditioning the light is presented only if the child responds appropriately to the sound and the child's response is rewarded or reinforced by the attractive visual presentation, thus maintaining stable conditioning. At this stage, the procedure appears more like operant conditioning.

The term 'visual reinforcement audiometry' was introduced by Liden and Kankkunen (1969) to describe a modified COR procedure. Although the apparatus was rather similar in size and distance from the child to that used by Suzuki and Ogiba, there were two important differences in overall technique.

1. The loudspeakers were mounted on moveable arms which allowed them to be placed at 15 cm from each of the child's ears, at 90° azimuth. Bearing in mind head-shadow effects, this enabled Liden and Kankkunen to determine thresholds for each ear separately. However, the crucial effect of moving the loudspeakers was that it separated the sound position from the position of the visual reinforcer (which remained at 30–45°). This emphasizes one of the principles of VRA: that, although sound and light should be adjacent in time, they need not be in the same spatial position; greater flexibility of test procedures thus becomes possible. When they are spatially separated, the classical conditioning of the orientation reflex begins to play a lesser role and the procedure appears more and more like an operant conditioning technique.

2. Liden and Kankkunen removed the necessity for adequate localization skills in the child, which were a requirement for the successful use of COR. Many children with impaired binaural or unilateral hearing will be rather poor at localizing sound (see, for example Durlach, Thompson and Colburn, 1981) and including a demand for successful localization in the COR task confounds basic sensitivity skills with higher-order localization skills; it is useful to have an assessment of both but they may need to be kept separate.

In terms of test procedure, what Liden and Kankkunen did to assess sensitivity uncontaminated by localization skills was to use sound and light always on one side, rather than randomly changing from side to side as Suzuki and Ogiba had done. This procedure is used in the protocol suggested later in this chapter.

Since VRA was first introduced it has been widened in its scope, and VRA is now used as a generic term to cover that class of behavioural audiometry procedures in which visual stimuli are specifically employed as reinforcers.

The Liden and Kankkunen procedure, like that of Suzuki and Ogiba, still involved one or two procedural disadvantages, which more recent approaches do not. In particular:

- pure tones were used which, despite the proximity of the loud-speakers to the ear, may have led to errors due to sound-field acoustics;
- the proximity of the apparatus itself presented problems, because small, not easily detected eye movements could be sufficient for the child to obtain the visual reward;
- proximal equipment can be daunting to a young infant; and
- the apparatus itself, albeit fairly simple, had to be constructed on a one-off basis.

Haug, Baccaro and Guilford (1967) described a version of VRA which is perhaps more similar to procedures now in use than those of Liden and Kankkunen or of Suzuki and Ogiba. They used a loud-speaker 2 m from the child, at 90° azimuth. The child was seated on the parent's knee, with its attention drawn by an assistant to a variety of toys in front of it on a table. The tester was situated in an adjoining room, with an observation window adjacent to the loudspeaker in the test room. When sounds elicited a gross head-turn response to the loudspeaker the visual reinforcer was a brightly illuminated moving glove-puppet, presented in the observation window by the tester. No attempt was made to assess localization (only one sound source was used), but after sound-field testing the status of each ear was assessed separately using headphone presentation (but still associated with the glove-puppet reinforcer in the observation window).

Basic principles of VRA

The essence of VRA is to reinforce an observable behavioural response (usually head turning) to frequency-specific sounds with a visual reward. The child's attention is attracted by the sound and it turns in order to see the visual reward. Sufficient trials are given in order to assess threshold responses to sounds accurately at a number of different frequencies.

Beyond this core, there may be facilities to assess localization, to assess each ear separately using headphones or tubephones (insert ear-phones), to assess thresholds under each earmould using tubephones, to assess the presence of an air–bone gap using a bone vibrator and to assess hearing for speech. In addition, it is always useful to obtain a general impression of auditory attention, listening skills, speech and language development and general development. With an appropriate-ly designed test set-up, and appropriately trained audiologists, such specific assessments and more general impressions are possible and necessary to any paediatric audiological assessment. Although the prime aim of VRA is to obtain an accurate assessment of frequency-specific thresholds, this must always be undertaken within the context of the whole child and the associated observations.

For different cases there will be different priorities for audiological and developmental assessment, and the precise VRA set-up will therefore vary from child to child. In later sections the detailed procedures for using VRA to determine thresholds in both sound field and 'closed-circuit' (i.e. with headphones, bone vibrator or tubephones) applications will be described. Assessing sound field thresholds can be performed with a child wearing hearing aids, if necessary.

Present a sound to a child in a sound field and it will tend to turn and locate (look at) the source. This is known as the orientation reflex (OR). Should the sound be presented repeatedly the OR will habituate and the child will cease to turn, unless there is something about the sound or its source that continues to interest: the sound of a familiar toy or voice might be sufficient to engage the child's interest and keep it turning to locate successive presentations, at least for a while. In audiology, however, we are interested in determining thresholds for narrow bandwidth stimuli of different frequencies. Such stimuli are not likely to continue to interest the child beyond the first few orientation reflex turns. This 'interest' is a function of bandwidth (see Thompson and Folsom, 1985).

In VRA a visually interesting stimulus is associated with the sound source in order to slow down the habituation of the OR and to enable more presentations to determine thresholds with reasonable accuracy. Thus,

SOUND elicits HEAD TURN

and the head turn at the correct moment allows the audiologist to infer that the child has heard the sound.

However, with narrow-band stimuli at least, this OR would soon habituate. In order to delay habituation, an interesting visual stimulus is associated with the sound presentation, thus:

NARROW BANDWIDTH
SOUND $\Big\}$ elicits HEAD TURN.
and
VISUAL STIMULUS

Associating a visual stimulus with the sound will also produce the OR. If the visual stimulus is interesting enough, and if the child is able to make the association between sound stimulus and visual stimulus, then *conditioning* has taken place and the child will turn to the sound alone in order to see the visual stimulus. This has been termed the conditioned orientation reflex, and is the basis of VRA:

SOUND elicits HEAD TURN reinforced by VISUAL STIMULUS.

In the first situation, when conditioning is taking place, the child is shown sound and visual stimulus together. When conditioning is secure (i.e. the child 'knows' that sound 'means' visual stimulus and turns correctly in response to the sound alone), the visual stimulus is presented as a *reinforcer* of the conditioning. Thus we can think of the sound stimulus producing a head turn, which is *rewarded* by a visual reinforcer; hence VRA.

Many suitable visual reinforcers exist, and the choice may depend upon budget, tester preference etc. Some people simply use flashing coloured lights; some use toy animals with eyes that light up, or a box which lights up to reveal the toy inside; some use toy animals which not only light up but which also move. One example of a visual reinforcer is shown in Figure 5.1. In this, the clown's face has lights that can be flashed as appropriate.

However, although a toy with eyes that light up may be sufficiently interesting for most children, it will not be suitable for all: children with Down's syndrome, for example, might find it not interesting enough, and children with visual impairment might require something

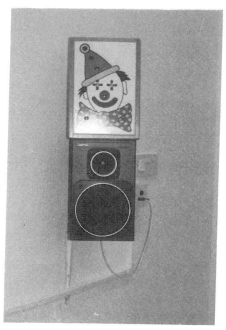

Figure 5.1 A loudspeaker and visual reinforcer.

more easily visible. This requires some equipment versatility, which may be achieved by interchangeable reinforcers or video screen reinforcers with programmable options. Common practice in Australia uses a glove-puppet reinforcer in a lit-up box operated by the tester at the observation window. The child faces 90° away from the observation window, and has to turn to locate loudspeaker and reinforcer by the observation window. Using a glove-puppet scheme allows the reinforcer to be changed.

Sound field testing

Given that the usual clinical goal is to define sensitivity primarily in the important speech frequency range, VRA becomes most powerful if it can be used to estimate thresholds at 0.5, 1, 2 and 4 kHz. With some severe hearing losses it may be useful to use 0.25 kHz, and occasionally (for example, when monitoring the high-frequency thresholds of children on ototoxic treatment) 3 and 6 kHz as well. Pure tones are *not* recommended for sound-field use; thus, if frequency-specific thresholds are to be estimated the stimuli of choice are warble tones (see Walker, Dillon and Byrne, 1984 for a detailed discussion of stimulus parameters). In certain circumstances narrow-band noise may be helpful but on most audiometers this has filter slopes of only 12 dB per octave, which may lead to invalid threshold estimates in the case of a steeply sloping high-frequency hearing loss.

The most sophisticated sound-field VRA set-ups will use an audiometer with warble tones, narrow-band noise and a microphone for voice located outside the test room. The tester (T_1) operates the audiometer, the sound-field outputs of which drive loudspeakers in the test room. T_1 observes the child and its responses through a one-way observation window. A second tester (T_2) sits in the test room with the child, managing the events and helping to control the child's attention. The usual position for the loudspeakers and associated visual reinforcers is 45, 60 or 90° azimuth from the centre forward. This positioning is quite sufficient for clear head turning responses; positions behind the child (greater than 90°) may cause difficulties for children with other handicaps, or may result in checking behaviour (turning to wait for the visual stimulus, in anticipation) which interferes with returning the child to a forward symmetrical position between stimuli. Figure 5.2 shows a diagram of such an arrangement.

This set-up can be modified or simplified in various ways to suit more modest budgets:

- it is possible to use only one loudspeaker, located at 45, 60 or 90°;
- it is possible to use only one room, in which case the audiometer and T_1 may sit in a suitably unobtrusive position and T_2 may observe the child's responses.

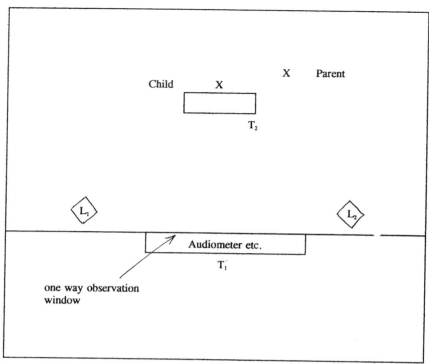

Figure 5.2 Possible two-room arrangement for VRA. T_1 and T_2 are testers, L_1 and L_2 are loudspeakers with visual reinforcers above.

A similar set-up using, for example, a hand-held warble tone generator (which could be operated by T_2 from the table top, using a foot switch to bring in the visual reinforcer at 45, 60 or 90° or by T_1 from a position of 45° behind the child, as in distraction testing), will dispense with the audiometer altogether. In the latter situation, the visual reinforcement contingent upon a correct head turn would be performed by T_2 operating a foot switch. In this case T_1 must sit at 45° behind the child to guard against the child picking up the visual cues present when the stimuli are presented.

In what follows, one possible detailed protocol for sound field testing is provided, with reference to the complete two-room set-up shown in Figure 5.2. This is not the only way of performing sound-field VRA, but the reader will see that such a protocol contains a number of important (and indeed essential) details that will of necessity form part of all VRA testing. There are few places, if any, in the literature to which the student or clinician can turn to check fine details of VRA testing procedure, and it is helpful – if perhaps a little tedious – to present such details here. It also serves as a useful reference for closed-circuit VRA testing, which will be considered later.

1. T_2 collects the child and its parent from the waiting room and settles them in the test room. It may be helpful with children over 1 year old to leave a small box of toys on the table for the child to explore as it settles down.

2. T_2 talks with the child's parent to a greater or lesser extent: relevant points of history may be taken, and the outline of the test explained briefly. T_2 (and T_1) will be making observations about the child's behaviour and development. T_2 may find it useful occasionally to engage the child with a smile or a passing comment.

3. T_2 chooses a toy or toys (the minimum necessary), which may be helpful to get the child to adopt the symmetrical forward position. These toys are left on the table and any others removed. The child's position immediately before the stimulus should be symmetrical, facing forward. Children aged between 6 months and a year or so (and possibly older) will be on the parent's knee, held gently and the parent is instructed not to give the child any clues. Older children will be best seated on a small chair, preferably one with arms tucked under the table. One parent should be seated close by and on the side opposite to that being used for the visual reinforcement.

4. T_1 presents a 1 kHz signal (well above presumed threshold) at the same time as a visual reinforcer. One loudspeaker is used (L_1 in Figure 5.2). It may be worth briefly delaying the onset of the visual reinforcer, because a clear head turn to the sound alone will provide useful information. However, the delay should be minimal, and the child should see clearly that sound and light appear at the same time. This can be emphasized by switching both off while the child is looking at the visual reinforcer. If the child does not turn to locate the sound and view the reinforcer, T_2 should draw the child's attention to the reinforcer when it is on.

5. Conditioning trials (step 4) are repeated as often as required to secure conditioning. This is shown by the child clearly turning in response to the sound alone.

Note that for young children (less than 1 year old) the conditioning may take many trials. A response time (the time taken to turn) of 1 or 2 s must be allowed for. Conditioning may be speeded up by using narrow-band noise; in which case T_1 should be sure to include *at least* a 4 kHz warble tone later, when the conditioning and responses are better and clearer. Whenever responses to warble tones at any level cannot be elicited narrow-band noise is worth trying .

6. T_2's task is to encourage the child gently to the forward-symmetrical position between trials. The child will be interested in the visual reinforcer and may keep looking at, or regularly checking, it. The best way to deal with this is to wait, and perhaps *gently* to engage interest in the table top by tapping or by moving the toys. Eventually, the checking will cease because it is not reinforced.

7. When conditioning is secure T_1 should proceed to the test trials proper, that is to trials in which sound only is presented (still from L_1). If T_1 judges that the child has turned in response to the sound, then visual reinforcement is presented. This judgement is crucial, and will depend on how good T_1 is as an observer of children and their development. The 'checking' responses may be mistakenly taken for real responses if the sound happens to be presented at the same time, causing false-negative assessments (that is, thresholds assessed as being better than they really are). These can be avoided by good and careful observation and by withholding the visual reinforcer for a moment or two after the child turns – this helps to distinguish checking glances, which are short-lived, from real responses. With a real response the child knows that the reinforcer will come and will tend to wait for it but the reinforcer should not be held off for more than a moment or two; if the child gives up and turns away before the visual reinforcer is given, this will tend to extinguish the conditioning. False-negative assessments may also be avoided by using variable (and often lengthy) inter-trial intervals.

8. There is no rigid '10 dB down, 5 dB up' rule for stimulus presentation. Depending upon the age of the child, its state and other factors concerned with time, T_1 may choose to present whatever stimulus will give the most information about possible thresholds. Depending upon the acoustics and calibration of the room no attempt is usually made to track thresholds below 25 or 30 dB SPL ('within normal limits').

9. With a child with hearing loss it may be helpful to return occasionally to a good clear suprathreshold signal with reinforcement. Similarly, it may be helpful to observe and repeat clearly a definite non-response (i.e. a sound below threshold).

10. T_2 should control events in the test room, taking responsibility for settling the child, for keeping the parents involved (see later section on family involvement), for choosing and changing suitable toys and for inducing the child to return to the front symmetrical position with minimal stimulation. The test room should be relatively quiet and uncluttered, and it is not helpful for T_2 to talk to the child continuously.

It is important, however, for them to 'join in' the turning response *after* the child has turned, to look at the reinforcer and to say 'isn't that fun?' or some such comment. If T_2 fails to do this, particularly with a child aged 1½ to 2½ years, the situation may frighten the child to the extent that testing becomes impossible.

Sometimes, particularly with children under 12 months, the child may become too interested in T_2, or may be too shy to participate, and it may help for T_2 to leave the test room completely. In such a situation the parent should join in with the 'isn't that fun?' remarks.

11. In assessing thresholds T_1 must leave variable and often lengthy gaps between stimuli. Such gaps act, in effect, as 'no stimulus control trials': too many stimuli presented frequently in the hope that the next one may produce a clear response are no use. Some workers favour a system in which both T_1 and T_2 independently judge the occurrence of a response; only if both agree (by pressing appropriate switches) would reinforcement be given. Further rigour has been suggested by the use of automated stimulus presentation sequences, keeping both T_1 and T_2 'blind' to whether a stimulus has been presented, and giving reinforcement only if both judge a response to have occurred. This 'double-blind' procedure is currently under investigation and would involve considerable changes in the protocol described here.

12. For most purposes it is safe and correct to assume that the procedure as described above is testing the better ear, which is not necessarily that on the side of the loudspeaker used. After determining better-ear thresholds across the range 0.5–4 kHz, judgement about localization skills may be made by presenting narrow-band noise (rather than warble tones) at suprathreshold levels from L_1 and L_2, with associated visual reinforcement (a live voice may also be used). Any doubt about localization should raise suspicion of unilateral hearing loss if the better-ear thresholds were within normal limits.

13. Voice detection using the child's name is a useful addition to confirm overall threshold estimates. Again, visual reinforcement and L_1 and L_2 may be used.

The procedures thus described will generally be sufficient to define or make useful observations on the history, general developmental progress, speech/language development, auditory attention and listening skills, localization ability and sound-field threshold sensitivity across frequencies. In the following sections, important extensions of the basic VRA protocols that allow the collection of more detailed audiometric information will be considered.

Closed-circuit VRA

Although a lack of audiometric data should not preclude provision of amplification, accurate frequency-specific estimates of threshold sensitivity for each ear are central to the successful selection and fitting of hearing aids for children. This is particularly difficult in the case of very young infants. Building up an accurate audiometric profile as early as possible is also vital to the recursive and dynamic nature of habilitation that integrates ongoing assessment and selection of aids, fitting and verification with appropriate, family driven, management and intervention strategies. The use of supra-aural headphones to obtain ear-specific threshold estimates from young infants using VRA has been documented in a number of studies (cited later in this chapter). However, traditional headphones tend to restrict head movements during VRA. Even with a shortened headband, headphones can fail to provide a good acoustic seal, because of the small size of the infant's head, thus introducing poor noise-exclusion properties at low frequencies. Another disadvantage is that interaural attenuation is limited, with a corresponding need for masking. There is also the possibility that infants with very small ears (such as those with Down's syndrome) may have collapsed ear canals.

Success with conventional headphones is possible, but our experience suggests that the use of lightweight insert earphones such as Etymotic ER-3A or Eartone 3A provides an alternative means of obtaining ear and frequency-specific data using VRA with fewer practical difficulties and with more potential for direct application to the selection of hearing aids for infants.

It is now generally accepted that children with unilateral hearing loss are at educational risk even when the hearing sensitivity is within normal limits in the other ear (ASHA, 1991). There is some evidence to suggest that children impaired in the right ear in particular may suffer adverse effects in the educational setting (Jensen, Borre and Johansen, 1989). The ASHA guidelines emphasize the importance of early ear-specific assessment, with effective masking of the non-test ear if necessary, and specify the use of VRA in combination with tympanometry. Closed-circuit application of VRA is essential for informing intervention decisions and for monitoring progressive or fluctuating hearing loss in infants with suspected asymmetrical hearing loss that may have been indicated by ABR or sound-field VRA results.

Insert earphones consist of a transducer coupled to the ear canal by a tube attached to a connecting nubbin and to a tube running through a disposable foam eartip. Advantages of insert earphones over traditional headphones include greater interaural attenuation with reduced need for masking, elimination of collapsed ear canal difficulties and reduction of ambient noise effects with increased accuracy of low frequency thresholds. (For a review of the clinical capability of insert earphones for audiometry see Borton et al., 1989.) During use the two plastic cases containing the receivers are clipped to the child's clothes, attached with small, double-sided Velcro discs or suspended from a loop around the child's neck (Figure 5.3). A foam eartip, with the foam trimmed to an appropriately small size if necessary, is attached to the connecting nubbin and rolled and compressed tightly. The eartip is then placed in the child's ear canal flush with the floor of the concha. Care must be taken to avoid blocking the sound tube with the foam plug, which is then held in place long enough for it to expand.

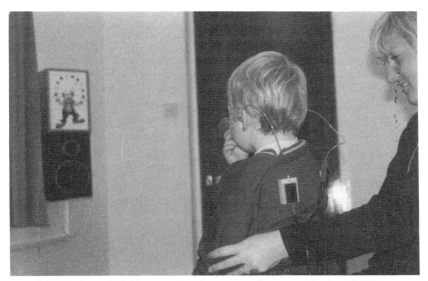

Figure 5.3 VRA/signal delivery using insert earphones with the child's own earmoulds.

The child is brought under stimulus control in the sound-field (following the procedure described earlier) before the insert earphones are placed. If necessary, the foam tips may be inserted one at a time, as this is more acceptable to some children: either way, time and skill is required for satisfactory placement. When changing the signal delivery transducer, for example the loudspeaker in the sound-field to insert earphones, some children unable to transfer the conditioning already established in the sound-field to the closed circuit mode may benefit from a brief re-shaping period. Stelmachowicz and Seewald (1991) have suggested that using narrow-band masking in the non-test ear via an insert earphone and presenting the stimulus to the test ear via a loudspeaker in the normal way may allow ear-specific data to be obtained from these children. Threshold estimation measures then proceed in the normal way. It may also be beneficial to use different visual reinforcers on either side of the child to maintain interest.

When using VRA for fitting a hearing aid, although the sound delivery tube of the insert earphone is designed to terminate in either an impedance probe or a foam plug, it is useful to deliver the signal via ER-3A insert earphones attached to the child's custom earmould once conditioning has been established in the sound-field. The foam eartip and sound tube are removed and the small plastic nubbin is inserted directly into the earmould tubing. The VRA protocol is then carried out in the conventional way. A button-type receiver may be used as the transducer if output levels above 110 dB HL are required.

For hearing-aid work the SPL in the child's ear canal corresponding to the threshold estimate obtained at each frequency must be ascertained. This can be achieved by measuring the SPL with a probe tube microphone in the ear canal at each threshold estimate. However, this procedure may not be optimal for a restless or uncooperative child because of the time required. For most young children of about 6–24 months, we apply 2 cm³ coupler conversion factors to the audiometer dial reading along with the real ear to coupler difference obtained using probe tube microphone measures, which is a much quicker process; the only extra time involved, in addition to the actual VRA procedure, being the few minutes necessary to obtain the real ear to coupler differences. The ear canal SPL estimates are then used to select gain and maximum output targets for selection and fitting of hearing aids. The targets are verified by probe tube microphone measurements and/or by sound-field-aided VRA.

Thus it is possible to collect ear and frequency-specific audiometric threshold data from young infants using the VRA paradigm in a form that is directly applicable to computer-assisted implementation of hearing-aid selection procedures (Seewald, 1992). Collection of audiometric data in this manner has the added advantage of avoiding some of the difficulties inherent in interfacing audiometric and electroacoustic information because all the data are expressed as dB SPL in the child's ear canal. In practice, attaching the insert earphones to the infant's earmoulds is simply accomplished in only a fraction of the time needed for insertion of foam eartips or for placement and acceptance of conventional headphones. Young infants invariably accept their first earmoulds without fuss and, provided that they are comfortable and well-fitting, they can be used with insert earphones as soon as the child is conditioned to respond to VRA in the sound-field. Other advantages of using the child's own moulds are that the cost of disposable eartips is avoided, insertion depth is constant, the insert earphones are less likely to be dislodged or pulled out and increased flexibility is possible with regard to parent/child positioning for VRA.

No studies on threshold estimation using insert earphones and custom earmoulds in infants have yet been published but clinical impressions so far suggest that threshold measures obtained in this manner closely agree with thresholds obtained using headphones. Further investigation is under way to determine the effects of mode of signal delivery on threshold estimation.

Efficacy of VRA

How successful is VRA for estimating infant hearing thresholds? Extensive literature reviews have been published elsewhere (e.g. Wilson and Thompson, 1984) and this section will therefore mention only a few relevant studies.

Using the VRA technique described above, Haug, Baccaro and

Guilford (1967) reported results from 54 infants aged 5–36 months. Sound-field (better-ear) threshold measurements were completed successfully on all but two children in the 19–24 month age range. Pure tone air and bone conduction thresholds were successfully assessed on all but five children, two from the 5–12 month age range ($n = 8$) and three from the 19–24 month range ($n = 23$). Of the 49 for whom both sound-field and headphone thresholds were assessed, the agreement (at 0.5, 1 and 4 kHz) was in all cases within 10 dB.

Moore, Thompson and Thompson (1975) studied infant sound localization behaviour as a function of four reinforcement conditions:

1. No reinforcement.
2. Social reinforcement (a smile, verbal praise and/or a pat on the shoulder).
3. Simple visual reinforcement (a flashing red light).
4. Complex visual reinforcement (a colourful animated toy bear).

Four groups of 12 children aged 12–18 months were examined. Each child, in a standard VRA paradigm using one loudspeaker at 45° azimuth, received 30 presentation trials of a complex noise at 70 dB SPL, and 10 control (no sound, no reinforcement) trials. The mean number of head-turn responses to the sounds were 27.3, 20.5, 15.2 and 9.7 for the complex, simple, social and 'no reinforcement' conditions respectively. The control trials resulted in turns towards the loudspeaker in only 4.8% of these (no sound) trials. The cumulative head-turn responses for the four groups are shown in Figure 5.4, which also shows that the 'no reinforcement' group habituated rapidly, and that auditory localization in this age group is strongly influenced by the type of reinforcement used.

In a further study, Moore, Wilson and Thompson (1977) used the complex reinforcer to examine the lower-age boundary of VRA. Ten infants in each of three age groups (4 months, 5–6 months and 7–11 months) were each given 30 visual reinforcement trials, and ten control infants were given trials with no reinforcement. The mean response rates (out of 30) for the groups are shown in Table 5.1. The difference between response rates with reinforcement and no reinforcement for the 5–6 and 7–11 month groups is significant, indicating that VRA is usable (at least at higher SPLs) for normal children from 6 months onwards.

Wilson, Moore and Thompson (1976) studied 90 normally developing infants of 5–18 months old. Using complex noise and complex reinforcement, they estimated auditory thresholds using a '20 dB down, 10 dB up' technique. Average thresholds across subjects fell in the 21–29 dB SPL range, with the 10th and 90th percentile points being 20 and 40 dB SPL for the 5 month olds ($n = 15$) and 20 and 30 dB SPL for the 6–18 month olds ($n = 75$). The variability of only 10 dB (one

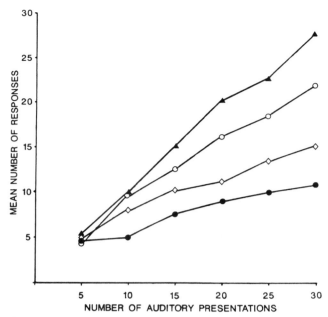

Figure 5.4 Cumulative mean head turn responses in blocks of stimulus trials as a function of reinforcement conditions in 48 children aged 12–18 months. ▲, complex visual reinforcement; ○, simple visual reinforcement; ◆, social reinforcement; ●, no reinforcement. (From Moore, Thompson and Thompson, 1975.)

Table 5.1. Mean response for the reinforcement and no reinforcement groups ($n = 10$) by age band

Age (months)	Reinforcement	No reinforcement
7–11	26.6	10.7
5–6	25.5	5.5
4	6.4	7.0

From Moore et al. (1977).

measurement step) for the children over 6 months old is very encouraging. All measurements were completed for all children except one in only one clinic visit.

Wilson and Moore (1978) and Goldman (1979) (cited by Wilson and Thompson, 1984) used VRA and warble tones to measure thresholds in normal infants aged 6–13 months. In most cases only one clinic visit was required. Wilson and Moore used the same signals and set-up to measure the thresholds of a group of otologically normal young adults. The mean results from these two studies are shown in Figure 5.5. It is apparent that

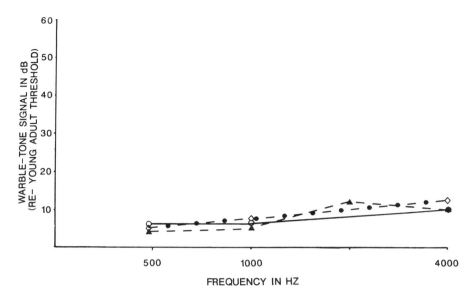

Figure 5.5 VRA warble tone sound-field thresholds for infants from two studies (♦–●–●–♦, Wilson and Moore, 1978, 6–7 months; ▲—▲, Goldman et al., 1979, ○—○, Wilson and moore, 1978, 12–13 months) compared with those of young adults.

- VRA can be used successfully for frequency-specific stimuli; and
- VRA can be used to track estimated thresholds in infants down to within 10 dB of adult thresholds.

Thompson and Folsom (1985) studied 30 normally developing 1-year-old infants and 63 premature children aged 8–24 months under conditions of visual and no visual reinforcement, using stimuli with bandwidths between 2 and 4 kHz. When no reinforcement was used, the wider-bandwidth stimuli resulted in more head-turn responses but visual reinforcement produced no difference in response behaviour across different bandwidths for suprathreshold or threshold stimulations. The results suggest that if conditioning can be established the bandwidth characteristics of the stimulus have no influence on the responsivity of infants, and that the examiner is therefore free to use auditory signals with a high degree of frequency specificity, such as warble tones.

J.S. Horner and J.P. Horner (1979, unpublished results) used a VRA technique to estimate headphone air conduction thresholds and bone conduction thresholds in 31 5–11-month-old infants. In six cases the procedure was unsuccessful: in the remaining 25 infants two 20-min sessions were required for 22 and one 35-min session for the other 3.

The average number of tone presentations required to establish any particular threshold was 8.7. Mean air conduction thresholds ranged from 0 to 30 dB HL.

Wilson and Moore (1978) also used VRA to estimate headphone thresholds in 30 normal infants aged 6–7 (n = 15) and 12–13 (n = 15) months. Thresholds were measured at 0.5, 1 and 4 kHz in two 15-min sessions using warble tones: average thresholds were 33 dB SPL for 0.5 kHz (at this frequency the younger age group gave thresholds 5 dB worse), and 24 dB SPL at 1 and 4 kHz (no difference between age groups).

Tolland (1992, unpublished data) obtained threshold measures using VRA in the sound-field and with appropriately calibrated insert earphones in a group of ten infants aged 6–19 months. Six children had hearing levels within normal limits and four showed varying degrees of hearing loss with normal middle ear function. Insert earphones were accepted by eight of the ten children tested. Ear- and frequency-specific threshold data at four frequencies were obtained for seven children, including one of 6 months, using insert earphones. The mean thresholds obtained from five infants with normal hearing levels were in agreement with those reported in the literature for sound-field testing and better than those reported for headphone testing. Although only a small sample of children was involved, this pilot study demonstrates the feasibility of using insert earphones with VRA procedures for ear-specific threshold estimation in infants.

Most of these data refer to children with (assumed) normal hearing – what of VRA with hearing-impaired children? Here the published studies are fewer. Because hearing-impaired children often exhibit poor listening skills, poor auditory attention and poor localization ability, the definition of thresholds for such cases may be more problematic, for VRA or indeed any technique. It appears that, provided time is allowed for suitable conditioning, VRA is just as successful at estimating thresholds with hearing-impaired children as with the normally hearing. Indeed, sound-field VRA may be more applicable than other methods for the hearing-impaired, because differential localization responses are not required and (as we know) localization skills are degraded in children with sensorineural hearing loss.

Rudmin (1984) reported two 11-month-old infants with severe sensorineural hearing losses in whom VRA was used to define headphone thresholds across the range 0.25–4 kHz for each ear. Test–retest reliability across two sessions (1 day in one case, 5 months in the other) was good, thresholds differing by no more than 15 dB.

Talbot (1987) reported a study of 17 hearing-impaired infants who were first tested using VRA procedures when aged between 6 and 27 (mean 14.6) months. Nine of the group were initially tested in the sound-field using VRA and warble tones, eight were tested using VRA and headphone pure tones. The same children were retested at between 25 and 41 (mean 32) months using conventional play audiometry at frequencies of 0.25, 0.5,1, 2 and 4 kHz, and a 'down 10 dB, up 5 dB' technique was used for both the VRA and play audiometry. All the children showed sensorineural impairments of a moderate or severe degree. Agreement between VRA thresholds and the later (confirmatory) play audiometry thresholds was very good, with no significant differences between test and retest at any frequency. Individual cases did not vary between VRA and play audiometry by more than 10 dB across all thresholds, except for two differences of 15 dB and one of 20 dB.

Primus and Thompson (1985) investigated the response strength of normally hearing 1- and 2-year-old children using VRA techniques. Results showed that the 2 year olds habituated more rapidly than the 1 year olds and that once habituation had occurred reconditioning with the same reinforcement was not possible. The use of novel reinforcers, introduced at appropriate times in the evaluation, resulted in significantly greater response recovery with a corresponding increase in the number of responses obtained.

Thompson, Thompson and McCall (1992) evaluated strategies for increasing the number of VRA responses before habituation obtained from normal 1- and 2-year old children in a single clinical visit. In agreement with previous studies, they found that the use of novel reinforcers significantly delayed the onset of habituation but that 2 year olds habituated more rapidly than 1 year olds and did not provide additional responses even after a short break, in contrast to the 1 year olds who provided on average, a further five responses after being given a short break from testing.

Primus (1988) modified the VRA procedure by introducing a pretrial alert to the impending auditory signal in order to investigate attention effects in infants. A comparison of conventional VRA and this modified VRA technique suggested a small but significant improvement in threshold levels in favour of the modified protocol.

VRA and children with other disabilities

Few studies have examined the use of VRA on children with other disabilities. Our clinical impression, however, is that it is a useful technique for auditory assessment in most children unless the disability is severe:

- motor control difficulties can obscure obvious head-turn responses;
- visual disability will interfere with responses if severe;
- general developmental delay or severe communication problems will often not interfere with VRA and it may prove to be a particularly useful test for these groups in which hearing impairment needs to be eliminated as a contributory factor;

- similarly, the hyperactive child who may be particularly difficult to test by other means will often respond very clearly to the VRA paradigm.

In all cases, the development of attention is a crucial constraining factor, and a 9-month-old child with developmental delay may not yet be ready for VRA. We have been able to use VRA with children with Down's syndrome, but rarely with those younger than 1 year. A range of flexible strategies and the use of other sensory reinforcers such as vibratory stimulation, puffs of air or music may be needed in addition to visual reinforcers in order to bring difficult-to-test children under stimulus control. (See Condon (1991) and Northern and Downs (1991) for practical strategies in using VRA procedures for assessment of children with additional disabilities.)

Greenberg et al. (1978) reported a study of the use of VRA with 41 children with Down's syndrome aged between 6 months and 6 years. Using complex noise stimuli, they found that about one-third of the children did not turn towards the sound spontaneously, nor could they be taught to turn for the visual reinforcement. Of the remaining two-thirds, thresholds were established for the complex noise in 81% in one clinic visit; threshold values ranged from 30 to 60 (mean 38) dB SPL. Interestingly, using a standard developmental assessment it was shown that Down's syndrome children with a developmental age of less than 10 months could generally not be tested with VRA procedures.

Gravel and Traquina (1992) used VRA to obtain threshold estimates for 211 babies and infants aged 6–24 months, with a range of conditions including sensorineural hearing loss, otitis media, craniofacial abnormalities and neurodevelopmental disorders. At the first assessment session frequency-specific data were obtained either under headphones or in the sound-field from 90% of the infants, with 84% providing ear-specific results. This study has clearly shown VRA to be a practical and efficient procedure for the routine assessment of most 6–24-month-old infants, including those considered difficult to test, because it provides ear- and frequency-specific estimates of hearing thresholds and therefore information as to the type, degree and configuration of hearing sensitivity.

Despite the known high prevalence of hearing loss in pre-term infants, few studies have addressed the question of VRA performance and age in such children. Moore, Thompson and Folsom (1992) examined the relationship between corrected and developmental age and auditory responsiveness as predictors of VRA performance in 60 pre-term infants. Individual corrected age was determined by subtracting the estimated weeks of prematurity in gestational age from chronological age, while developmental age was derived using the Bayley Scales of

Infant Development (Bayley, 1969). Developmental age and corrected age were significantly related to VRA performance. The results indicated that, in contrast to the results of studies using VRA with full-term infants, which have shown good response to VRA by a chronological age of 6 months, the same level of response is not achieved by pre-term infants until approximately 8 months corrected age (6 months developmental age).

The possible adverse effects of unilateral hearing loss are increasingly being recognized but detection tends to be late because of such factors as lack of early parental concern. Few studies of localization abilities have been conducted in infants with unilateral hearing loss. A recent feasibility study by Auslander et al. (1991) examined use of a localization task to detect unilateral hearing loss in infants. Four-corner localization ability was assessed in a group of adults and in 29 normally hearing infants aged 9–20 months using routine VRA procedures. A mild unilateral hearing loss was then simulated using a foam earplug. Analysis of the data indicated the feasibility of using a simple horizontal localization task as a screening procedure for unilateral hearing loss even at levels as low as 25 dB HL. The authors point out the need for further studies on the effects of degree, type and configuration of hearing loss on localization abilities.

Future developments

There is at present no standard protocol for VRA. Among the many factors and variables that need to be considered are, for example:

- numbers of examiners;
- test signals and reinforcer properties;
- psychometric procedures;
- effects of infant behaviour and attention level;
- observer bias;
- response latency criteria; and
- use of control trials.

A number of recent studies have addressed questions in some of these areas in an attempt to improve the rigour and efficiency of VRA in threshold estimation.

Bernstein and Gravel (1990) investigated what they identified as one of the main limitations of the VRA paradigm, namely the systematic decline in motivation of the infant to see the reinforcers as the number of trials increases, with the consequence that results may be compromised by the 'order' effect inherent in the traditional protocol of establishing threshold for one frequency and then another. They developed a single-examiner, computer-assisted staircase protocol (ISP) that interwove three adaptive threshold searches, using trial-by-trial randomization of the test frequency in a single test run to obtain threshold estimates at all three frequencies tested and a measure of motivation effects. The accuracy and efficiency of their procedure was demonstrated by comparing conventional pure tone audiometry and ISP threshold estimates in a group of adults and a group of infants aged 9–18 months with normal cochlear sensitivity, including a number with otitis media on the day of testing. The effects of learning and motivation were assessed by monitoring responses to catch trials (no signal presented) and probe trials (clearly audible signals presented). Consideration of such information is important because a high rate of response on catch trials indicates that the child is not under stimulus control, and failure to respond on probe trials indicates possible momentary inattentiveness, distraction or a lack of motivation.

Eilers et al. (1991a) investigated the interaction of test parameters with infant behaviour and hearing status in an attempt to devise an automated, four-frequency threshold estimation procedure capable of being completed in a single session with a single examiner. A computer-implemented model designed to simulate infant responses using VRA was developed. Results indicated that accuracy was most influenced by the probability of task orientation, which reflects factors such as attention, state and responsiveness in infants, and is minimally affected by stopping rules. The results also suggested that accuracy and test length were adversely affected by starting levels: starting levels close to threshold result in more accurate estimates of threshold than those further from threshold. Test length, used in this simulation as a measure of efficiency, was affected most by the stopping rule (defined by the number of reversals used) and to a lesser extent by starting intensity. In order to assess the adequacy of the model used in the simulation, a follow-up investigation (Eilers et al., 1991b) compared results of VRA from 146 infants aged 6–24 months, with normal and abnormal tympanograms, with simulation results. The comparison indicated that the procedure successfully distinguished between the two groups of children.

Automated VRA facilities are extremely rare at present in the UK. A manual system in which reliability of response is judged subjectively, one or two testers are used and fewer trials are run to establish thresholds, is adequate for most situations. However, technological advances, increased knowledge of infant learning and behaviour and a desire to improve accuracy and efficiency is leading to the development of expanded, automated versions, including computer-assisted portable systems. An automated version of VRA may be implemented using an audiometer in the test room to access a computer interfaced to a logic system outside the test room; communication with the computer from the test room may also be accomplished by activating switches connected to the interface. The equipment selects trial type, stimulus presentation and level, activates reinforcers and provides a trial by trial record of the infant's responses. A computer-assisted system can be programmed to present a variety of digitized signals, to include pre-programmed control and probe trials, to limit the time window of the child's response and to reduce observer bias by introducing masking noise at the onset of every trial interval. Future applications of automated versions using modified VRA protocols may include interactive video techniques such as those being developed by Boothroyd (1991) for speech pattern contrast work with young children.

The robust nature and proven efficacy of VRA means that the procedure can be used for increasingly more detailed study of other dimensions of the auditory function in young infants. In addition to measuring sensitivity thresholds, the VRA paradigm has been used extensively in suprathreshold tasks such as speech discrimination ability. For example, using a procedure known as the Visually Reinforced Infant Speech Discrimination (VRISD) paradigm, Eilers, Wilson and Moore (1977) were able to demonstrate that a high percentage of infants aged 6–14 months could discriminate subtle speech contrasts. The VRISD paradigm was also used by Nozza et al. (1990) to investigate the effects of noise on the speech/sound discrimination of a group of infants 7–11 months old. Their data suggest that infant speech processing abilities are more susceptible to noise than those of adults.

The application of computer-based VRA and rigorous psychophysical procedures in the area of auditory prelinguistic behaviour need to be developed further and exploited fully in the search for early predictors of amplification benefit for very young children and for validation of fitting of the hearing aid. This is a particularly urgent need because of the inappropriateness and inadequacy of present speech discrimination tests that tend to highlight reduced hearing ability in young children rather than provide evidence of the acoustic information actually available to them.

The VRA paradigm has been further expanded to such areas as masked thresholds and frequency selectivity (Nozza and Wilson, 1984), critical bands (Schneider, Morrongiello and Trehub, 1990), binaural release from masking (Nozza, Wagner and Crandell, 1988) and frequency resolution (Spetner and Olsho, 1990).

Family involvement

Behavioural assessment of hearing sensitivity in the sound-field using VRA is often the first opportunity that families have to begin to understand the extent of their child's hearing impairment, especially if previous information has been obtained by electric response audiometry. In our clinical practice once a child has been confirmed as having a hearing loss we adopt a collaborative, family-focused approach to the habilitative process. The first step in this process is to involve family members in the assessment procedures. Because of its robust nature, and because the child actively participates in the assessment, the VRA paradigm provides parents with the opportunity to exercise their expertise as reliable, informed observers of their child's behaviour in the test situation.

Nevertheless, it is vital for audiologists to be aware that this 'confirmation' of the hearing loss can be a traumatic experience for many parents, especially in cases where high levels of sound are required to elicit a response or where no response is obtained at any frequency. (Note that family members should be provided with earplugs or defenders when exposed to high levels of sound in the test room.) It is vital to allow time and opportunity for feelings, needs and opinions to be expressed to help parents come to terms with the child's hearing impairment.

Strong feelings may be experienced in every repeat test situation. Parents of very severely hearing-impaired young children are particularly vulnerable in spite of being warned of the likelihood of no response occurring during aided sound-field VRA. It is not uncommon for 'no response' to be the norm for 4 or 5 months following optimal hearing aid fitting and use. In a few cases it then becomes apparent that there is no useful residual hearing. Parents of children in whom no response to sound can be elicited should be assured that VRA response behaviour can be established by conditioning with vibrotactile stimulation using a bone conductor.

The sharing of information and open communication should be the norm for clinical practice from the point of identification of hearing loss, so that the parents can integrate the results of ongoing assessments and their implications into their perceptions of the whole child. Factors affecting management are thus seen as part of the family decision-making process rather than as the consequence of professional actions and directions. This early intervention is crucial to the beginnings of empowerment of the infant's caregivers as the main agents affecting development and optimal growth of family/professional relationships.

This process is facilitated by involving family members as coassessors in the early VRA procedures. The parents or caregivers participate alternately in the darkened instrumentation/observation room and in the VRA test room as co-assessors. Observations of the child's attention state and response behaviour are shared and results agreed and recorded. For example, the parent or caregiver in the test room is involved in shaping the behaviour of the child by pacing and controlling activities, and in making on-line decisions with the second tester timing the introduction of novel reinforcers or the need for a short break. If only one adult accompanies the child, it is useful to video part of the procedure and to discuss it with the parent. Other family members (grandparents for example) often comment on the usefulness of this participation, with its opportunities to gain different perspectives and a greater understanding of hearing assessment procedures. This helps to establish open communication between family and professionals. Families need to make informed decisions about their child, and this approach helps them in their attempts to construct a framework for thinking about and discussing such concepts as communication, residual hearing, aided listening levels, sound perception, the benefits and limitations of amplification and the need for change or modification of a hearing aid as more accurate data are obtained.

Calibration

When VRA is used with standard earphones, IEC calibration procedures and standards apply for specifying the pure tone stimuli in terms of dB HL. For VRA used with insert earphones, typical earphone to headphone correction factors provided by the manufacturers may be used for insert earphones plugged directly into the output of the audiometer without recalibrating the audiometer.

However, it is suggested that insert earphones to be used as the main transducer should be calibrated to the interim insert earphone reference equivalent threshold sound pressure levels (RETSPLs) specified by ANSI (S 3.6 – 1989, Appendix G) corrected for a B & K dB-0138 HA-2 coupler (Frank and Richards, 1991). Although insert earphone RETSPLs have also been specified by ISO (389, DAD – 3,1990), mean insert earphone thresholds, averaged over the existing database, are in closer agreement with the interim ANSI than the ISO RETSPLs (Frank and Vavrek, 1992).

For sound-field VRA there are, however, no national or international standards regarding normal threshold values. Sound-field SPLs may vary from clinic to clinic, depending upon room acoustics, stimulus generators etc. and ideally the minimum audible field (MAF) curve should be defined, using a group of otologically normal young adults, for each sound-field room. In addition the sound-field SPL should be defined using the substitution method. In this way, sound-field thresholds from any room can be converted to (or compared with) dB HL values. If such 'biological calibration' (MAF curve) has not been defined, use can be made of the equivalent threshold sound pressure levels (ETSPLs) suggested by ASHA (1991). These are based upon the published work by, for example, Morgan, Dirks and Bower (1979). The ASHA suggested ETSPLs for speech and for frequency specific stimuli, for three alternative loudspeaker locations (0, 45 and 90° azimuth) are reproduced in Table 5.2.

Table 5.2. Monaural sound field equivalent threshold sound pressure levels (ETSPLs) for frequency specific stimuli of comparable bandwidth and for speech at three azimuth locations

Stimulus (Hz)	Azimuth (°)		
	0	45	90
125	32.0	—	32.0
250	16.0	20.0	16.0
500	9.5	9.0	7.5
750	—	0.5	—
1000	5.5	0.9	3.5
1500	4.5	2.0	2.0
2000	2.5	–0.5	4.0
3000	0.5	–4.1	0.5
4000	1.5	–3.1	1.0
6000	7.5	3.8	1.5
8000	13.0	—	9.0
Speech	16.5	12.5	15.0

From ASHA (1991).

Cox and McCormick (1987) used these values to compare thresholds obtained in the sound-field to those measured under earphones for a group of normally hearing listeners. As the ASHA (1991) working group point out:

> Their data suggest that these ETSPLs are appropriate for the calibration of sound-field warble tones. As such, the levels may be used as reference for determination of deviation from normal hearing sensitivity in the sound-field. These ETSPLs have not been accepted as a national or international standard. Consequently the values cannot be called reference ETSPLs. However, the ETSPLs reflect the most current data available. (ASHA, 1991, p.35)

The ASHA (1991) report represents the conclusions of a working group set up to consider sound-field calibration. It is probably the most detailed and comprehensive summary available, and until national or international procedures are agreed this report should be adopted as the basis for sound-field calibration in the UK. The report further reinforces the efficacy of linear SPL as the measurement mode of choice, for both speech- and frequency-specific stimuli, and recourse to weighted scales (such as dB (A)) should no longer be necessary – and indeed simply introduces further inconsistencies.

Conclusion

VRA is a powerful means of establishing ear and frequency-specific auditory threshold information in infants of 6–7 months of age and those older children who are difficult to test. Further research is needed to improve the efficiency of VRA in threshold estimation and to develop the paradigm to investigate other dimensions of auditory functioning in young infants. Finally, VRA plays a central role in informing parents of the early management of hearing-impaired infants and has great potential for family involvement in the habilitation process

References

American Speech–Language–Hearing Association (1991). Guidelines for the audiological assessment of children from birth through 36 months of age. *ASHA* **33**, 37–43.

Auslander, M.C., Lewis, D.E., Schulte, L. and Stelmachowicz, P.G. (1991). Localization ability in infants with simulated unilateral hearing loss. *Ear and Hearing* **12**, 371–376.

Barr, B. (1955). Pure tone audiometry for preschool children. *Acta Otolaryngologica Supplementum*, 121.

Bayley, N. (1969). *Bayley Scales of Infant Development: Birth to Two Years*. San Antonio, TX: Psychological Corp.

Bench, J. and Menk, L. (1975). Stimulus complexity, state and infants' auditory behavioral responses. *British Journal of Communication Disorders* **10**, 52–60.

Bernstein, R.S. and Gravel, J.S. (1990). A method for determining hearing sensitivity in infants: the interweaving staircase procedure (ISP). *Journal of the American Academy of Audiology* **1**, 138–145.

Boothroyd, A. (1991). Speech perception measures and their role in the evaluation of hearing aid performance. In: Geigin, J. and Stelmachowicz, P.G. (eds). *Pediatric Amplification. Proceedings of the 1991 National Conference*, pp. 77–91. Omaha, NB: Boys Town National Research Hospital.

Borton, T. E., Nolen, B.L., Luks, S.B. and Meline, N.C. (1989). Clinical applicability of insert earphones for audiometry. *Audiology* **28**, 61–70.

Condon, M.C. (1991). Unique challenges: children with multiple handicaps. In: Geigin, J. and Stelmachowicz, P.G. (eds). *Pediatric Amplification. Proceedings of the 1991 National Conference*, pp. 183–194. Omaha, NB: Boys Town National Research Hospital.

Cooper, J., Moodley, M. and Reynell, J. (1978). *Helping Language Development*. London: Edward Arnold.

Cox, R.M. and McCormick, B. (1987). Electroacoustic calibration for sound field warble tone thresholds. *Journal of Speech and Hearing Disorders* **52**, 388–392.

Dix, M. and Hallpike, C. (1947). Peep-show: new technique for pure tone audiometry in young children. *British Medical Journal* **719**, 719–723.

Durlach, N.I., Thompson, C.L. and Colburn, H.S. (1981). Binaural interaction in impaired listeners. *Audiology* 20, 181–211.

Eilers, R. E., Wilson, W. R. and Moore, J. M. (1977). Developmental changes in speech discrimination in infants. *Journal of Speech and Hearing Research* 20, 766–780.

Eilers, R. E., Miskiel, E., Ozdamar, O., Urbano, R. and Widen, J. E. (1991a). Optimization of automated hearing test algorithms: simulations using an infant response model. *Ear and Hearing* 12, 191–198.

Eilers, R., Widen, J.E., Urbano, R., Hudson, T. and Gonzales, L. (1991b). Optimization of automated hearing test algorithms: A comparison of data from simulations and young children. *Ear and Hearing* 3, 199–204

Frank, T. and Richards, W.D. (1991). Hearing aid coupler output level variability and coupler correction levels for insert earphones. *Ear and Hearing* 12, 221–227.

Frank, T. and Vavrek, M.J. (1992). Reference threshold levels for an ER–3A insert earphone. *Journal of the American Academy of Audiology* 3, 51–59.

Goldman, T.M. (1979). Response of infants to warble-tone signals presented in soundfield using visual reinforcement audiometry. MSc Thesis, University of Cincinnati.

Gravel, J.S. and Traquina, D.N. (1992). Experience with the audiological assessment of infants and toddlers. *International Journal of Pediatric Otorhinolaryngology* 23, 59–71.

Greenberg, D.B., Wilson, W.R., Moore, J.M. and Thompson, G. (1978). Visual reinforcement audiometry (VRA) with young Down's syndrome children. *Journal of Speech and Hearing Disorders* 43, 448–458.

Haug, O., Baccaro, M.A. and Guilford, R. (1967). A pure-tone audiogram on the infant: the PIWI technique. *Archives of Otolaryngology* 86, 101–106.

Jensen, J., Borre, S. and Johansen, P. (1989). Unilateral sensorineural hearing loss in children: cognitive abilities with respect to right/left ear differences. *British Journal of Audiology* 23, 215–220.

Kankkunen, A. (1982). Pre-school children with impaired hearing. *Acta Otolaryngologica Supplementum*, 391.

Kaplan, P.S., Fox, K.B. and Huckeby, E.R. (1992). Faces and reinforcers: effects of pairing condition and facial expression. *Developmental Psychobiology* 25, 299–312.

Liden, G. and Kankkunen, A. (1969). Visual reinforcement audiometry. *Acta Otolaryngologica* 67, 281–292.

Moore, J.M., Thompson, G. and Thompson, M. (1975). Auditory localization of infants as a function of reinforcement conditions. *Journal of Speech and Hearing Disorders* 40, 29–34.

Moore, J.M., Thompson, G. and Folsom, R.C. (1992). Auditory responsiveness of premature infants utilizing visual reinforcement audiometry (VRA). *Ear and Hearing* 13, 187–194.

Moore, J.M., Wilson, W.R. and Thompson, G. (1977). Visual reinforcement of head-turn responses in infants under 12 months of age. *Journal of Speech and Hearing Disorders* 42, 328–334.

Morgan, D.E., Dirks, D.D. and Bower, D.R. (1979). Suggested threshold sound pressure levels for frequency-modulated (warble) tones in the sound field. *Journal of Speech and Hearing Disorders* 44, 37–54.

Northern, J.L. and Downs, M.P. (1991). *Hearing in Children*, 4th edn. Baltimore, MD: Williams and Wilkins.

Nozza, R. J. and Wilson, W.R. (1984). Masked and unmasked pure tone thresholds of infants and adults: development of auditory frequency selectivity and sensitivity. *Journal of Speech and Hearing Research* 27, 613–622.

Nozza, R.J., Wagner, E.F. and Crandell, M.A. (1988). Binaural release from masking for a speech sound in infants, preschoolers and adults. *Journal of Speech and Hearing Research* 31, 212–218.

Nozza, R.J., Rossman, R.N., Bond, L.C. and Miller, S.L. (1990). Infant speech sound discrimination in noise. *Journal of the Acoustical Society of America* 87, 339–349.

Primus, M. A. (1988). Infant thresholds with enhanced attention to the signal in visual reinforcement audiometry. *Journal of Speech and Hearing Research* 31, 480–484.

Primus, M. and Thompson, G. (1985). Response strength of young children in operant audiometry. *Journal of Speech and Hearing Research* 28, 539–547.

Rudmin, F.W. (1984). Brief clinical report on visual reinforcement audiometry with deaf infants. *Journal of Otolaryngology* 13, 367–369.

Seewald, R.C. (1992). The desired sensation level method for fitting children: Version 3.0. *The Hearing Journal* 45, 36–41.

Schneider, B.A., Morrongiello, B.A. and Trehub, S.E. (1990). Size of critical band in infants, children and adults. *Journal of Experimental Psychology: Human Perception Performance* 16, 642–652.

Spetner, N.B. and Olsho, L.W. (1990). Auditory frequency resolution in human infancy. *Child Development* 61, 632–642.

Stelmachowicz, P.G. and Seewald, R.C. (1991). Probe tube microphone measures in children. *Seminars in Hearing* 12, 62–72.

Suzuki, T. and Ogiba, Y. (1961). Conditioned orientation reflex audiometry. *Archives of Otolaryngology* 74, 84–90.

Talbot, C.B. (1987). A longitudinal study comparing responses of hearing-impaired infants to pure tones using visual reinforcement and play audiometry. *Ear and Hearing* 8, 175–179.

Thompson, G. and Folsom, R.C. (1985). Reinforced and nonreinforced head-turn responses of infants as a function of stimulus bandwidth. *Ear and Hearing* 6, 125–129.

Thompson, G., Thompson, M. and McCall, A. (1992). Strategies for increasing response behaviour of 1 and 2-year-old children using visual reinforcement audiometry (VRA). *Ear and Hearing* 13, 236–240.

Walker, G., Dillon, H. and Byrne, D. (1984). Sound field audiometry: Recommended stimuli and procedures. *Ear and Hearing* 5, 13–21.

Wilson, W.R. and Moore, J.M. (1978). Pure-tone earphone thresholds of infants utilizing VRA. *Proceedings of the American Speech and Hearing Association, San Francisco, USA*.

Wilson, W.R. and Thompson, G. (1984). Behavioural audiometry. In: Jerger, J. (Ed.). *Pediatric Audiology*, pp. 1–44. London: Taylor & Francis.

Wilson, W.R., Moore, J.M. and Thompson, G. (1976). Soundfield auditory thresholds of infants utilizing VRA. *Proceedings of the American Speech and Hearing Association*. Houston, USA.

Chapter 6
Pure tone audiometry

SALLY WOOD

Introduction

Pure tone audiometry is the procedure most commonly used for the measurement of hearing impairment. Pure tones, that is tones with a single frequency of vibration, are presented via headphones (air conduction) or via a bone vibrator (bone conduction) and the patient's sensitivity at discrete frequencies is measured. When stimuli are presented through headphones the sound travels through the outer and middle ear – the conducting mechanism – before reaching the cochlea and auditory nerve. Abnormal pathology at any stage in this pathway may affect air conduction sensitivity. When stimuli are presented via the bone conductor it is assumed that the stimulus reaches the cochlea through vibration of bone and soft tissue. Abnormal pathology occurring at or beyond the cochlea may affect sensitivity of bone conduction. The lowest level at which a pure tone stimulus can be heard through the headphone is known as the *air conduction threshold* at that frequency and the quietest stimulus that can be heard when the bone vibrator is placed on the mastoid bone is known as the *bone conduction threshold* for that frequency. *Threshold* is defined precisely later in this chapter. Comparison of air and bone conduction thresholds (the air–bone gap) provides a means of quantifying the amount of conductive hearing impairment. Some important provisos to the assumptions relating to bone conduction will be discussed later.

The purpose of pure tone audiometry is to measure the threshold of hearing using both air and bone conduction and thus to arrive at a description of the degree and type of hearing impairment.

The audiometer

Audiometers range from the simple screening types, with a facility for air conduction measurement at a restricted range of frequencies and intensities, to the complex clinical types with facility for a range of clinical tests as well as measurement of pure tone threshold. For clinical purposes the frequency range usually extends from 125 Hz to 8 kHz in octave intervals, the octave increase corresponding to a doubling of the previous frequency. The steps are therefore:

125 Hz   250 Hz   500 Hz   1 kHz   2 kHz   4 kHz   8 kHz

The following intermediate frequencies are also included in most clinical audiometers:

750 Hz   1.5 Hz   3 kHz   6 kHz

The intensity is calibrated in steps of 5 dB and extends from −10 dB up to a maximum value which varies with frequency but is most commonly 120 dB in the mid frequencies for air conduction. This decibel scale is known as dB HL and has been especially constructed for pure tone audiometric measurements. The sensitivity of the human ear varies with frequency, being most sensitive in the mid frequencies. It would be clumsy and inconvenient to have a normal value for threshold that varies with the frequency under test and, therefore, the dB HL scale was constructed such that 0 dB HL corresponds to the normal threshold (for young adults with no history of ear disease or noise exposure) at each frequency. The actual output sound pressure level from the headphone (or bone vibrator) at a dial setting of 0 dB HL will be different at different frequencies. Any pure tone threshold measurement is, therefore, a statement of how many decibels better or worse the hearing is than normal.

Standards for audiometers

The standard that governs the specification of audiometers is BS 5966 (1980), which is equivalent to IEC 645 (1988). Audiometers are divided into five types, IEC types 1-5, according to the facilities that they possess. For each type the standard defines the test frequencies that must be available, together with the maximum and minimum hearing levels for air and bone conduction at each frequency. It also defines the centre and cut-off frequencies for narrow-band masking noise at each frequency and acceptable deviations from nominal performance in terms of frequency, output, harmonic distortion levels and rise and fall time for pure tone stimuli.

Air conduction

BS 2497 (1972) (and its equivalent ISO 389 (1991)) give values for the sound pressure levels produced in the acoustic coupler or artificial ear that correspond to the average normal threshold of hearing. These values (known as reference equivalent threshold sound pressure levels – RETSPL) vary with frequency and are measured either in an acoustic coupler or in an artificial ear. They are a function of the precise earphone/cushion combination used. The most common combination in the UK is the TDH 39 or 49 earphone with MX 41 AR supra-aural cushion. The acoustic coupler is used for the calibration of Telephonics TDH-39 and Beyer DT-048 earphones used with MX 41 AR supra-aural cushions. The characteristics of the acoustic coupler are given in BS 4668 (1971), which is technically equivalent to IEC 303 (1970a). All other types of earphone or earphone/cushion combinations are calibrated with an artificial ear complying with BS 4669 (1971), which is technically equivalent to IEC 318 (1970b). There are as yet no internationally accepted standards for circumaural cushions.

In recent years interest in the use of insert earphones has increased. Insert earphones do not require the use of a headband, prevent the problem of collapsing ear canals, allow audiometry to be carried out in higher ambient noise levels (Berger and Killion, 1989) and provide increased intra-aural attenuation ,thus reducing the need for masking (Frank and Richards, 1991). Several studies (Wilber, Kruger and Killion, 1988; Frank and Richards, 1991) have investigated the calibration of insert earphones and RETSPLs have been specified by the International Organization for Standardization (ISO 389, 1989).

Bone conduction

The bone vibrator is calibrated in terms of the vibratory force levels transmitted to the mechanical coupler when the vibrator is excited electrically at the level corresponding to normal hearing threshold. These values (known as reference equivalent threshold force levels – RETFL) are given in BS 6950 (1988), which is technically equivalent to ISO 7566 (1987), and refer to a vibrator applied to the mastoid process with a static force of 5.4 N with the non-test ear being masked by a narrow-band noise at a level of 35 dB above the pure tone threshold of that ear. The vibrator should have a plane circular driving face with an area of 150–200 mm². The Radioear B-71 and B-72 are widely used bone vibrators that comply with the standard. The characteristics of the mechanical coupler used for bone conduction calibration are given in BS 4009 (1991), which is equivalent to IEC 373 (second edition) (1990).

Calibration of audiometers

Several studies (Martin, 1968; Fearn, 1976) have highlighted the variation in performance of audiometers in regular clinical use. Regular objective checks of performance are essential and should be undertaken at least every 12 months (preferably every 6 months) and at any time there is a possibility that the equipment has been damaged or its performance has changed. Regular subjective checks, as detailed below, should enable problems to be detected early. Detailed recommendations for calibration arrangements are discussed by Shipton (1987).

Regular checks

Before any checks are made the equipment should be allowed to warm up for 15 min. The following routine checks are recommended by the Department of Health and Social Security (DHSS) (1978).

- The earphone and vibrator serial numbers should be checked; the transducers should be unique to a particular audiometer – they cannot be exchanged between audiometers without full recalibration.
- All dials and switches should be checked for clean and silent operation.
- The tester should listen to the output from both headphones and the bone vibrator at all frequencies at about threshold to ensure that output is audible and that no spurious signals or noise are present.
- The interrupter switch should be checked for silent operation.
- The listening check should be repeated for a high-level output.
- Narrow-band masking should be checked through both headphones and the insert receiver to ensure that the signal level is correct, the output is free from spurious signals and noise and that the frequency of the output changes with dial frequency.
- Any other functions provided, e.g. Stenger, wide-band masking should be checked.

Weekly checks should also include a more thorough examination of leads and headbands. Signal attenuators should be checked over the whole intensity range for linearity and silent operation of interrupters.

The audiogram

This is a graphical representation of the results obtained in pure tone audiometry. Figure 6.1 shows the standard format recommended by the British Society of Audiology (BSA) (1989).

The ordinate extends from –10 to +140 dB and is marked 'Hearing Level (dB)'. The scale is not specific to a particular calibration standard but a space is included at the bottom of the standard form for this information. The abscissa extends from 125 Hz to 8000 Hz and is marked at octave intervals. Dotted vertical lines represent the fre-

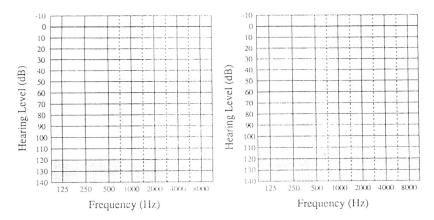

Figure 6.1 The audiogram format recommended by BSA.

quencies 750, 1500, 3000 and 6000 Hz. The scale is marked 'Frequency (Hz)'. The symbols recommended by the BSA for use in pure tone audiometry are shown in Figure 6.2.

Threshold measurement

The definition of auditory threshold is to some extent arbitrary. As with any psychophysical measurement there will be an intensity above which the patient responds on all presentations and a lower intensity below which the patient will fail to do so. Between the two intensities

O	Right ear - air conduction
●	Right ear - air conduction - not masked (possible shadow threshold)
◒	Right ear - air conduction - masked but no change on masking
X	Left ear - air conduction
𝐗	Left ear - air conduction - not masked (possible shadow threshold)
X̲	Left ear - air conduction - masked but no change on masking
△	Bone conduction - not masked
[	Right ear bone conduction
]	Left ear bone conduction

Figure 6.2 Recommended symbols for use in pure tone audiometry.

is a region wherein lies the threshold. The precise value of threshold obtained may be affected by a number of variables, as discussed below.

Patient variables

The attention, motivation and ability of the patient to concentrate may affect the measurement procedure. It is important that the patient is comfortable and the temperature and ventilation of the test room may affect performance: Wilber (1979) quotes an example of children tested at a temperature of 90°F whose thresholds were as much as 15 dB poorer than at a more comfortable temperature. The patient should be free from visual and auditory distractions and background noise must be controlled to avoid masking effects.

Equipment variables

Regular calibration and checking of equipment is necessary. The possibility of error, when using audiometers with gross calibration errors is obvious (e.g. an audiometer whose attenuator is not functioning below a dial setting of 30 dB will result in losses of up to 30 dB being recorded as normal). Cross-talk between earphones may result in false thresholds being recorded in patients with unilateral losses. However, problems may arise even in audiometers that are calibrated to the relevant standard because of the variability that is permitted. For example, at 3 kHz the tolerance on frequency is ± 3% and so two audiometers, one with an output of 2910 Hz and one with an output of 3090 Hz, will both be considered to be within calibration standards. However, if a patient with a very steeply sloping high frequency loss is tested, the thresholds as measured by the two audiometers at a nominal setting of 3 kHz could be significantly different. Woodford (1984) reports that in some cases the variability could be as much as 20 dB.

Background noise

Background noise may exert a masking effect and cause raised (that is worse) thresholds to be recorded. This is dependent upon several factors:

- the frequency characteristics and intensity of the background noise;
- the frequency of the test tones used;
- the lowest threshold it is desired to measure;
- the mode of presentation.

Bone conduction measurements require more stringent criteria for background noise because the supra-aural cushions used in air conduction audiometry have some sound attenuation properties, particularly at high frequencies (Berry, 1973). The effects of background noise are discussed in detail by Shipton and Robinson (1975), who conclude that a frequency analysis of the noise is necessary (a single dB A measurement is insufficient as threshold elevation varies greatly with the frequency distribution of the noise). Standards exist (BS 6655, 1986; ISO 8253-1, 1989) for the maximum acceptable levels of background noise in audiometric test rooms.

Procedural variables

These include:

- the instructions given to the patient;
- the threshold measurement procedure adopted;
- the attenuator step size; and
- the criterion adopted for threshold.

Instructions given to the patient can be an important variable. A patient who is instructed to respond only when he or she is *sure* that the tone is present is likely to respond differently from one instructed to respond if he or she *thinks* the tone is present.

The numerous ways in which the threshold could be traced vary from a simple descending procedure (starting from a level at which the signal is clearly audible and reducing it until the patient no longer responds), to more sophisticated forced-choice procedures in which the patient is instructed that a tone is present in one of two or three intervals and that the task is to indicate which interval contained the tone. Marshall and Jesteadt (1986) showed that the use of a forced-choice procedure resulted in thresholds which were on average 6.5 dB better than those obtained with a clinical audiological procedure. Arlinger (1979) reported a multicentre study comparing an ascending and a bracketing method. He found no significant difference in threshold but the bracketing procedure took an average of 5 minutes longer per patient. Tyler and Wood (1980) compared three manual methods of pure tone audiometry and found no significant differences in threshold, but one method did take significantly longer to establish threshold. Time, of course, is an important factor in clinical procedures.

In another study Jervall and Arlinger (1986) compared step sizes of 2 and 5 dB in manual audiometry. They found slightly higher (that is worse) thresholds with the step size of 5 dB but use of the lower step size resulted in a 30–40% increase in time required to establish threshold. Leijon (1992) points out that the measurement error involved in pure tone audiometric threshold determination includes a quantization component due to attenuator step size. An increase in step size may decrease the standard deviation of repeated thresholds while at the same time increasing the true measurement error.

It is clear, therefore, that in order to minimize variability a standard procedure for threshold measurement should be adopted. The most commonly used procedure is known as the 'Method of Limits' (in which the stimulus is systematically varied). It is based on the Hughson and Westlake ascending technique described by Carhart and Jerger (1959) and modified by the American Speech and Hearing Association (ASHA). This has been adopted as one of two standard procedures by the BSA. The attenuator step size is 5 dB and the criterion for threshold is that the patient responds on 50% of ascending presentations with a minimum of two responses at that level. The Method of Limits is briefly described below. Readers are strongly advised to read the original procedures as described by BSA (1981, 1985).

Determination of threshold in adults

The procedure is explained to the patient and he or she is instructed to make the desired response whenever they hear the test tone, no matter how faintly. Ideally, the patient's response should be silent and indicate the duration of the test tone by, for example, pressing a button (or raising a finger) when the tone appears and releasing the button (lowering the finger) when the tone is no longer heard. Older children and adults are usually tested in a sound-proof booth so that auditory and other distractions are kept to a minimum. The tester should be able to observe the subject. The test tones should have a duration of 1–3 s and it is important to avoid a rhythmical presentation, which may allow the patient to anticipate the tone. Equally, it is important to avoid very long silent intervals, which will give rise to false responses.

The better hearing ear is usually tested first at 1 kHz, proceeding to higher and then to lower frequencies with a retest at 1 kHz. If the retest value at 1 kHz is more than 5 dB better than the original threshold the next frequency is retested, and so on. The opposite ear is then tested in the same order but without the retest at 1 kHz.

Initially, the tone is presented at about 40 dB above the estimated threshold and the patient's response checked. If there is no response, successive increments of 20 dB are used until there is a response. Once this familiarization has been achieved, measurement of threshold begins. The intensity is reduced in steps of 10 dB until the patient no longer responds, at which point the intensity is increased in steps of 5 dB until the patient responds. After a positive response the intensity is reduced in 10 dB increments until no response occurs and then again raised 5 dB at a time. Threshold is defined as the lowest level at which a response occurs in at least one-half of a series of ascending trials with a minimum of two responses at that level: if a patient responds at a particular level on two out of three ascending presentations the criterion is met. This method is often referred to as the '10 down, 5 up' procedure for obvious reasons.

Pure tone audiometry in young children

Preliminaries

Most normally developing children of 3;6 years and above (and many between 2;6 and 3;6) will be able to cooperate successfully with pure tone audiometric testing using toy material if the tester is sufficiently skilled. The initial approach to the child is very important and he or she should be accompanied into the clinic by their parent or carer. It is not advisable, and is rarely necessary, to separate children of this age from the parent for the purpose of audiological assessment. The child should be tested in a clinic room that has been treated to reduce background noise to acceptable levels, or in a sound-proof booth which is large enough to accommodate tester, child, parent and equipment. The room should be as free as possible from visual distractions; toys and games should be kept out of sight until required, as should medical and other equipment not in frequent use. The child is seated in a small chair at a low table with the parent seated next to them. The tester then kneels beside the child keeping the audiometer behind and out of his or her vision, as shown in Figure 6.3.

Young children can be very adept at picking up extraneous cues and even with this arrangement the tester must take great care that the subject does not see the tester's arm move in depressing the switch, as this can alert the child to the presentation of a signal. For a skilled tester

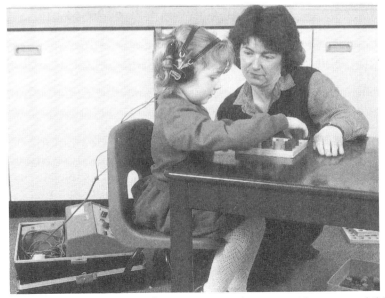

Figure 6.3 Suitable arrangement for pure tone audiometry with a young child.

familiar with the audiometer, manipulation of the controls should become second nature so they can direct their attention wholly to working with the child.

This arrangement has the advantage that the tester has direct control over the timing of signal presentation and of either the response reward or the correction of invalid responses. Optimum synchrony of the stimulus/reward (or correction) can be difficult to achieve if two testers are involved.

With children between the ages of 3;6 and 5 years it is a matter for the tester's discretion whether to start with a sound-field performance test (see Chapter 4) or with pure tone audiometry. If the child appears in any way 'clingy' or anxious it is often advisable to start with a performance test. This gives the child a chance to relax and cooperate without imposing headphones.

Conditioning procedure

The initial stage involves conditioning the child to make a simple response on the presentation of an auditory signal. This initial signal can be a pure or warble tone produced by a sound-field audiometer or a pure tone through the headphones, which can be held near the child or worn by the child. Whichever is chosen it is imperative that this initial signal be well above the child's threshold – a child cannot be conditioned to respond to a signal that he or she cannot hear. Informal observation when the child enters the clinic and during history taking should give some indication of their hearing – as will the history and parent's opinion. In cases of children with severe hearing loss it is often useful to use a vibratory signal from the bone conductor as the initial signal. The principles of conditioning and response reinforcement utilizing play materials (discussed in Chapter 4) should be applied to pure tone audiometry at this stage.

Having achieved reliable responses to sound-field stimuli most children will accept the headphones. The tester should wear them for a brief listening check, in case an unexpected fault has developed, and then place each headphone (normally colour-coded red for the right ear and blue for the left ear) centrally over the child's external auditory meatus (after moving the hair out of the way), adjusting the headband to fit. The child is immediately given something (for example, a peg) to hold to occupy the hands and prevent him or her fiddling with the head set, and one or two supra-threshold signals are given to remind the child of the task. Some children become upset or worried at this stage and reject the headphones, in which case it may be helpful to have the parent or a cooperative sibling wear the headphones and participate briefly in the task or to detach one headphone and hold it close to the child's ear, encouraging him or her to listen and make the appropriate response. In extreme cases an approximate threshold measurement may be possible in this way, but it must be noted on the audiogram as this may introduce error in the measurement.

Suitable activities for pure tone audiometry

When testing children under 5 years the most suitable activities involve a simple motor response, e.g. placing a peg in a board or stacking beakers (as described in Chapter 4). If the response required is too complicated or the game is too interesting the child may become absorbed in the activity rather than listening for the auditory stimulus. The activities must, therefore, be as simple as possible while providing some interest. A very fiddly response may slow the procedure down and could be difficult for children with poor fine motor skills. For such children a more appropriate response is to drop an object into a box or to knock it off the table or the arm of a chair. A selection of activities is needed, so that the child's interest and motivation is maintained by switching to a new activity if necessary. The advantages in using this type of activity (rather than have the child say 'yes' or press a button) are:

1. The response in itself is rewarding for the child and is reinforced by praise from the tester.
2. A false positive response can be corrected by the tester (for example, the peg can be removed from the board).
3. The procedure can be carried out without, or with a minimum of, verbal instruction as appropriate for the child's language level.

Threshold measurement in children

Generally speaking, the threshold measurement procedure used with children should be the same as that used with adults (i.e. '10 down, 5 up'). With young children however, it is particularly necessary to work rapidly while at the same time trying to avoid unnecessary sacrifice in accuracy. It is essential to vary the inter-stimulus interval with occasional fairly long intervals (more than 5 s), particularly if there is a suspicion that the child is anticipating the signal, but long silent intervals can result in the child losing concentration and it may be necessary to give occasional supra-threshold signals during the process of threshold exploration in order to retain the subject's attention. If a child is making a rather hesitant response to a particular signal and the tester is not sure whether this is a genuine response, increasing the dial setting by 5 dB and presenting this signal should result in a very positive response from the child if the previous response was genuine.

If it appears that the child's concentration will not permit the measurement of the minimum of three air conduction thresholds for each ear using the standard procedure it may be necessary to modify the procedure by using a '20 down, 10 up' procedure; an alternative is to test down to a level of 15 or 20 dB and accept two positive responses at this level rather than measuring thresholds of 0–5 dB more accurately. If either of these modifications is used the fact should be noted on the audiogram. However, this should not be used as an excuse for sloppy techniques or for using such modifications with children who are capable of carrying out standard threshold measurement procedures: information may be lost in this way, particularly with regard to the need for masking if true thresholds of –5 dB, for example, are not measured.

Order of test

Older children and adults may reasonably be expected to cooperate for the number of threshold measurements that are deemed to be necessary, but with young children the tester is working with a shorter concentration span and only a limited number of thresholds can be obtained. Therefore, it is necessary to choose the next threshold measurement on the basis that it may be the last one obtained in that session. It is generally advisable to obtain air conduction thresholds at 500 Hz, 1 kHz and 4 kHz in both ears first and to fill in other frequencies later depending upon the results obtained. Generally, the convention is to test air conduction first and then bone conduction as required; however, there is room for discretion with young children. For example, if sound-field results have been obtained and show some hearing loss, it may be sensible to test bone conduction first as this will indicate whether there is any sensorineural component in the better hearing ear at each frequency. Experience shows that some young children respond more reliably to bone conduction stimuli than they do to air conduction stimuli. The reason for this is not clear, although it seems that the child feels less 'cut off' when wearing the bone conductor than when wearing a set of headphones. If bone conduction measurements are obtained first it also means that vibrotactile conditioning can be used to greater effect. However, if sound-field results have been normal it is more sensible to aim first for air conduction thresholds in both ears to explore the possibility of a unilateral loss which may be missed by sound-field tests.

Other methods

If a child is not developmentally ready for the conditioning and cooperation described above and in Chapter 4, other methods may be used to obtain pure tone thresholds. Visual reinforcement audiometry (as described in Chapter 5) may be carried out with the child wearing supra-aural or insert earphones and/or bone vibrator. In these cases the sort of procedures outlined in Chapter 5 may be utilized. Other techniques such as Tangible Reinforcement Operant Conditioning Audiometry (TROCA) (Hodgson, 1985) may also be used. Interest in the use of 'computer games' to provide positive reinforcement in the response task is also likely to be increased over the next few years (see Chapter 4).

Influence of age on pure tone thresholds

The deterioration in sensitivity of hearing with age (presbyacusis) is well known and standard values for the threshold of hearing by air conduction as a function of age and sex are available in ISO 7029 (1984). This standard gives the median values for otologically normal subjects in the age range 18–70 years. No standard exists for those under 18 years but there has been increased interest in the question of appropriate normal threshold values for infants and children and in the age at which normal adult values are attained.

It is generally accepted that hearing sensitivity is lower in infants than in adults (Wilson and Thompson, 1984) and that it improves during childhood. However, there does not appear to be agreement upon the age at which adult values are attained. Some authors (Fior, 1972; Maxon and Hochberg, 1982) have suggested that adult values are attained at around 11–13 years of age but others (Roche et al., 1978) have demonstrated that improvement continues between 12 and 17 years. The mechanism for this improvement is not clear, although studies by Elliott and Katz (1980) and Yoneshige and Elliott (1981) appear to have ruled out factors such as mild middle ear disorders and acoustic leakage caused by poor ear/earphone coupling. It is not clear whether the change results from some form of physiological maturation or maturation of the child in terms of attention and listening skills. The amount of improvement in threshold reported varies across studies that have used different measurement procedures, stimuli and step sizes. Orchik and Rintelmann (1978) used an ascending procedure with a step size of 5 dB and reported an improvement of the order of 5 dB between 3;6 and 6;6-year-old children for pure tones at 0.5, 1 and 2 kHz. Buren, Solem and Laukli (1992) found no change in sensitivity in three groups of children aged 10, 14 and 18 years but they did find that mean thresholds differed from the RETSPL values of ISO 389 by up to 4.1 dB in the frequency range 0.5–4 kHz. This raises questions about the choice of population upon which to base standard threshold data, which are discussed in some detail by these authors and also by Robinson (1988).

Reliability of threshold measurement

A number of studies (Hickling, 1966; Jervall and Arlinger, 1986; Robinson, 1991) have examined the repeatability of threshold measurement in adults. The general consensus is that for air conduction measurements repeatability is best at 1 and 2 kHz and progressively less good at frequencies outside this range. Threshold measurements in adults typically show standard deviations of about 5 dB for air conduction and 8 dB for bone conduction (Robinson and Shipton, 1982). Atherley and Lord (1965) showed that variability at high frequencies is due to the effect of altered earphone placement on standing wave formation. Variability in low frequency threshold is thought to be due to leakage of sound through the imperfect seal between the headphone cushion and the ear. Several studies (Shaw, 1966; Dillon, 1977; Lippman, 1981) have shown that use of circumaural earphones can reduce this problem.

Reliability in children

Surprisingly little has been written about the reliability of repeated pure tone threshold measurement in young children. Lowell et al. (1956) followed a group of 21 hearing-impaired children from 3;6 to 6;11 and compared results of initial and final tests: 66% of threshold pairs were within 5 dB and 89% within 10 dB. During the course of their study with normal hearing children from 3;6–6;6 years of age, Orchik and Rintelmann (1978) looked at test–retest threshold comparisons and found that 93% of threshold comparisons were within 5 dB.

Masking in pure tone audiometry

One of the main problems in pure tone audiometry arises from the ability of sound to cross the head: if a sound presented to one ear, the test ear, is sufficiently intense it may cross the skull and be perceived by the contralateral or non-test ear. If the patient responds positively to this auditory signal a false threshold will be recorded for the test ear. The crucial factor in determining whether this 'cross hearing' is occurring is the amount of sound lost in crossing the skull. This is known as the transcranial transmission loss (transcranial attenuation, interaural attenuation) and is different for air and bone conduction stimuli. If the not masked thresholds indicate that cross hearing has occurred then masking procedures should be used. Masking is the process by which the threshold of audibility for one sound is raised by the presence of another sound, the masking sound. In clinical practice the masking sound is introduced to the non-test ear and the test ear threshold redetermined. It is necessary to ensure that the correct level of masking is used; too little and the non-test ear may still perceive the test tone; too much and the masking sound may cross over and raise the threshold in the test ear.

Considerations in masking

Previous studies (Zwislocki, 1953; Coles and Priede, 1970; Snyder, 1973; Smith and Markides, 1981) have investigated the value of trans-cranial transmission loss for both air and bone conduction stimuli and found some intersubject variability. However, in setting up criteria for masking, it is the minimum level at which this occurs that is of interest. For air conduction stimuli using MX 41 AR cushions the minimum value has been found to be 40 dB. Therefore, if any air conduction threshold exceeds the contralateral bone conduction threshold (because it is the contralateral cochlea in which the tone will be perceived) by 40 dB or more, then there is a possibility of cross hearing. This should be indicated on the audiogram by use of the appropriate symbol (●, x) and consideration given as to whether masking procedures are needed. For bone conduction stimuli the minimum value of transcranial transmission loss has been found to be 0 dB, which means that any bone conduction threshold obtained without masking cannot clearly be attributed to either ear. The necessity for masking procedures is based on an assessment of the significance of any possible air–bone gap. A number of examples are given below to illustrate these points.

Examples of cross hearing

In the audiogram shown in Figure 6.4 the naive tester may well interpret the configuration to show normal hearing in the left ear with a

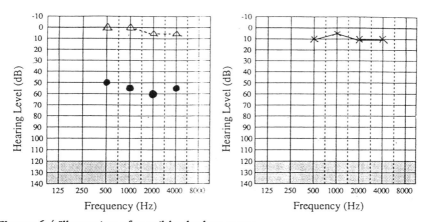

Figure 6.4 Illustration of possible shadow curve.

moderate conductive loss in the right ear. However, upon consideration it is clear that the not-masked bone conduction thresholds could
refer to either ear and, without masking, it is impossible to assign them
to a particular ear. Further, because the left ear air conduction thresholds are normal, the left ear bone conduction thresholds will theoretically be at least as good, and therefore it is possible that the right ear
air conduction thresholds are 'shadow thresholds' from the left
cochlea. In this case the true audiogram could be either that shown in
Figure 6.5 (a profound loss on the right) or that shown in Figure 6.6 (a
moderate mixed loss on the right).

Figure 6.7 shows another audiogram obtained without masking. In
this case it is not possible for the air conduction thresholds to be a
result of cross hearing because, whichever ear the bone conduction
thresholds refer to, there is no difference of 40 dB or more at any fre-

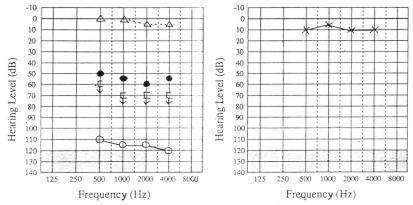

Figure 6.5 Possible true picture – a profound loss on the right.

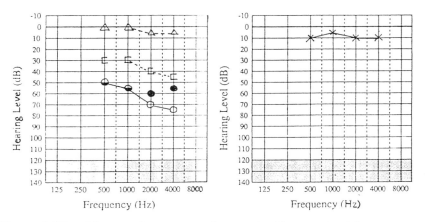

Figure 6.6 Possible true picture – a moderate mixed loss on the right.

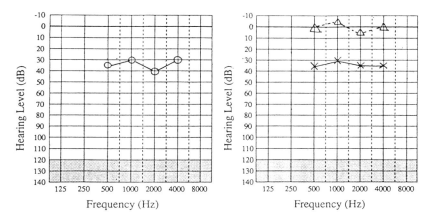

Figure 6.7 Example of an audiogram obtained without masking.

quency. However, without masking it is not possible to assign the bone conduction thresholds to a particular ear. A significant air–bone gap is clearly possible in either ear but without masking it is not possible to quantify the size of the gap. It may be that in one ear the loss is wholly or partly sensorineural.

In obtaining masked bone conduction thresholds there is no clear indication about which ear to start with. Initially, one could decide to obtain masked thresholds for the left ear, masking the right ear. If the masked bone conduction thresholds shift by more than 10 dB it is reasonable to assume that the not masked thresholds refer to the right ear. However, if they do not shift, it will be necessary to obtain masked thresholds for the right ear, masking the left ear. This situation, which necessitates masking both ears for bone conduction, arises commonly in patients with bilateral conductive losses.

Another example is shown in Figure 6.8. In this case, having already obtained the not-masked air conduction audiogram, there is no indication to mask at this stage. When the not masked bone conduction thresholds are obtained at 500 Hz and 1 kHz a significant air–bone gap could be present in both ears and, therefore, masking is necessary. When the masked bone conduction thresholds are obtained for the right ear it is clear that the not masked bone conduction thresholds refer to the left ear and, therefore, no further bone conduction masking is necessary. However, having obtained this information, it is now clear that the right ear air conduction thresholds at 500 Hz and 1 kHz could be shadow thresholds from the left cochlea and therefore masking of the air conduction thresholds at 500 Hz and 1 kHz on the right is necessary.

In the case shown in Figure 6.9, there is a definite possibility of a significant air–bone gap in the left ear at all frequencies. It is necessary

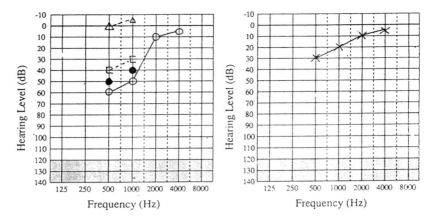

Figure 6.8 Cross hearing in air and bone conduction.

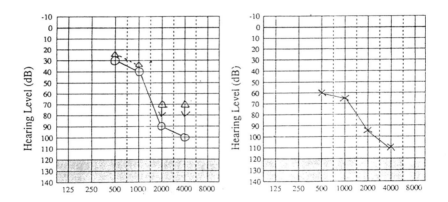

Figure 6.9 A further example of an audiogram obtained without masking.

to attempt to obtain masked bone conduction thresholds at 500 Hz and 1 kHz for the left ear. There is no point in masking at higher frequencies because the not masked thresholds for bone conduction are beyond the maximum output of the audiometer (and masked thresholds must be the same as, or greater than, not masked thresholds).

Summary

The above examples show that consideration of the minimum values of transcranial transmission loss (40 dB for air conduction, 0 dB for bone conduction), together with the not masked thresholds obtained, indicates when cross hearing may be occurring and therefore when masking is necessary. Masking is necessary in the following circumstances.

Air conduction

Whenever a threshold exceeds the contralateral bone conduction threshold by 40 dB or more.

Bone conduction

Whenever a significant air–bone gap may be present. In clinical practice a gap of 15 dB or more is generally considered significant.

Nature of masking stimuli

Masking is the process by which the threshold of audibility for one sound is raised by the presence of another – the masking sound. This was first studied in depth by Wegel and Lane (1929) who looked at the masking of one pure tone by another. Fletcher (1940) investigated the masking of pure tones by bands of noise and concluded that only a narrow band of frequencies surrounding the tone – the critical band – contributes to the masking of a tone. In terms of masking efficiency a band width equal to the critical band is the most efficient. However, this noise would have considerable tonal quality and, therefore, band widths of 0.33–0.5 octaves are normally used in clinical audiometry. For a further discussion of this see Scharf (1970).

Clinical masking procedures

Studebaker (1979) has classified the approaches to the problem of clinical masking into two groups – psychoacoustic and acoustic methods. The psychoacoustic method is based on the shadow or plateau technique described by Hood (1960) and is the type most commonly used in the UK. The acoustic or formula method is more often described in American texts (Studebaker, 1979; Katz, 1985). A third method, which involves simply presenting a fixed level of masking to the non-test ear and re-measuring the test ear threshold frequency, gives erroneous results (Coles and Priede, 1970) because it is not possible with this method to ensure that insufficient or excessive masking has not been used.

Plateau technique (Hood's shadow technique)

A hypothetical masking function is shown in Figure 6.10 (the pure tone threshold in the test ear is shown on the vertical scale and the level of masking in the non-test ear on the horizontal scale). The masking stimulus is presented to the non-test ear and its threshold, M, is determined. The masking stimulus is increased in steps of 10 dB and at each

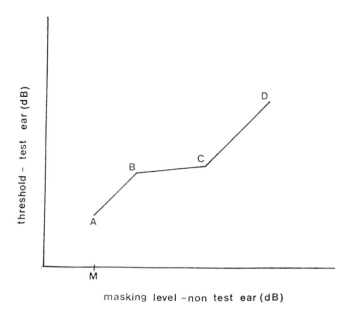

Figure 6.10 Hypothetical masking function.

increment the pure tone threshold in the test ear is determined. The resulting masking function falls into three phases. In the initial phase A–B increases in masking result in equal increments in measured threshold because both stimuli are being perceived in the non-test cochlea. During stage B–C increases in masking do not produce equal increases in measured threshold. The two are largely independent although a small increase in threshold due to the phenomenon of central masking is often seen. This is the plateau, at which a 20-dB increment in masking results in a change in threshold of 5 dB or less, and indicates that the test tone is perceived in the test ear and the masking noise in the non-test ear. At stage C–D further increases in masking produce equal increments in threshold, indicating that both stimuli are being perceived in the same (test) ear (that is, the masking noise has now crossed over and is being perceived in the test ear). In practice it is not always possible to obtain such a plateau: the maximum masking level may be reached before a plateau is obtained, or the maximum output of the pure tone may be reached before a plateau is seen (in this case the masked threshold is designated by the appropriate symbol with a downward arrow).

   In the case of bilateral conductive losses the so-called 'masking dilemma' can occur. This is because once the masking is of sufficient intensity to mask the non-test cochlea it also reaches the test cochlea and therefore no plateau can be obtained.

Recommended procedure for clinical masking

The method described below is that recommended by the BSA (1986) and readers are strongly advised to refer to the original for full details.

The narrow-band masking noise is presented to the contralateral (non-test) ear via headphones for air conduction audiometry or insert receiver for bone conduction audiometry. The threshold of masking, M, is determined in the usual way. If no interrupter switch is provided for the masking channel an ascending threshold is established. The patient is next instructed to respond to the test tone as usual and to ignore the masking noise. The masking is increased by 10 dB to ensure effectiveness, and the pure tone threshold redetermined. The results are plotted on a masking chart as shown in Figure 6.11.

This procedure is continued until the masking function is obtained and a plateau seen. This is usually defined as the level over which a 20-dB change in masking results in an increase in threshold of 5 dB or less. In the example shown in Figure 6.11 the pure tone threshold is 60 dB. In some cases it may be necessary to check intermediate steps until a plateau is clearly defined.

In some cases of more severe loss the limit of masking may be reached before a clear plateau is defined. This should be indicated on the masking chart and no clear conclusions about the threshold can be drawn. In other cases the pure tone threshold may exceed the maximum output of the audiometer at some point in the masking function

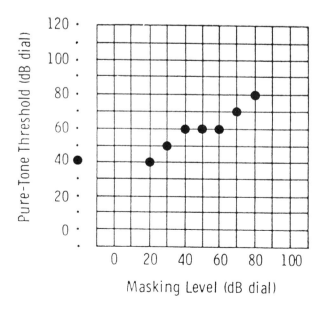

Figure 6.11 Example of a masking function.

and the conclusion in such a case is that the tone threshold exceeds this level: this should be indicated on the audiogram.

Minimum effective masking level

This is the level of masking, above the threshold of masking, which is required to ensure that the masker is effective (i.e. that a 10-dB increase in masking will result in a 10-dB increase in threshold). The value varies between individuals (Coles and Priede, 1970; Barret and Rowson, 1982) but generally a level of 10–20 dB SL is sufficient to ensure effective masking.

Effective masking

Effective masking refers to the level of the test tone that the masker will *just* mask, for example a narrow-band noise masker set to 40 dB effective masking should just mask a pure tone signal at 40 dB HL. Some audiometers have masking dials which are claimed to be calibrated in effective masking. Before relying on this claim it is wise to check the calibration using one of the methods described by Studebaker (1979) or Coles and Priede (1970). In the case of insert earphones, which are often used to deliver masking in bone conduction measurements, this type of calibration is not accurate because of the wide variability in sound pressure levels achieved in the ear.

Masking procedures for children

Many children who are able to cooperate sufficiently to obtain reliable pure tone audiograms will also be able to respond reliably when masking procedures are used. The age at which a child will respond reliably in this way is variable but between 3 and 5 years of age an increasing number of children are able to do this.

First, the threshold for the masking noise in the non-test ear (M) must be determined. The child is instructed to listen for the 'rushing noise' or the 'noise like the sea' and when this is presented at a supra-threshold level the child is guided in making an appropriate response and rewarded for doing so. When he or she is responding reliably at supra-threshold levels the threshold of masking can be measured. If several masked thresholds are required it is advisable to obtain M at all frequencies first to avoid constantly changing the listening task and possibly confusing the subject. Once it has been obtained the child is instructed to listen for the 'whistle' and to ignore the masking noise. The masking noise is presented at a level of 10 dB above the recorded threshold. At this point the child is likely to respond to the masking noise and needs to be reminded to wait for the 'whistle', which is then presented at a supra-threshold level and the child guided/rewarded for the correct response. Two or three responses at this level will retrain the patient to respond upon presentation of the pure tone.

The threshold for the pure tone can now be redetermined in the normal way, again using the technique of demonstrating and guiding the child in the correct response with appropriate reward. This is more likely to be successful than giving complex verbal instructions about ignoring one sound and listening for another, which tend to confuse young children. As the masking levels are increased it is important to observe the patient carefully because high levels of masking may cause distress: if this occurs the procedure should be terminated and an appropriate note made on the masking chart and the audiogram.

Frequencies to be masked

A clear understanding of the mechanism of cross hearing and the levels at which it may occur is necessary for the correct interpretation of audiometric results. However, a literal adherence to the masking rules may result in a very large number of frequencies that require masking. This is rarely possible in children and it is preferable to obtain a small number of masked thresholds reliably. The frequencies and mode of presentation will depend upon the possibilities presented by the not-masked audiogram and when testing children it may be useful to carry out impedance measurements before deciding which frequencies to mask.

Impedance measurements are not a substitute for bone conduction measurements; they can show the existence of a conductive problem but not its magnitude: take, for example, the audiogram shown in Figure 6.7. If middle ear impedance measurements showed a normal tympanogram and stapedial reflexes in the right ear but a flat tympanogram in the left, it would be advisable to obtain masked bone conduction thresholds for the right ear first, because this ear is most likely to have a sensorineural loss. Without the impedance results there is no clear indication to mask one ear rather than the other; if masked bone conduction thresholds were obtained first for the left ear and these were no different from the not-masked thresholds, this would indicate a need to obtain masked bone conduction thresholds for the right ear. However, by this time the child is likely to have lost concentration. Although this example may be unlikely in practice it illustrates the potential usefulness of impedance measurement in making informed decisions about masking.

Interpretation of audiograms

The purpose of pure tone audiometry is to quantify the degree, and if possible the type, of hearing loss based upon comparison of the air and bone conduction thresholds for each ear at each frequency (assuming that all necessary masking has been carried out). However, a number of factors must be understood in order to ensure that results are interpreted correctly.

Collapse of the ear canal during audiometry

This problem was first identified by Ventry, Chaiklin and Boyle (1961) and has been investigated by a number of workers including Creston (1965), who studied the problem in children. It is caused by pressure of the supra-aural cushion on the pinna resulting in some degree of occlusion of the canal, which gives rise to artefactually depressed air conduction thresholds. Creston reported that this occurred in 3.5% of 282 6–9-year-old children who underwent pure tone audiometric testing at school. Most authors agree that the higher frequencies (1 kHz and above) are usually affected and that threshold shifts of the order of 15 dB are common, although shifts as large as 30 dB have been observed. The solutions that have been suggested include:

- use of circumaural earphones;
- sound-field audiometry;
- holding the supra-aural cushion and phone against the child's ear;
- use of rubber inserts to maintain canal patency; and
- use of insert earphones.

In children, indication of a conductive problem on pure tone audiometry without such indications on either sound-field testing or impedance measurement should alert the tester to this problem: it may be more common than has been previously thought.

Vibrotactile thresholds in air and bone conduction

The phenomenon of vibrotactile perception of auditory stimuli has been known for many years and has been investigated by a number of workers (Nober, 1964, 1967, 1970; Boothroyd and Cawkwell, 1970). Most authors agree that it does not occur at frequencies above 1000 Hz and that areas other than the mastoid (e.g. palm of hand, fingertips, wrist) may be marginally more sensitive to vibratory stimuli. Boothroyd and Cawkwell compared their results with those of previous investigations and arrived at a range of levels at which there is a possibility of tactile rather than auditory perception. These are shown in Table 6.1.

Boothroyd and Cawkwell support the finding of other workers that there is considerable inter-subject variability and that for this reason it is not possible simply to draw a line on an audiogram that will separate tactile and auditory thresholds. Rather, it is necessary to be aware of a range of values over which the possibility of vibrotactile perception must be considered.

Table 6.1. Vibrotactile thresholds (dB HL)

Frequency (Hz)	250	500	1000
a–c	80–110	100–120	120–130
b–c	20–40	55–70	80–85

The audiogram shown in Figure 6.12 illustrates the problem. This audiogram could well be interpreted as showing a mixed loss at low frequencies, when in fact the bone conduction thresholds could be vibrotactile rather than auditory and the loss entirely sensorineural.

This is another example of the possibility of impedance measurements contributing to the interpretation of pure tone audiometric results.

Bone conduction measurements

Measurements of hearing by bone conduction are usually more problematic and subject to error than air conduction measurements. These problems arise from the difficulties associated with calibration and other equipment variables. There has been debate about the relative merits of forehead and mastoid placement of the bone vibrator: the test–retest reliability has been found to be better with forehead placement, and inter-subject variability is smaller. However, Dirks (1964) concluded that the differences are not large enough to be of great practical advantage. It has also been suggested that bone conduction measurements at the forehead are less influenced by the status of the middle ear than are mastoid measurements. The main advantage of mastoid placement is its greater sensitivity; a less intense signal is needed to reach threshold, which means that a greater dynamic range is

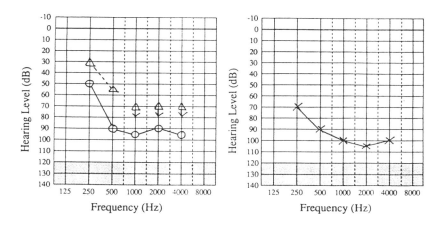

Figure 6.12 Example of vibrotactile thresholds.

available and therefore a greater range of hearing levels can be measured.

The force with which the vibrator is applied and its surface area may also affect measured thresholds. The British Standard refers to measurements at the mastoid with a vibrator area of 150–200 mm² applied with a force of 5.4 (± 0.5) N. From published reports it is not clear whether increasing the force of application has a significant effect on threshold, and if so at what point this effect occurs. It seems likely that headbands designed for adults may not apply the vibrator with the force required for small children but this does not seem to have been investigated in any detail.

The limited accuracy of bone conduction audiometry is discussed in detail by Coles, Lutman and Robinson (1991). Their prime concern is with the significance and interpretation of air–bone gaps in medicolegal assessment. They point out that bone conduction thresholds have a greater degree of variability than air conduction thresholds and that calibration is more problematic for bone conduction than for air conduction. The mechanical coupler is required to be stabilized at a temperature of 23°C – a condition that can be difficult to achieve in practice – and a deviation of 2 °C can produce a calibration error of about 1 dB. Also, bone conduction calibration standards are based on thresholds obtained with 35 dB of effective masking in the non-test ear to ensure a strictly unilateral measurement; inevitably an element of central masking is introduced, which tends to elevate the measured threshold. If masking is then not used in the clinical situation there is inevitably a bias towards better (i.e. lower) thresholds.

Air-borne radiation in bone conduction audiometry

Several studies (Lightfoot, 1979; Bell, Goodsell and Thornton, 1980; Shipton, John and Robinson, 1980) have highlighted the problem of air-borne radiation of sound during bone conduction measurements at high frequencies (3 and 4 kHz). This air-borne sound may enter the normal pathway of the external and middle ear and if it is subjectively louder than the vibratory sensation a false bone conduction threshold (and hence a false air–bone gap) will be recorded. This problem may be overcome by the use of sound-attenuating earplugs in the test ear at these frequencies. However, the plugs should not be in place for all bone conduction testing because at lower frequencies the occlusion effect (an improvement in bone conduction thresholds when the test ear is occluded) may occur.

Influence of the middle ear on bone conduction

In some instances the influence of the middle ear status on bone conduction measurements is well known. For example, Carhart (1962) described the depression in bone conduction thresholds in patients with otosclerosis and the subsequent improvement in these thresholds after stapes mobilization. He quantified the artefactual depression of bone conduction thresholds as 5 dB at 500 Hz, 10 dB at 1 kHz, 15 dB at 2 kHz and 5 dB at 4 kHz: this is now known as the Carhart notch.

Other types of middle ear impairment have been shown to influence bone conduction thresholds. Hulka (1941), Huizing (1960), Carhart (1962) and Dirks and Malmquist (1969) have all reported changes in bone conduction threshold in patients with secretory otitis media and other middle ear problems. Their results tend to show an improvement in low-frequency bone conduction response and a slight loss in the high-frequency response.

Similarly, experimental work in animals has shown that various alterations to the middle and external ear (such as loading the tympanic membrane, pressure changes in the external canal or fixation of middle ear structures) result in changes in bone conduction thresholds (Huizing, 1960; Tonndorf, 1966).

In clinical practice, children with otitis media with effusion often show depressed bone conduction thresholds at high frequencies (15–20 dB at 4 kHz), with subsequent improvement when the condition resolves.

The occlusion effect

The occlusion effect is the improvement in bone conduction threshold obtained when the external auditory meatus is occluded. It occurs in ears with normal hearing or sensorineural losses but is absent in conductive losses. The improvement in threshold is about 25 dB at 250 Hz, 20 dB at 500 Hz, 5–10 dB at 1 kHz and is generally absent at frequencies above this. It is often seen clinically when masked bone conduction thresholds are measured. Initially, the bone conduction threshold is not masked and not occluded but insertion of the insert receiver provides occlusion and therefore the not-masked threshold may improve. It is advisable to re-measure the not-masked occluded bone conduction threshold with the insert receiver in place before proceeding with masking.

The occlusion effect is another example of the ability of changes in the external canal and middle ear to influence bone conduction thresholds. For a fuller discussion of the mechanisms of bone conduction and the way in which they are influenced by the external and middle ears, readers are referred to Dirks (1985) or Tonndorf (1972).

Limited output on bone conduction

The maximum output available from the bone vibrator is limited, particularly at low frequencies, because of problems in producing high level outputs without distortion. Typically, the maximum output at 500 Hz is 60 dB and at 1 kHz 70 dB. Care should be taken not to exceed the maximum output (many audiometers permit the dial setting to be increased beyond this level with no comparable increase in output). This limited output means that in children with more severe losses bone conduction measurements may not contribute much useful information. In such cases impedance measurements are extremely useful in identifying conductive problems although they do not provide any measure of the degree of any conductive loss.

Conclusion

Obtaining and interpreting pure tone audiograms from young children is a skilled activity. In practice it is often not possible to carry out extensive masked threshold measurement but because of this it is essential to have a thorough understanding of the problems and pitfalls in order to interpret correctly the results from pure tone audiometric testing.

References

Arlinger, S. D. (1979). Comparison of ascending and bracketing methods in pure tone audiometry. *Scandinavian Audiology* 8, 247–251.

Atherley, C. and Lord, P. (1965). A preliminary study of the effect of earphone position on the reliability of repeated auditory threshold determination. *International Audiology* 4, 161–166.

Barret, H. and Rowson, V. (1982). Normal variation in the masking effectiveness of the narrow band noises of one audiometer. *British Journal of Audiology* 16, 159–165.

Bell, I., Goodsell, S. and Thornton, A.R.D. (1980). A brief communication on bone conduction artefacts. *British Journal of Audiology* 14, 73–75.

Berger, E.H. and Killion, M.C. (1989). Comparison of the noise attenuation of three audiometric earphones with additional data on masking near threshold. *Journal of the Acoustical Society of America* 86, 1392–1403.

Berry, B.F. (1973). *Ambient Noise Limits for Audiometry.* National Physical Laboratory Acoustics Report AC60.

Boothroyd, A. and Cawkwell, S. (1970). Vibrotactile thresholds in pure tone audiometry. *Acta Oto-Laryngologica* 69, 381–387.

British Society of Audiology (1981). Recommended procedures for pure tone audiometry using a manually operated instrument. *British Journal of Audiology* 15, 213–216.

British Society of Audiology (1985). Recommended procedures for pure tone bone-conduction audiometry without masking using a manually operated instrument. *British Journal of Audiology* 19, 281–282.

British Society of Audiology (1986). Recommendations for masking in pure tone threshold audiometry. *British Journal of Audiology* 20, 307–314.

British Society of Audiology (1989). Recommended format for audiogram forms. *British Journal of Audiology* 23, 265–266.

BS 4668 (1971). *An Acoustic Coupler for the Calibration of Earphones Used in*

Audiometry. London: British Standards Institution.

BS 4669 (1971). *Specification for an Artificial Ear of the Wide Band Type for the Calibration of Earphones used in Audiometry*. London: British Standards Institution.

BS 2497 (1972). *Specification for a Reference Zero for the Calibration of Pure tone Audiometers*. London: British Standards Institution.

BS 5966 (1980). *Specification for Audiometers*. London: British Standards Institution.

BS 6655 (1986). *Pure Tone Air Conduction Threshold Audiometry for Hearing Conservation Purposes*. London: British Standards Institution.

BS 6950 (1988). *A Standard Reference Zero for the Calibration of Pure Tone Bone Conduction Audiometers*. London: British Standards Institution.

BS 4009 (1991). *An IEC Mechanical Coupler for the Calibration of Bone Vibrators Having a Specified Contact Area and Being Applied with a Specified Static Force*. London: British Standards Institution.

Buren, M., Solem, B.S. and Laukli, E. (1992). Threshold of hearing (0.125–20 kHz) in children and youngsters. *British Journal of Audiology* 26, 23–31.

Carhart, R. (1962). Effect of stapes fixation on bone conduction. In: Ventry, I.M., Chaiklin, J.B. and Dixon, R.F. (Eds). *Hearing Measurement*, pp .116-129. New York: Appleton-Century-Crofts.

Carhart, R. and Jerger, J.F. (1959). Preferred method for clinical determination of pure tone thresholds. *Journal of Speech and Hearing Disorders* 24, 330–345.

Coles, R.R.A. and Priede, V.M. (1970). On the misdiagnoses resulting from incorrect use of masking. *Journal of Laryngology and Otology* 84, 41–63.

Coles, R.R.A., Lutman, M.E. and Robinson, D.W. (1991). The limited accuracy of bone conduction audiometry: its significance in medicolegal assessments. *The Journal of Laryngology and Otology* 105, 518–521.

Creston, J.E. (1965). Collapse of the ear canal during routine audiometry. *Journal of Laryngology and Otology* 79, 893–901.

Department of Health and Social Security (1978). *Routine Checking of Audiometric Equipment: Recommended Procedures for Daily and Weekly Checks*. Services for Hearing Impaired People – Information Sheet Number B701.

Dillon, H. (1977). Effect of leakage on the low frequency calibration of supra-aural headphones. *Journal of the Acoustical Society of America* 61b, 1383–1386.

Dirks, D. (1964). Factors related to bone conduction reliability. *Archives of Otolaryngology* 79, 551–558.

Dirks, D. (1985). Bone conduction testing. In: Katz, J. (Ed.) *Handbook of Clinical Audiology*, 3rd edn, pp. 202–223. Baltimore: Williams and Wilkins.

Dirks, E. and Malmquist, C.M. (1969). Comparison of frontal and mastoid bone conduction thresholds in various conductive lesions. *Journal of Speech and Hearing Research* 12, 725–746.

Elliott, L. and Katz, D. (1980). Children's pure tone detection. *Journal of the Acoustical Society of America* 67, 343–344.

Fearn, R.W. (1976). Calibration of audiometers. *Journal of Sound and Vibration* 46, 151–153.

Fior, R. (1972). Physiological maturation of auditory function between 3 and 13 years of age. *Audiology* 11, 317–321.

Fletcher, H. (1940). Auditory patterns. *Review Modern Physics* 12, 47–65.

Frank, T. and Richards, W.D. (1991). Hearing aid coupler output level variability and coupler correction levels for insert earphones. *Ear and Hearing* 12, 221–227.

Hickling, S. (1966). Studies on the reliability of auditory threshold values. *Journal of Auditory Research* 6, 39–46.

Hodgson, R. (1985). Testing infants and young children. In : Katz, J. (Ed.) *Handbook of Clinical Audiology*, 3rd edn, pp. 642–663. Baltimore: Williams and Wilkins.

Hood, J.D. (1960). The principles and practice of bone conduction audiometry. *Laryngoscope* LXX, 1211–1228.

Huizing, E.H. (1960). Bone conduction, the influence of the middle ear. *Acta Otolaryngologica (Suppl.)* 155, 1–99.

Hulka, J. (1941). Bone conduction changes in acute otitis media. *Archives of Otolaryngology* 33, 333–346.

IEC (1970a). *An Acoustic Coupler for the Calibration of Earphones Used in Audiometry, IEC 303*. Geneva: International Electrotechnical Commission.

IEC (1970b). *An IEC Artificial Ear, of the Wide Band Type, for the Calibration of Earphones used in Audiometry, IEC 318*. Geneva: International Electrotechnical Commission.

IEC (1990). *An IEC Mechanical Coupler for the Calibration of Bone Vibrators Having a Specified Contact Area and Being Applied With a Specified Static Force, IEC 373*. Geneva: International Electrotechnical Commission.

IEC (1988). *Audiometers – Part 1 Pure Tone Audiometers, IEC 645*. Geneva: International Electrotechnical Commission.

ISO (1984). *Acoustics – Threshold of Hearing by Air Conduction as a Function of Age and Sex for Otologically Normal Persons, ISO 7029*. Geneva: International Organisation for Standardisation.

ISO (1987). *Acoustics – Standard Reference Zero for the Calibration of Pure Tone Bone Conduction Audiometers, ISO 7566*. Geneva: International Organisation for Standardisation.

ISO (1989). *Acoustics – Audiometric Test Methods – Part 1: Basic Pure Tone Air and Bone Conduction Threshold Audiometry, ISO 8253-1*. Geneva: International Organisation for Standardisation.

ISO (1991). *Acoustics – Standard Reference Zero for the Calibration of Pure Tone Air Conduction Audiometers, ISO 389*. Geneva: International Organisation for Standardisation.

Jervall, L. and Arlinger, S. (1986). A comparison of 2 dB and 5 dB step size in pure tone audiometry. *Scandinavian Audiology* 15, 51–56.

Katz, J., Ed. (1985). *Handbook of Clinical Audiology*, 3rd edn. Baltimore: Williams and Wilkins.

Leijon, A. (1992). Quantization error in clinical pure tone audiometry. *Scandinavian Audiology* 21, 103–108.

Lightfoot, G.R. (1979). Air-borne radiation from bone conduction transducers. *British Journal of Audiology* 13, 53–56.

Lippman, P.R. (1981). MX41/AR ear phone cushions versus a new circumaural mounting. *Journal of the Acoustical Society of America* 69, 589–592.

Lowell, E., Rushford, G., Hoversten, G. and Stoner, M. (1956). Evaluation of pure tone audiometry with pre school age children. *Journal of Speech and Hearing Disorders* 21, 292–302.

Marshall, L. and Jesteadt, W. (1986). Comparison of pure tone audibility thresholds obtained with audiological and two interval forced choice procedures. *Journal of Speech and Hearing Research* 29, 82–91.

Martin, M.C. (1968). The routine calibration of audiometers. *Sound* 2, 106–109.

Maxon, A. and Hochberg, I. (1982). Development of psychoacoustic behaviour:

sensitivity and discrimination. *Ear and Hearing* 3, 301–308.

Nober, E.H. (1964). Pseudoauditory bone conduction thresholds. *Journal of Speech and Hearing Disorders* 29, 469–476.

Nober, E.H. (1967). Vibrotactile sensitivity of deaf children to high intensity sound. *Laryngoscope* 77, 2128–2146.

Nober, E.H. (1970). Cutile air and bone conduction thresholds of the deaf. *Exceptional Children* 56, 571–579.

Orchik, D.J. and Rintelmann, W.F. (1978). Comparison of pure tone, warble tone and narrow band noise thresholds of young normal hearing children. *Journal of the American Audiology Society* 3, 214–220.

Robinson, D.W. (1988). Threshold of hearing as a function of age and sex for the typical unscreened population. *British Journal of Audiology* 22, 5–20.

Robinson, D.W. (1991). Lon-term repeatability of the pure-tone hearing threshold and its relation to noise exposure. *British Journal of Audiology* 25, 219–236.

Robinson, D.W. and Shipton, M.S. (1982). A standard determination of paired air- and bone-conduction thresholds under different masking noise conditions. *Audiology* 21, 61–62.

Roche, A.F., Siervogel, R.M., Himes, R.M. and Johnson, J.H. (1978). Longitudinal study of hearing in children: Baseline data concerning auditory thresholds, noise exposure, and biological factors. *Journal of the Acoustical Society of America* 64, 1593–1601.

Scharf, B. (1970). Critical bands. In: Tobias, J. V. (Ed.), *Foundations of Modern Auditory Theory, Vol. 1*, pp. 159–202. London: Academic Press.

Shaw, E. (1966). Ear canal pressure generated by circumaural and supra-aural earphones. *Journal of the Acoustic Society of America* 39, 471–479.

Shipton, M.S. (1987). *Recommendations for Organising the Calibration of Pure Tone Audiometers*. National Physical Laboratory Acoustic Report AC 112.

Shipton, M.S. and Robinson, D.W. (1975). *Ambient Noise Limits for Industrial Audiometry*. National Physical Laboratory Acoustics Report AC 69.

Shipton, M.S., John, A.J. and Robinson, D.W. (1980). Air radiated sound from bone vibration transducers and its implications for bone conduction audiometry. *British Journal of Audiology* 14, 86–99.

Smith, B.L. and Markides, A. (1981). Interaural attenuation for pure tones and speech. *British Journal of Audiology* 15, 49–54.

Snyder, J.M. (1973). Interaural attenuation characteristics in audiometry. *Laryngoscope* 83, 1847–1855.

Studebaker, G.A. (1979). Clinical masking. In: Rintelmann, W. F. (Ed.), *Hearing Assessment*, pp. 51–100. Baltimore: University Park Press.

Tonndorf, J. (1966). Bone conduction studies in experimental animals. *Acta Otolaryngologica Supplementum* 213, 1–132.

Tonndorf, J. (1972). Bone conduction. In: Tobias, J. V. (Ed.), *Foundations of Modern Auditory Theory, Volume 2*, pp. 197–237. New York: Academic Press.

Tyler, R.S. and Wood, E.J. (1980). A comparison of manual methods for measuring hearing levels. *Audiology* 19, 316–329.

Ventry, I.M., Chaiklin, J.B. and Boyle, W.F. (1961). Collapse of the ear canal during audiometry. *Archives of Otolaryngology* 73, 727–731.

Wegel, R.L. and Lane, C.E. (1929). The auditory masking of one pure tone by another and its probable relations to the dynamics of the inner ear. *Physical Review* 23, 266–285.

Wilber, L. (1979). Pure tone audiometry. In: Rintelmann, W.F. (Ed.), *Hearing Assessment*, pp.1–38. Baltimore: University Park Press.

Wilber, L.A., Kruger, B. and Killion, M.C. (1988). Reference thresholds for the ER-3A insert earphone. *Journal of the Acoustical Society of America* **83**, 669–676.

Wilson, W.K. and Thompson, G. (1984). Behavioural audiometry. In: Jerger J. (Ed.), *Paediatric Audiology*, pp. 1–44. San Diego: College Hill.

Woodford, C.M. (1984). The effect of small changes in frequency on clinically determined estimates of auditory threshold. *ASHA* **April**, 25–30.

Yoneshige, Y. and Elliott, L.L. (1981). Pure tone sensitivity and ear canal pressure at threshold in children and adults. *Journal of the Acoustical Society of America* **70**, 1272–1276.

Zwislocki, J. (1953). Acoustical attenuation between the ears. *Journal of the Acoustical Society of America* **25**, 752–759.

Chapter 7
Electric response audiometry

STEVE MASON

Introduction

The functioning of the auditory system at different levels of the pathway has been extensively investigated in humans and other animals using recordings of electrical activity evoked by sounds. The electroencephalogram (EEG) was first recorded from the intact human scalp by Berger in 1929 and in the following year he described changes in the rhythm of the EEG to loud sounds (Berger, 1929, 1930). This was the birth of electric response audiometry (ERA). The next significant contribution to the field was by P.A. Davis (1939) and H. Davis and co-workers (1939), who described more specific changes in the EEG. All these early investigations, however, encountered the problem of detecting the response to a stimulus when the background noise was high. The only method of detection available to these workers was a simple superimposition of 10–20 EEG traces in order to identify the response. It was the introduction of signal averaging by Dawson in 1951, and the subsequent development of the electronic averaging computer (Clark, 1958), which completely revolutionized the field of ERA. Further improvements in technology and recording techniques have allowed the measurement of electrical responses to sound from the entire length of the auditory pathway (Picton et al., 1974).

The auditory pathway

Auditory evoked potentials may be recorded from the ear, brain stem and cortex of the auditory pathway. A brief summary of the anatomy and functioning of these structures, described in more detail by Abbas (1988) and Pickles (1988), is given as a basis for discussion.

Ear

The peripheral organ of hearing may be divided structurally into three distinct parts:

- the external ear;
- the middle ear;
- the internal ear.

The *external ear* consists of the pinna and the external auditory meatus and its function is to transmit acoustic signals into the *middle ear*, which is a small narrow cavity in the lateral part of the temporal bone. Inside this cavity is the articular chain of three small bones: the malleus, incus and stapes. These serve to transmit sounds into the cochlea, which is the receptor organ for hearing in the *inner ear*. The cochlea is a membranous spiral structure and along its length on the basilar membrane lie the sensory inner and outer hair cells and their supporting structures, known as the organ of Corti. Stereocilia project upwards from each hair cell; those on the outer hair cells are embedded into the underside of a jelly-like structure called the tectorial membrane, whereas those on the inner hair cells do not make a firm connection. The auditory nerve (VIII, cranial) originates from these hair cells. The majority of the auditory nerve fibres (90–95%) innervate the inner hair cells directly and are described as *radial fibres*. The remaining fibres (5–10%) innervate the more numerous outer hair cells and are known as *spiral fibres*. Each radial fibre innervates only two or three adjacent cells while the spiral fibres run for a considerable distance along the length of the cochlea, making contact with many outer hair cells. A human ear possesses about 30 000 auditory nerve fibres and ganglion cells.

Brain stem

The neural pathway extends from the cochlea to the auditory cortex and is illustrated in Figure 7.1. The auditory nerve leaves the cochlea through the internal auditory meatus, reaching the ipsilateral cochlear nuclei that lie at the dorsolateral border of the ponto-medullary junction. All incoming auditory nerve fibres terminate on cells within the cochlear nucleus complex. This acts as the first coding and sorting centre for auditory impulses, helping to isolate the most important impulses and dispatch them to various other centres in the brain stem. The dorsal region of the nucleus projects a number of fibres to the lateral lemniscus and inferior colliculus directly, while the ventral region communicates with the superior olivary complex. Both contralateral and ipsilateral projections exist, although the contralateral are more numerous. The medial superior olive has remarkable sensitivity to the relative time of arrival of stimuli from the two ears, suggesting that it is con-

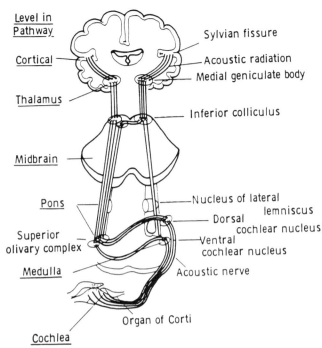

Figure 7.1 The auditory pathway including the cochlea, brain stem and cortex (adapted from Stockard, Stockard and Sharbrough, 1977).

cerned especially with the processing of directional information. This is the first level at which interaction can occur between the two ears. The short tract of the lateral lemniscus delivers the main fibres to the inferior colliculus; these are at least third-order neurones from the cochlea. The inferior colliculi then give rise to nerve fibres, the majority of which pass to the medial geniculate body of the same side. A few, however, cross to the opposite side, the highest level at which fibres cross in the auditory pathway. The inferior colliculus acts as a relay station, but also has a role in the localization of sounds. The medial geniculate body is functionally part of the thalamus and its main output is an ordered tonotopic distribution of nerve fibres to the primary auditory cortex.

Cortex

The human primary auditory cortex (AI) lies in the superior gyri of each temporal lobe. Secondary auditory areas (AII) are present in parts of the temporal, parietal and frontal cortex. The main language-processing cortex (Wernicke's area) is usually located in the superior part of the left temporal lobe adjacent to the primary auditory cortex, whereas the cortex responsible for the generation of language (Broca's area) is located in the posterior part of the inferior frontal gyrus.

Mechanism of hearing

Sound waves in the air enter the external auditory meatus and are transmitted via the tympanic membrane and the middle ear bones into the cochlea. Resultant pressure changes in the fluid in the scala vestibuli provide the mechanical drive for the basilar membrane which in turn stimulates the hair cells. This results in the generation of the receptor AC and DC electrical potentials, the cochlear microphonics (CM) and the summating potential (SP).

The mode of fluid vibration in the cochlea is a travelling wave pattern (Békésy, 1947), beginning at the base and travelling towards the apex. The envelope of the travelling wave pattern is not symmetrical; it rises slowly on the basal side and falls abruptly on the apical side. The point of maximum excursion of the wave occurs at progressively more apical locations along the basilar membrane as the frequency of a steady-state stimulus is lowered. A transient stimulus produces a travelling wave that starts at the basal end and moves up the cochlea. The most apical point reached by the wave depends upon the rise time, duration and frequency content of the stimulus. The wave takes about 5 ms to travel from the base to the apex in the human cochlea.

The characteristics of the travelling wave are determined by the physical properties of the basilar membrane, which results in a broad mechanical tuning of the cochlea with maximum sensitivity for high-frequency tones at the base and low-frequency tones at the apex. This broad tuning is complemented by a 'second process' that makes the neuronal responses more specific to one characteristic frequency than would be expected from just the simple travelling wave theory. This sharper tuning of the basilar membrane is thought to arise from complex interaction between the inner and outer hair cells (Brownell, 1986), the outer hair cells having an active control of the mechanics of the basilar membrane due to their electromotility. The overall result of this filtering is that the frequency response of each hair cell and afferent neurone can be described by a tuning curve sharply tuned to a characteristic frequency for low-intensity tones and broadly tuned for high intensity tones.

Action potentials are initiated in the auditory nerve by the cochlea and travel through various structures in the brain stem before reaching the primary auditory cortex. Auditory information is processed in the brain stem. There is a degree of sorting and coding of the stronger and earlier auditory signals at the cochlear nucleus and processing of directional information of sounds at both the superior olivary complex and the inferior colliculus.

The primary auditory cortex analyses the auditory information in terms of discrimination of pitch and intensity and the perception of auditory sequence and pattern. Further processing of this information for the understanding of language and the production of speech depends on highly integrated cortical activity within the primary and secondary auditory cortices including Wernicke's and Broca's areas.

Auditory evoked potentials

An auditory evoked potential (AEP) in humans is usually measured from the differential signal across a pair of surface recording electrodes on the scalp. One electrode is positioned over an area of high response activity (active) and a second over an area of low response activity (reference). When the active electrode is positioned close to the site of generation of the response this is termed a near-field recording; one sited some distance away is often called far-field. The optimum stimulus characteristics for evoking an AEP depend on the recording level of the auditory pathway. The stimulus to evoke a well-defined response from the ear and brain stem pathways must be fairly abrupt so as to produce a good degree of synchrony of firing of the nerve fibres, whereas much slower stimuli can be used to evoke a response from the cortex. The response at cortical level represents high level processing activity and is less dependent on the rise time of the stimulus. All AEPs are invariably small compared with the background electrical noise and a repetitive stimulus is required so that the response to noise amplitude ratio can be improved by use of signal averaging.

The evoked electrical activity in the auditory pathway is often described in terms of the time at which the response occurs after the auditory stimulus: early, middle or late latency responses (as shown in Figure 7.2). Each time period represents electrical activity from a progressively higher level of the auditory pathway. Many of these responses are valuable in otological and neurological investigation of the pathway as well as in the assessment of hearing acuity (Thornton, 1987).

Early latency responses

Electrical activity originating in the ear, auditory nerve and brain stem pathways is known collectively as the early components of the AEP and arises in the first 10 ms after an auditory stimulus. These early components may be further subdivided into those arising from the cochlea and auditory nerve – electrocochleography (ECochG) – and those recorded predominantly from the brain stem pathways – the auditory brain stem response.

Electrocochleography

Two techniques are used commonly for positioning the recording electrode in ECochG: trans-tympanic and extra-tympanic.

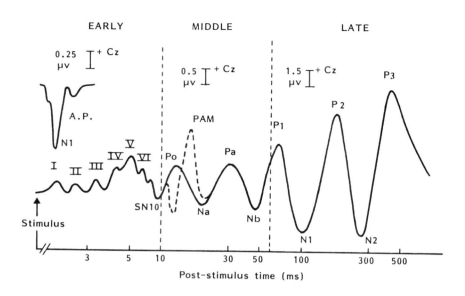

Figure 7.2 Early, middle and late latency components of the auditory evoked potential. The time following the stimulus is presented on a logarithmic scale.

The trans-tympanic method, first described by Portmann, Lebert and Aran in 1967, involves placing a needle electrode through the tympanic membrane, coming to rest on the promontory in the middle ear. This technique gives large, well-defined responses, but it is invasive and may require general anaesthesia.

The extra-tympanic technique involves positioning an electrode in the external auditory meatus close to the tympanic membrane (Mason, Singh and Brown, 1980). This technique is non-invasive and has wider applicability than the trans-tympanic method. Three response components are recorded in ECochG: cochlear microphonics (CM); summating potential (SP); and the compound auditory nerve action potential (AP). The CM and SP are predominantly receptor potentials, and reflect activity of the hair cells. The AP is the summation of electrical activity from a large number of individual nerve fibres originating from close to the cochlea. It is the only component from ECochG that has good threshold sensitivity and that can be used for assessment of hearing acuity.

Auditory brain stem response

The electrical activity evoked in the auditory nerve and brain stem pathways is known collectively as the auditory brain stem response (ABR).

The first definitive description of the ABR in humans was given by Jewett and Williston (1971), although Sohmer and Feinmesser first recorded these neurogenic responses in 1967. Jewett showed that the response evoked by a high-intensity click stimulus and recorded from a vertex and ipsilateral mastoid electrode configuration consists of a series of up to seven waves (designated I–VII in the Jewett classification), occurring in the first 10 ms after a stimulus (Figure 7.2). These waves are a far-field recording of the electrical activity from sequentially activated neurones of the ascending auditory nerve and brain stem pathways.

The precise origins of these waves are difficult to define and are complicated by the interaction between different generator sites. Proposed origins are based largely on animal studies (Achor and Starr, 1980), patients with brain stem disorders (Stockard and Rossiter, 1977) or comparative studies of surface and depth recorded ABRs in patients undergoing surgery (Moller and Jannetta, 1984).

Wave I is known to be the compound action potential of the auditory nerve and is the far-field equivalent of the AP component in ECochG. Wave II is thought to arise predominantly from proximal regions of the auditory nerve and wave III from the cochlear nucleus. The superior olivary complex is considered to be the main source of wave IV and the lateral lemniscus wave V. Waves VI and VII are thought to arise mainly from the inferior colliculus. The proposed generator sites for waves II to VII are slightly more distal than in early studies of the ABR.

As well as these fast individual waves of the ABR, as described by Jewett and Williston, a slow wave is associated with wave V and a negative component at a latency of about 10 ms. This slow negative response is often called SN10 after Davis and Hirsh (1979) and is thought to originate in the mid-brain, probably representing post-synaptic activity within the inferior colliculus (Hashimoto, 1982).

Middle latency responses

Auditory evoked potentials with latencies of 10–60 ms are termed the middle latency responses (MLR) and were first reported by Geisler, Frishkopf and Rosenblith (1958). They are generally accepted as being neurogenic in origin but can easily become contaminated with myogenic components (Bickford, Galbraith and Jacobson, 1963). The precise origin of the MLR is uncertain but most studies suggest that it arises mainly from the thalamus and primary auditory cortex (Parving et al., 1980; Kraus et al., 1982). The typical MLR waveform consists of three sequential waves with the peaks and troughs labelled Po, Na, Pa, Nb and Pb at latencies of 12, 20, 30, 45 and 60 ms respectively, as shown in Figure 7.3. It is recorded from a standard electrode configuration of vertex (active) and ipsilateral mastoid (reference) using a click or tone-pip stimulus. The waveform has sinusoidal characteristics, which are produced by using a restricted filter bandwidth that shapes the waveform. However, with a wide filter bandwidth the peak latencies are shortened and the waveform becomes less rounded (Figure 7.3). The slow wave V and SN10 components of the ABR, which contribute to the MLR, are then apparent (Kavanagh, Harker and Tyler, 1982).

The MLR is potentially useful for the assessment of hearing acuity. In conscious subjects it is well defined and reliable close to hearing threshold. However, it must be employed with caution during sleep and sedation because significant reductions in response amplitude, particularly the Pa, Nb and Pb components, have been reported (Brown, 1982; Okitsu, 1984).

A variant on the MLR is a steady-state response recorded with a stimulus rate of 40/s. At this repetition rate the ABR and MLR components overlap in-phase during signal averaging, to produce a 40 Hz compound sinusoidal waveform (this has been termed the '40 Hz' response by Galambos, Makeig and Talamachoff (1981)). It can be used for the assessment of hearing acuity but is reduced in amplitude by the effects of natural sleep and sedation (Brown, 1982).

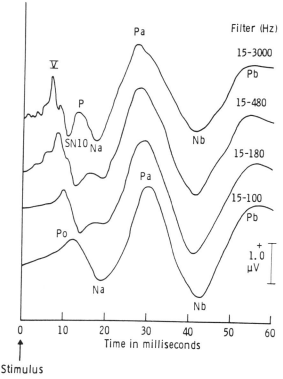

Figure 7.3 ABR and MLR components of the AEP evoked by a 60 dB nHL click stimulus, showing the effects of different high frequency filter settings.

During this middle time course myogenic activity arises from muscles in the body that react to sound (Bickford, Galbraith and Jacobson, 1963). The most clinically useful is the post-auricular muscle, which attempts to move the pinna in order to localize a sound: the post-auricular myogenic response (PAM), first described by Kiang et al. in 1963. This is a near-field response recorded from an electrode positioned directly over the muscle. It is a reflex response resulting from the passage of neural impulses through a reflex arc involving afferent pathways in the cochlea and brain stem and an efferent pathway in the facial nerve.

The PAM response comprises a complex waveform with five positive and negative peaks occurring between 10 and 24 ms. The most prominent components are a negative trough at 12 ms, a positive peak at 17 ms, and a second negative trough at 21 ms. At high click stimulus intensities a large amplitude response is often evoked but close to hearing threshold the response becomes small, variable, and more difficult to identify (Gibson, 1978). Most reduction and variability in amplitude can be related to loss of muscle tone. Some workers have recorded the response from right and left post-auricular muscles simultaneously (the crossed acoustic response) in an attempt to improve the detection of the response (Douek, Gibson and Humphries, 1975). Both muscles are often activated even if only a monaural stimulus is presented.

Late latency responses

The late or slow auditory evoked cortical response (ACR), also sometimes called the vertex potential, arises 50–500 ms after the stimulus and was first identified in the EEG by P.A. Davis (1939). It can be evoked reliably by a frequency-specific tone-burst, in contrast to the earlier responses which require a transient stimulus such as a click or tone-pip. The typical adult response, recorded from a standard electrode configuration of vertex (active) and ipsilateral mastoid (reference), consists of a small positive peak (P1) at approximately 50 ms, a large negative peak (N1) at about 100 ms and a large positive peak (P2) at around 175 ms after the stimulus. An occasional low-amplitude negative component (N2) appears at about 300 ms; this is inconsistent in adults but often dominates the immature response up to the age of about 8 years (Beagley and Kellogg, 1968). The N1 component of the ACR is thought to originate from auditory cortical areas in the temporal lobes (Picton and Scherg, 1991) with additional components possibly arising from non-specific frontal association cortex.

Several factors restrict the application of the ACR in young children. The stability of the ACR is dependent on subject maturity (Davis et al., 1967) and is affected by the level of attention and habituation to the stimulus (Davis and Zerlin, 1966).

ABR: the optimum choice for paediatric ERA

Children are usually referred for ERA because conventional behavioural audiometric tests have failed to provide reliable or adequate information about hearing acuity. The decision of which AEP to record in young children requires the consideration of a number of factors:

- practical aspects of the test procedure;
- threshold sensitivity and reliability of the response;
- the level of patient cooperation required;
- effect of sleep or sedation on the response;
- maturation of the response waveform;
- information required from the test.

Most AEP recording techniques, except for ECochG, involve placing surface recording electrodes on the scalp and are therefore acceptable for testing young patients, but electrode placement in both the trans- and extra-tympanic methods of ECochG requires general anaesthesia or at least sedation in a young child. Historically, ECochG was used extensively for assessment of hearing acuity in both adults and children but because alternative choices of AEP are now available it is difficult to justify the routine use of ECochG for this particular application except for the occasional special case (for example in a child with a suspected progressive sensorineural hearing loss with possible endolymphatic hydrops). A more detailed discussion of the clinical application of ECochG is given by Gibson (1978) and Abramovich (1990).

Each AEP has a number of advantages and drawbacks with respect to its suitability in young children.

ACR

The ACR is very variable in a young child which, combined with an active EEG, may lead to unacceptable loss of reliability. The response can be difficult to identify close to the threshold, leading to a lack of sensitivity of 20–30 dB when compared with the true behavioural threshold (Beagley, 1972). Response stability is decreased further by natural sleep and sedation, the conditions under which babies and young children often have to be tested. The ACR is more acceptable for use in children over the age of about 8 years and is ideal for adults who are more reliable in their response identification.

PAM

The PAM response should not be relied upon to give accurate information about hearing threshold because its sensitivity and consistency close to threshold is poor. It may occasionally be helpful in identifying a response from an active child during recordings of the ABR and MLR. High muscle tone often generates a large and easily identified PAM waveform.

MLR

The MLR gives a sensitive estimate of hearing threshold in older children and adults (Musiek and Geurkink, 1981) but is less reliable in young children (Okitsu, 1984; Stapells et al., 1988), and reduction in response amplitude during sleep and sedation has been observed. The steady-state variant of the MLR (the '40 Hz' response) is similarly affected by sleep and sedation and must be used with caution. An additional drawback of MLR is that the response amplitude at a stimulus rate of 40 Hz is not enhanced in very young infants (Suzuki and Kobayashi, 1984), probably because of the immature configuration of the response waveform.

ABR

The AEP preferred by most workers for audiological ERA assessment in young children is the ABR (Davis, 1976; Mokotoff, Schulman-Galambos and Galambos, 1977; Klein, 1983; Mason, McCormick and Wood, 1988). The wave V and SN10 components are stable and may be recorded reliably with stimulus levels close to the threshold of hearing, as illustrated in Figure 7.4. These components are resilient to the effects of adaptation and habituation and are not affected significantly by sleep, sedation or anaesthesia. Although the ABR is not able to give precise information about hearing loss at specific frequencies of sound, particularly mid to low tone frequencies, it is still the preferred response for a young child.

Instrumentation for ERA

A schematic diagram of the equipment required for ERA is shown in Figure 7.5. It consists of essentially two parts:

- an auditory stimulator to provide the necessary sounds to evoke the response;
- a signal amplifier/processor to capture and display the response.

The environment in which the ERA test is to be performed should provide low levels of background electrical interference and acoustical noise.

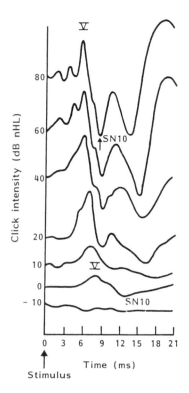

Figure 7.4 ABR waveforms recorded down to hearing threshold in a normally hearing child.

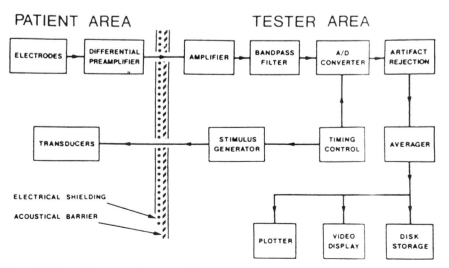

Figure 7.5 A schematic diagram of the stimulating and recording equipment for ERA (from Lightfoot and Mason, 1992).

Test environment

Careful consideration must be given to the site of the test room. It is necessary to sound treat the room or install a sound-proof enclosure to the same standard as for conventional audiological investigations. If a child has to be sedated or anaesthetized for the test, the ERA is usually carried out using portable equipment, and if the child is on the ward for sedation then a quiet side room, where the level of background noise should not exceed 40 dBA, is preferable.

In a hospital there are many sources of electrical interference, particularly related to the 50 Hz mains, arising from transformers, wiring, fluorescent lights and adjacent plant machinery such as lifts. Hospital 'bleep' systems can also introduce significant levels of high-frequency interference. In order to reduce the problems of electrical interference care should be taken in siting the clinic. Tungsten filament lights should be used rather than fluorescent tubes, and a filtered mains supply for the clinic taken as a spur off the ring main is preferred. Good attachment of the recording electrodes to the patient, with low and balanced contact impedances, will significantly improve the performance of the pre-amplifier in rejecting any interference.

Auditory stimulator

The generator of the auditory stimulus must be accurately linked in time with the recording equipment. A trigger pulse synchronizes the stimulator with the signal processor thereby time-locking the onset of the stimulus with data collection. The stimulus generator produces an electrical signal which is transduced into an acoustic waveform by the headphone or loudspeaker. An accurately calibrated attenuator allows selection of the intensity of this sound, typically in steps of 5 dB. Characteristics of the stimuli are often pre-programmed into a test menu.

Signal amplifier

The front end of the amplifier, the differential pre-amplifier, is the all-important first stage of the system. It measures the difference in the signal from a pair of recording electrodes and is very effective at rejecting interference (e.g. 50 Hz mains). Other important operating characteristics are a low level of amplifier noise and a high input impedance. The pre-amplifier must also provide a high level of electrical isolation of the patient from the mains-driven equipment and should comply with current safety standards in BS5724.

The pre-amplifier is positioned close to the patient so that electrode leads attached to the scalp are less than 1 m long. At this stage, before amplification, the signal is easily contaminated with interference. In many ERA systems the overall level of amplifier gain will often determine the amplitude at which artefacts are rejected from the signal (amplitude artefact rejection). The amplified electrical signal from the patient will contain a wide spectrum of frequencies relating to both the ABR waveform and noise: filtering is therefore required to exclude signals with frequency components outside the lower and upper limits of the spectrum of the ABR. In most ERA equipment this is an analogue filter with a bandwidth for passing signals defined by a low and high cut-off frequency. The cut-off frequency is usually specified at the point at which the signal is attenuated by 3 dB, and the rate of attenuation outside the pass band is typically in the range of 12–24 dB per octave.

Signal processor

The evoked potential in the signal baseline is very small compared with the background electrical activity and signal averaging is required in order to improve the response to noise amplitude ratio and enable identification of the response waveform. In addition to signal averaging most ERA equipment often has a number of other analysis routines available (such as a three- or five-point smoothing routine for removal of high-frequency noise on the averaged waveform) and cursor points for latency and amplitude measurement of the response. More sophisticated systems may have frequency analysis software and digital filters; however, these techniques are not essential for routine ERA.

Data display and storage

During signal averaging it is essential to be able to monitor both the on-line signal baseline and the ongoing averaged waveform in order to assess the reliability of the recordings. Averaged waveforms for estimation of a response threshold should be displayed in order of descending stimulus intensity: this will enable a more reliable assessment of the changes in amplitude and latency of the response. The ability to superimpose waveforms to check for repeatability of genuine response components is also essential. An on-line print-out of waveforms recorded during the test gives the opportunity to compare current waveforms with those recorded earlier in the test. This on-line plot of waveforms, however, must be quick and convenient so as not to hinder the progress of the investigation. Most ERA systems have the ability to store averaged waveforms on computer disk so that more detailed analysis of data can be carried out after the test.

Methodology

The stimulus and recording parameters for the ABR need to be specifically chosen for audiological application, in contrast to an oto-neurological investigation as emphasized in Figure 7.6. For assessment of hearing threshold or screening hearing the slow components of wave V and SN10 must be recorded because they provide the most reliable indicator of hearing acuity. Identification and measurement of waves I to V for an oto-neurological investigation will be more accurate and reliable when the slower components of the response are removed using signal filtering (Jacobson, 1985; Glasscock, Jackson and Josey, 1987). The methodology for audiological investigation will be described including discussion of the three main parameters that differentiate the application of the ABR: the stimulus repetition rate, signal filter and analysis time.

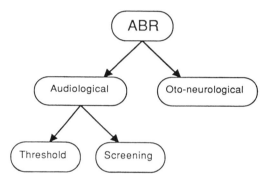

Figure 7.6 Different applications of the ABR that necessitate appropriate stimulus and recording parameters, and test procedures.

Stimulus

The characteristics of the stimuli most often used to evoke the ABR are shown in Figure 7.7. A stimulus with a fast rise time, such as a click, evokes a well-defined response waveform because a large number of auditory nerve fibres are fired in close synchrony. The disadvantage of the click stimulus, however, is that it has poor frequency specificity having acoustic energy over a wide range of frequencies. The frequency specificity may be improved using a short-duration tone-pip, which concentrates more energy at one tone frequency. The typical configuration of the tone-pip has a rise and fall time of 2 cycles of the tone with an on-time of 2 cycles (Figure 7.7). However, the use of tone-pips, particularly at tone frequencies below 2 kHz, is at the expense of significant degradation of the response waveform and makes identification of the response waveform close-to-threshold more difficult (Hawes and Greenberg, 1981). Most degradation arises from a reduction in the synchronization of firing of nerve fibres. Many workers therefore still use the click stimulus as first choice (Kileny, 1982; Don, Elberling and Waring, 1984).

The acoustic click stimulus is generated by passing a short-duration electrical pulse (100 μs) through a headphone transducer. It can be

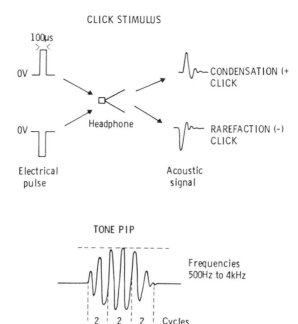

Figure 7.7 The standard click and tone-pip stimuli.

presented as a predominantly condensation pressure wave (+) or as a rarefaction wave (–), depending on the polarity of the electrical pulse presented to the transducer. Small amplitude and latency differences in the fast waveform components of the ABR are evoked by condensation and rarefaction click stimuli but the slow components and detection of the response threshold are not significantly affected by the click polarity (Mason, 1985; Sininger and Masuda, 1990). The use of a stimulus with alternating polarity for assessment of hearing acuity is therefore justified and is to be preferred because it cancels stimulus artefact at high intensity levels.

Transducers

The frequency content of the acoustic stimulus, particularly for the click, is controlled to a large extent by the transducer. Different types of transducers, such as headphones and loudspeakers, have characteristic frequency responses and will therefore modify the stimulus accordingly. The typical click generated by a Telephonics TDH39 or TDH49-type headphone produces a spread of frequency components in the acoustic waveform, as shown in Figure 7.8 . The TDH39 shows a slight peak in energy at around 3 kHz but this may differ slightly for other types of transducer. For example, a small earpiece used for testing infants in the Evoked Potentials Clinic in Nottingham has peak power

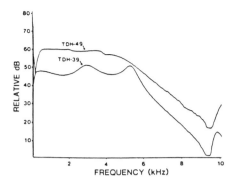

Figure 7.8 Acoustic spectra of l00 μs click stimuli presented through Telephonics TDH39 and TDH49 headphones.

for the click at a frequency of 2.5 kHz. This earpiece was designed for young babies and neonates because it is small and lightweight and reduces the risk of collapsing the ear canal, a problem that can occur when using standard headphones (Hosford-Dunn et al., 1983). Other techniques for presentation of the auditory stimuli include using a bone conductor (Schwartz and Berry, 1985) and sound-field via the hearing aid in a deaf child (Mahoney, 1985), but in both of these techniques the characteristics of the stimuli are changed from the conventional air-conducted stimuli presented through headphones and the response may not be as well defined.

Repetition rate

The rate chosen at which to present the stimulus to the patient must be a compromise between a fast rate (to minimize the recording time) and a slow rate (to maintain the required characteristics of the response). There is marked contrast in the degree of effect of the stimulus repetition rate on different components of the ABR. The wave V and SN10 components of the ABR are very resilient to increased rates of stimulation of 30/s or more, as shown in Figure 7.9 (Hyde, Stephens and Thornton, 1976; Mason, 1985), in contrast to the fast waves I, II and III. In general the more central nuclei show less adaptation than that found at the periphery (Thornton and Coleman, 1975). Relatively fast stimulus rates may therefore be employed for evoking the slow-wave components of the ABR. A stimulus rate of 40/s or more should be avoided, however, because of the problems of overlap of successive response waveforms (Figure 7.9), which is analogous to the '40 Hz' response. The maximum length sequence (MLS) technique (Picton, Champagne and Kellett, 1992) offers the possibility of unscrambling the responses with very rapid rates of pseudo-random stimulation but

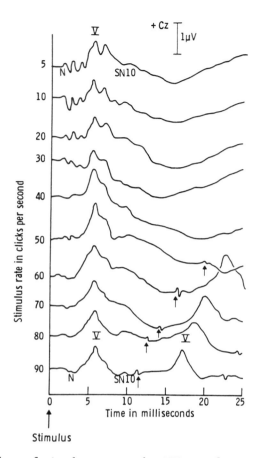

Figure 7.9 Effects of stimulus rate on the ABR waveform at a click intensity of 60 dB nHL.

this technique may significantly adapt the ABR waveform and may cause difficulties with identification of the response close-to-threshold. The typical rate employed for conventional stimulation and averaging is about 31/s. An exact fraction or multiple of 50 should not be used in order to avoid time-locked interference from the 50 Hz mains.

Stimulus intensity and calibration

The auditory stimulus must be accurately calibrated in terms of its characteristics, particularly the intensity level. For short-duration transient stimuli such as clicks and tone-pips the psychoacoustic threshold is raised compared with a continuous pure tone with the same peak sound pressure level (SPL). This is caused by the effects of temporal summation and spectral spread, and such stimuli require a special calibration procedure. The peak or peak-to-peak SPL of the transient stimulus is equated to a known calibrated pure tone on an oscilloscope using the electrical output from a sound level meter (Figures 7.10 and 7.11). The intensity of the stimulus may then be expressed in peak equivalent sound pressure level (peSPL).

Once the relationship between the transient stimulus and the calibrated pure tone has been fixed, a biological calibration of the stimulus in at least ten otologically and audiologically normal subjects should be established. Normal hearing threshold for the click (0 dB nHL) usually has a peak equivalent SPL of 30 dB peSPL compared with a 3 kHz pure tone. This offset may be allowed for in the calibration of the output level from the audiometer (so that a dial reading of 0 dB represents normal threshold for the click (0 dB nHL)) or may simply be subtracted from the existing SPL dial reading by the operator. In either case the intensity of the transient stimulus is subsequently expressed in decibels

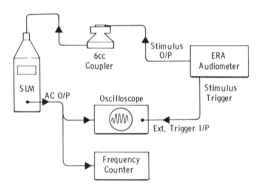

Figure 7.10 The measurement and calibration system for auditory stimuli in ERA.

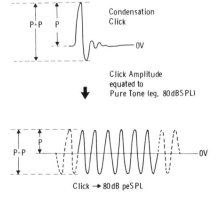

Figure 7.11 The amplitude of the click is equated to a pure tone using either a peak or peak-to-peak measurement.

above normal hearing threshold (dB nHL). A similar calibration technique is required for the tone-pip stimulus.

Contralateral masking

The possibility of cross-over of the test stimulus to the non-test ear exists in ABR investigations as it does in clinical audiology. In patients with a profound unilateral hearing loss, delayed but repeatable click ABR waveforms have been observed from stimulation of the deaf ear but were absent when masking was presented to the non-test normal ear (Chiappi, Gladstone and Young, 1979).

The inter-aural attenuation for the click is about 50 dB (Reid and Thornton, 1983) and therefore contralateral masking of the non-test ear should be employed when the difference in hearing loss between the test ear and the bone-conduction thresholds in the non-test ear is 50 dB or more across 2000 to 4000 Hz. A white noise masking sound is usually employed for the click stimulus and a narrow-band noise for the tone-pip centred at the tone frequency.

A reliable pure tone audiogram is generally not available for children referred for ERA and therefore the decision of when to use masking and at what intensity is difficult using standard methods (Sanders, 1978). Masking should be used whenever the evoked response thresholds on each ear differ by 50 dB or more. The level of masking is directly related to the intensity of the test stimulus, remembering that any adjustment of the stimulus must be accompanied by a similar change in the masking level. Chiappi, Gladstone and Young (1979) used the same intensity level for both the masking and the stimulus (e.g. 60 dB nHL) because they found that the masking had very little effect on the response waveform, even at high intensity levels (90 dB nHL). Reid and Thornton (1983) hypothesized that the click stimulus and masker follow different afferent pathways, explaining the apparent lack of interaction between the two sounds. A conservative protocol is to set the masking level at about 30 dB down on the test stimulus in order to reduce the risk of any over-masking.

Data capture

Recording electrodes

The ABR is recorded from the surface of the scalp using EEG-type electrodes, which consist of a silver dome (6 or 9 mm in diameter) coated in silver chloride. The standard electrode configuration for recording the ABR is to place an active electrode on the vertex of the head (where there is maximal response activity), and a reference electrode on either the ipsilateral earlobe or mastoid (where there is low response activity), as shown in Figure 7.12. A third electrode, the earth or guard, is required for proper functioning of the amplifier and is often positioned on the forehead or contralateral mastoid. Careful application of the recording electrodes on the scalp achieving a low contact impedance (less than 5kΩ) is essential for optimum performance of the pre-amplifier. The skin should be cleaned thoroughly with surgical spirit before attaching the electrodes with collodion glue, electrode paste, sticky discs or adhesive tape. Conductive electrode jelly is used to achieve good contact between the electrode and scalp. In very young babies and neonates particular care should be taken concerning the application of electrodes to the delicate skin, and the use of collodion glue for example is not recommended. Electrodes and associated equipment must be thoroughly washed or sterilized (particularly blunt-ended needles) in order to minimize the risk of cross-infection. The surface of the skin should not be broken during routine application of EEG-type electrodes

The ABR is a far-field recording and the response is present over a large area of the scalp, although maximal at the vertex. Davis and Hirsh (1979) used a high forehead electrode as the active site in young children and infants. This is particularly useful for very young babies because a low contact impedance at the vertex is occasionally difficult to achieve with the delicate fontanelle. There is only a small reduction (18%) in response amplitude of the slow wave components at a high forehead site compared with the vertex, as shown in Figure 7.13 (Mason, 1985).

The reference electrode site (ipsilateral mastoid or earlobe) is not completely inactive and records the early waves I and II (and to some extent wave III). The general configuration of the wave V and SN10 components (which are recorded predominantly from the vertex) is also affected to some extent by the site of the reference electrode, and the ipsilateral mastoid or earlobe is recommended. A single data

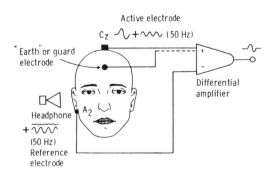

Figure 7.12 The standard electrode configuration for recording the ABR.

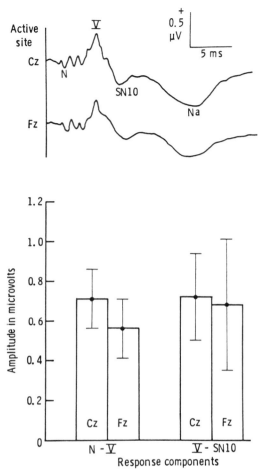

Figure 7.13 Comparison of the amplitude (mean ± 1 s.d., *n* = 8) of the ABR waveform for vertex and forehead active electrode sites recorded at a click intensity of 60 dB nHL.

channel is adequate for the estimation of hearing thresholds, which is fortunate because the application of more than one array of electrodes to a young child is often difficult and time consuming, and should be avoided wherever possible.

Signal amplification and filtering

The amplitude of the ABR is typically in the range 0.1–1 μV, often superimposed on a background activity level of 20–50 μV: amplification gain of around 100 000 is therefore required to bring the signal amplitude up towards the 5 V typical of the input range of the analogue to digital converter in the signal processor. Significant improvement in the amplitude of the response relative to the background noise (R/N ratio) may be achieved with appropriate selection of signal filtering. The amplitude of the slow (low-frequency) wave V and SN10 components is most affected by the level of high-pass filtering (low cut-off frequency) of the filter but the low-pass (high cut-off frequency) filter is less critical. In early studies a wide range of different filter settings have been employed including those which have severely attenuated the slow wave components. However, it is now generally accepted that a bandwidth in the range of 20, 30 or 50 Hz up to 1 or 3 kHz is recommended (Davis and Hirsh, 1976; Klein, 1983). The optimum low cut-off frequency is dependent on the attenuation slope (dB/octave) of the filters in the amplifier. A 20-Hz cut-off has been reported as optimum by Mason (1984a) with a filter slope of 36 dB/octave. The typical click-evoked ABR waveforms recorded in that study with different high-pass filter settings are shown in Figure 7.14. For a shallow filter slope (12 dB/octave), a cut-off frequency of 30 or 50 Hz is more appropriate. Similar filter settings are essential for recording responses to tone-pip stimuli (Yamada et al., 1983).

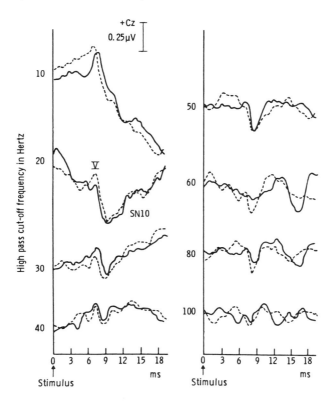

Figure 7.14 Effects of high-pass filtering on the close-to-threshold (20 dB nHL) click ABR waveform.

Analysis window

The signal data are recorded for a set period of time after onset of the stimulus – this is often termed the analysis window, sweep time or epoch. The length of this analysis window for audiological application of the ABR is typically 20 ms: this keeps the slow SN10 component of the waveform well within the window, particularly if the response occurs late due to immaturity of the waveform and if the stimulus level is close-to-threshold. This contrasts with oto-neurological application in which a time window of 12 ms is typically employed.

Artefact rejection

Large fluctuations of the on-line signal baseline, which can occur during signal averaging, have considerable influence on the detection of a response in the final averaged waveform, particularly with low-amplitude response waveforms. The technique for excluding individual sweeps of data containing gross electrical activity arising from movement, myogenic activity and excessive EEG activity is a rejection routine based simply on amplitude: if the incoming signal exceeds a predetermined level, it is excluded from the average.

The rejection level is chosen to allow all normal baseline signals, but to reject high levels of activity. In an active child the amplitude of electrical activity often exceeds ± 100 μv and a large number of sweeps are rejected: this effectively necessitates abandoning the test. The baseline signal from a child sitting quietly in a chair may approach an amplitude of ± 25 or ± 50 μv but will exceed it only occasionally, allowing a reliable response waveform to be recorded. A sedated or sleeping child has a baseline signal at least below ± 25 μv and sometimes below ± 10 μv in amplitude. A rejection level of ± 25 μv (referred to the input) is therefore optimal. Upper and lower limits of ± 50 μv and ± 10 μv should not be exceeded because the averaged waveform may be excessively contaminated with noise or the number of rejected sweeps will be unacceptably high (over 50%).

Signal extraction and processing

The presentation of a single stimulus will evoke a response that is indistinguishable from the background noise. To make the response apparent, a method of signal extraction is necessary in order to improve the R/N ratio.

Several techniques of signal extraction and processing have been proposed, the most common of which is signal averaging. This technique relies on synchronization of the evoked potential to the stimulus with random background electrical activity. Individual sweeps of the signal are averaged which results in enhancement of the response relative to the background noise. Theoretically, the R/N ratio is improved by a factor equal to the square root of the number of sweeps taken into the average but this increase ratio will be strictly adhered to only if there is an invariant response and normally distributed random noise. In most situations for the ABR these assumptions are sufficiently satisfied: one notable exception, however, is when the stimulus rate accidentally locks on to some residual interference, such as the 50 Hz mains and for this reason exact multiples or fractions of 50 Hz should not be used for the stimulus rate.

It is possible to improve the R/N ratio greatly by acquiring many sweeps, although the most efficient increase is in the early stage of the averaging process because of the relationship to the square root of the number of sweeps: in clinical practice there is also a practical limit caused by cooperation of the patient and test time available. There is therefore a law of diminishing return. The number of individual sweeps that must be averaged to enable reliable identification of a response waveform, particularly at low stimulus intensities, depends to a great extent on the quality of the on-line signal baseline. In most recording situations 2000 sweeps should be adequate, but in a sedated or sleeping child it may be possible to finish the average at 1000 sweeps if a well-defined response is present, and 4000 sweeps may be required to achieve the same level of reliability with a slightly noisier signal baseline.

Test conditions

Reliable assessment using the ABR requires good recording conditions, which are achieved when a child is asleep or sitting quietly during the test. This will minimize noise on the signal baseline arising from myogenic activity and movement artefacts. It is important that a report on ERA should include some indication of the level of reliability that can be attached to the interpretation of the waveforms. An appointment letter for ERA should advise the parents to try to keep the child awake before the test so that he or she falls asleep soon after they arrive at the clinic. Any disturbance of the child for the test should be kept to a minimum: if a child is asleep on arrival then attempts should be made to carry out the test without moving them. A cooperative, conscious child of 4 or 5 years of age will often sit in a comfortable chair or lie on a couch for the test: a younger child or baby is best either placed on the parent's knee or cradled in their arms. If a child is prepared to sit still for 20–30 min useful recordings with the click stimulus may be achieved without the need for sedation.

The frequency of use of sedation varies considerably between centres and may depend on the facilities available. Some workers use sedation and even general anaesthesia for almost all young children but other centres use sedation more selectively. The children that present the most difficulty in testing are 1–3 years old. In Nottingham about 30% of the children in this age range are sedated, and very rarely a baby under 6 months.

In Nottingham trimeprazine is used for sedation – an initial oral dose of 4 mg/kg body weight with a follow-up dose of 2 mg/kg about an hour later if the child is still very active. Chloral hydrate is one of a number of alternative sedatives. Sedation is administered on the ENT ward and the ERA test carried out in a quiet side room when the child is asleep. Usually the child is admitted the day before and is given the sedation the morning of the test: in our experience the overnight stay makes the child more likely to sleep during the test than admission on the same day. The effects of trimeprazine last 2–3 h and the patient has recovered sufficiently to be allowed home by about mid-afternoon. General anaesthesia is an alternative approach to sedation, carried out in theatre or in the clinic by special arrangement with the anaesthetist: in the latter situation it may be appropriate to use a non-gaseous anaesthetic such as intramuscular ketamine.

Interpretation of the ABR

Estimation of hearing threshold

Identification of a response in the averaged waveform can be difficult in ERA and is a potential source of gross error regarding the accuracy of threshold estimation. Careful attention should therefore be paid to the level of reliability that can be attached to the interpretation. Reliability may be improved by adopting certain recording protocols. Two averaged waveforms recorded with the same stimulus intensity (Figure 7.15) will check the reproducibility of the response waveform and will help to identify random noise components. This replication procedure is very important in ERA investigations. Subsequent addition and subtraction of the two averaged waveforms may help further in the differential identification of residual noise and true response components. Although two averaged waveforms can be recorded sequentially, an improved technique records them almost simultaneously by averaging the odd- and even-numbered individual sweeps separately (Mason, 1985).

Waveform scores

Averaged waveforms at each stimulus intensity need to be assessed for presence of a response and three decision levels or waveform scores are applicable:

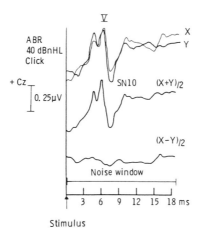

Figure 7.15 Recording protocols for the ABR to assist identification of a genuine response waveform.

1. Definite response present (++).
2. Probable response present (+).
3. No response (–).

These scores have been used routinely for observer scoring in the ERA clinic at Nottingham for several years. Some workers have used five scores, including those given above and questionable decisions for the positive (+?) and negative (–?) scores (Schimmel, Rapin and Cohen, 1974). In our experience five decision levels in a threshold protocol are difficult to implement in a routine clinical situation.

Threshold protocol

An efficient ERA test requires the minimum number of averaged waveforms in order to define the ABR threshold accurately and reliably. The operator of the test should follow a protocol that controls the order in which runs at different stimulus intensities are presented to the child (Mason, 1984b). In a typical protocol each estimate of a threshold requires a number of supra- and sub-threshold waveform scores. Two typical sequences of stimulus runs in order to estimate response threshold are shown in Figure 7.16. The stimulus intensity for the first run of a threshold is set at 40, 30 or 20 dB above the suspected hearing threshold, depending on the degree of hearing loss; for example +40 dB for suspected thresholds of better than 40 dB HL, +30 dB for hearing loss up to 50 dB HL, and +20 dB for a loss of 60 dB. It is advisable not to exceed a stimulus level of 80 dB nHL (or possibly 90 dB nHL for the first stimulus run) at the risk of disturbing a young child or

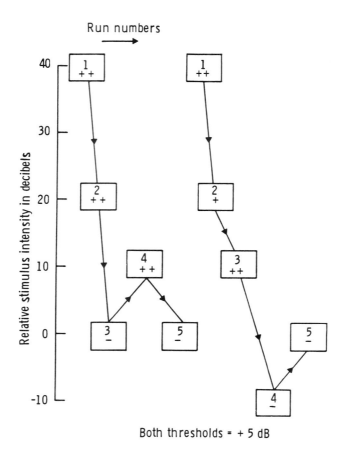

Run numbers

Both thresholds = + 5 dB

Figure 7.16 Two typical sequences of stimulus runs and subsequent waveform scores that define the evoked response threshold.

baby. High-intensity stimuli should be used cautiously throughout the investigation in order minimize discomfort, particularly if a recruiting-type cochlear loss is suspected.

The stimulus intensity order of subsequent runs is dependent upon the previous waveform scores. In general, the stimulus intensity should be decreased by 20 dB after a + + score, 10 dB after a + score, and increased by 20 dB following a – score. These changes are then modified close-to-threshold until a clear 'no response' and 'response present over a 10 dB interval' can be defined. In routine ERA, there is usually insufficient time to record at intensity intervals of 5 dB and therefore an interpolation procedure needs to be adopted to estimate the threshold to the nearest 5 dB. If the waveform score immediately above the response threshold is +, the threshold is positioned at that stimulus level; a + + score gives a threshold 5 dB better (Figure 7.16).

In routine ERA investigations ++ response at 20 dB nHL is usually acceptable to define normal hearing without proceeding to lower stimulus levels.

Accuracy of the threshold

Accuracy of the estimation of response threshold is very dependent on the recording conditions. A high percentage of click-evoked ABR thresholds should be within 10 dB of the behavioural threshold when a child is either asleep or sitting quietly. In a study of 25 normally hearing adults (Mason, 1985) in whom a reliable estimate of the subjective hearing threshold could be ascertained, 92% of the click-evoked ABR thresholds were within 10 dB of the subjective click threshold, as shown in Figure 7.17. The recording conditions in that study were equivalent to a child sitting quietly for the test and give good threshold sensitivity for the click-evoked ABR. The sensitivity of the tone-pip ABR, however, may be reduced with the same recording conditions because of loss of definition of the response waveform, particularly with tone frequencies in the mid- to low-frequency range.

Input/output functions

In the audiological application of the ABR the amplitude and latency of the wave V and SN10 components are usually measured according to

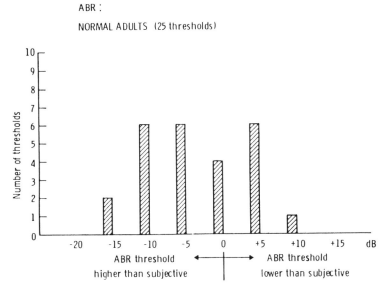

Figure 7.17 The agreement between the click ABR and subjective hearing threshold.

Figure 7.18. The changes in amplitude and latency of these components with stimulus intensity are described as the input/output (I/O) functions, and can give a useful insight into the characteristics of a hearing loss (as discussed later). The typical I/O functions in normally hearing young children, showing the effects of maturation, are given in Figure 7.19. In general response amplitude is reduced and latency increased with reduced stimulus intensity. The rate of this change is dependent on the relative level of the stimulus intensity; rapid increase in wave V latency is observed close-to-threshold, particularly in normal hearing.

Maturation of the waveform

The ABR is affected systematically by maturation of the peripheral and brain stem pathways (as shown in Figures 7.20 and 7.21). These effects are thought to be caused predominantly by increased myelination of nerve fibres, although other processes cannot be ruled out. Only waves I, III and V are apparent at birth and these components are delayed and broadened. The waveform begins to resemble the adult response by the age of 18 months, with waves II, IV, VI and VII becoming identifiable (Salamy and McKean, 1976). The latencies and inter-peak latencies of waves I, III and V decrease progressively with maturation. Hawes and Greenberg (1981) reported that the latency of the SN10 component in new-borns is about 12.5 ms, compared with 10 ms in adults. The overall amplitude of the response in the full-term new-born is only slightly lower than the adult response and as result the response may be identified in very young babies with relatively low stimulus levels. It is generally accepted that click-evoked response thresholds of better

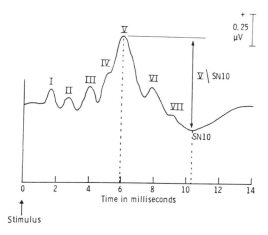

Figure 7.18 Measurement of the amplitude and latency of the wave V and SN10 components of the ABR.

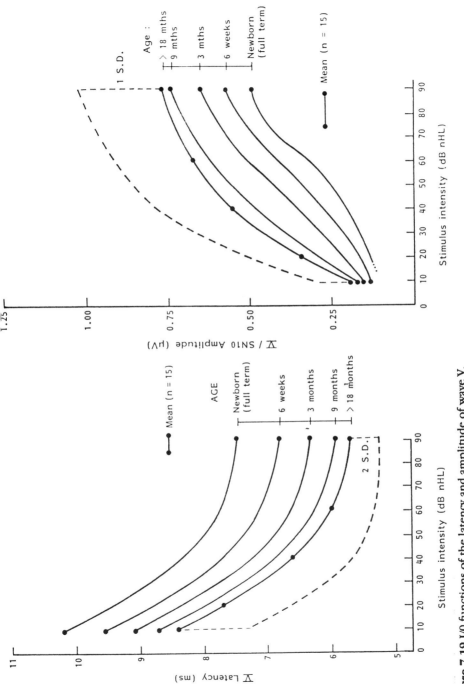

Figure 7.19 I/O functions of the latency and amplitude of wave V.

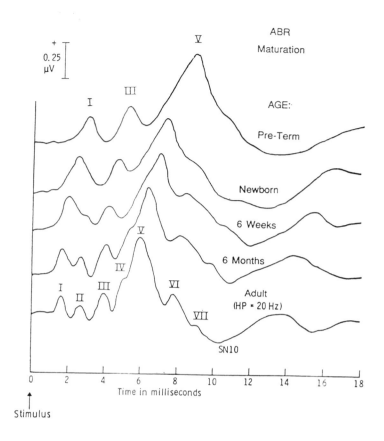

Figure 7.20 Effects of maturation on the amplitude and latency of the high-intensity ABR waveform.

than 20 dB nHL can be achieved in normally hearing babies when they have reached an age of 4–6 weeks past their expected date of delivery. Preterm babies further lack maturation of the latency and amplitude of the ABR waveform compared with full-term new-borns, which may result in a raised ABR threshold.

Frequency specificity

How closely does a measure of hearing threshold using the ABR correspond to behavioural hearing at a specific sound frequency? The degree of specificity depends initially on the characteristics of the auditory stimulus and subsequently on the generation of the response by the cochlea. The ABR is evoked predominantly by the onset of the

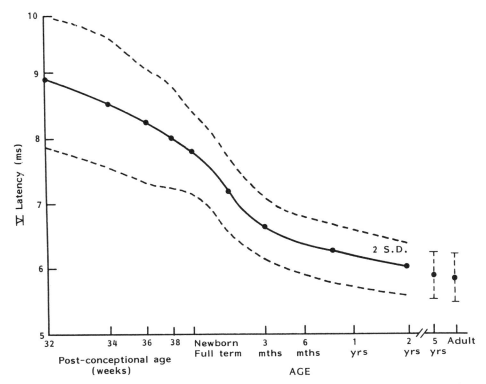

Figure 7.21 The relationship between wave V latency and subject age for a click stimulus of 60 dB nHL.

stimulus rather than by its continuation and therefore the rise time of the stimulus is an important characteristic.

Click-evoked ABR

The click is acoustically a wide-band stimulus but it generates maximal response activity from the basal high-frequency turn of the cochlea, and the resultant ABR threshold generally correlates with behavioural hearing across 2–4 kHz (Coats and Martin, 1977; van der Drift, Brocaar and van Zanten, 1987). An approximate translation of the frequency dependency of the click-evoked ABR with respect to the subjective pure tone audiogram is shown in Figure 7.22. Attempts to improve the frequency specificity of the click-evoked ABR have involved the presentation of ipsilateral masking sound to the cochlea (Teas, Eldridge and Davis, 1962). Those neurones sensitive to the frequency components of the masking are activated and are then unable to respond when the stimulus sound is presented, causing a response to the click stimulus to arise from restricted regions along the basilar membrane.

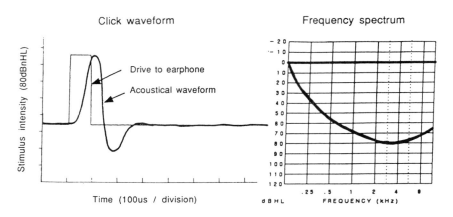

Figure 7.22 The approximate relationship between the frequency dependency of the click-evoked ABR and the subjective pure tone audiogram (from Lightfoot and Mason, 1992).

Two appropriate types of masking sound are high-frequency and notched noise.

High-frequency noise will selectively mask the response from high-frequency fibres. Using different cut-off frequencies the contribution from different regions of the basilar membrane to the click-evoked ABR can be established. This technique is known as derived response measurement (Parker and Thornton, 1978). In routine clinical testing, however, these derived responses are difficult to implement. The technique is time-consuming and often gives low amplitude responses, which results in poor threshold sensitivity.

Notched noise is an alternative method of presenting the masking sound in conjunction with the click stimulus. In this type of masker a narrow band of frequencies of sound has been stopped or rejected from a broad band noise, which theoretically allows response to frequencies of the click that are within the notch while all other activity is masked. In practice the click-evoked response in notched noise can be difficult to interpret because the origin of some components, particularly with a 500 Hz notch, is difficult to explain (Stapells et al., 1985). Response amplitude is often small and identification of responses close-to-threshold can be very difficult. Stapells et al. (1985) concluded that the click-evoked ABR in notched noise does not hold much promise as a viable routine tool in ERA.

Tone-pip ABR

A better degree of frequency specificity for ABR thresholds can be achieved using tone-pip stimuli, which concentrate more energy at one tone frequency (demonstrated in Figure 7.23). The configuration of the frequency spectrum depends on the characteristics of the tone-pip (e.g. rise, fall and on time, tone frequency). Typical configurations of the tone-pip ABR waveforms are shown in Figure 7.24. The slower components dominate the response waveform at 500 Hz and 1 kHz tone frequencies and there is an increase in wave V latency with lower tone frequency. This latency change reflects, in part, the time taken by the travelling wave to reach the more apical regions of the cochlea. There is also a spread of energy in both the tone and the travelling wave in the cochlea. Early responses evoked by high-intensity, low-frequency tone-pips are probably mediated to some extent by the high-frequency region of the cochlea. This spread of energy away from the nominal frequency of the tone pip becomes sub-threshold as the stimulus intensity is decreased and the pip then evokes a response more specific to its frequency. Studies by Klein (1983) and Folsom (1984) suggest that adequate frequency specificity of the ABR can be achieved for routine ERA when the intensity of the tone-pip is less than about 60 dB nHL at tone frequencies of 1 kHz and above. A typical intensity series of the 1-kHz tone-pip ABR recorded in normal hearing is shown in Figure 7.25. It is important to note the smaller and much broader response waveform than in the click-evoked ABR, particularly with stimulus intensity close to threshold.

Masking noises, similar to those described for the click (notched and high frequency), can be used to improve the frequency specificity of the response, particularly for high-intensity tone-pips (Picton et al., 1979; Jacobson, 1983; Fjermedal and Laukli, 1989). However, the optimum choice of which to apply depends on the tone frequency of the

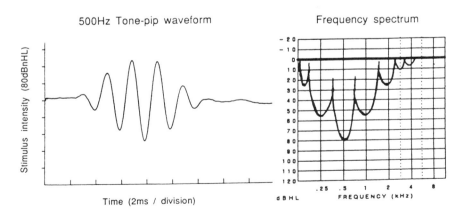

Figure 7.23 The approximate relationship between the frequency dependency of the tone-pip ABR and the subjective pure tone audiogram (e.g. 500 Hz tone-pip). A pip with higher tone frequency and/or slower time characteristics would have less spread of energy across the PTA (from Lightfoot and Mason, 1992).

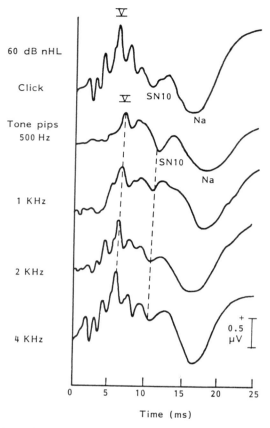

Figure 7.24 Typical configurations of the tone-pip ABR waveform with tone frequencies ranging from 500 Hz to 4 kHz.

stimulus. Responses to low-frequency tone-pips are probably best recorded with high-frequency masking because spread of masking into the lower frequency region of the cochlea is minimal in contrast to notched noise. For high-frequency tone-pip responses the optimal type of masker is notched noise. Although low-frequency noise might appear the best choice, the specificity of this type of masker is poor because energy spreads into the high-frequency basal end of the cochlea.

Any technique for improving the frequency specificity of the audiological ABR investigation must also take into consideration the recording efficiency. This reflects how quickly a recognizable response can be identified through signal averaging and improves if response amplitude increases or background noise decreases. All masking techniques result in a loss of efficiency due to a decrease in response amplitude at the expense of improved frequency specificity. Some workers recommend

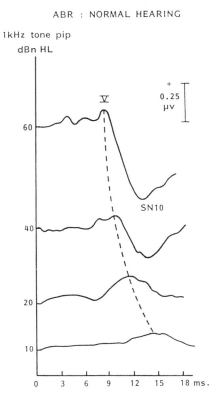

ABR : NORMAL HEARING

Figure 7.25 An intensity series of ABR waveforms in normal hearing evoked by a tone-pip stimulus of 1 kHz.

the use of tone-pips with notched noise (Picton et al., 1979); others consider tone-pips without masking to be acceptable for routine ERA (Davis et al., 1985). Discussion of the relationship of the tone-pip ABR threshold to the pure tone audiogram later in this chapter will apply to responses recorded without ipsilateral masking because this facility is not available on most commercial ERA equipment.

Application in the routine clinic

Referral category

The ABR has become a valuable tool for audiological assessment in an increasing number of young children over the last 15 years. It is applicable for the difficult to test child, the very young infant at risk of congenital hearing loss or the child who is too physically or mentally impaired to cooperate for behavioural testing. Special populations will include children with Down's syndrome, the deaf–blind child, those with virus infections such as meningitis and patients with chronic otitis media. A congenital or acquired hearing loss constitutes a significant threat to a child's ability to develop effectively.

Interpretation of hearing loss

Conductive hearing loss

The external and middle ear comprise the conductive mechanism. Developmental and pathological conditions of the external and middle ears can interrupt the efficiency of the transfer of sounds into the inner ear and impair the generation of an evoked potential. Audiometrically a conductive loss is characterized by elevated thresholds for air-conducted sounds and relatively normal thresholds with bone conduction.

The effect of conductive pathology on the air-conducted ABR is to prolong the latencies of all components of the ABR, including wave V (Hecox and Galambos, 1974). Essentially the latency I/O function for wave V is shifted from the normal curve by an amount equivalent to the level of conductive hearing loss but maintains the same gradient – as shown in Figure 7.26. Although this shift can be used as an approximate predictor of the level of hearing loss (Fria and Sabo, 1980) the most accurate assessment is derived from the ABR threshold (Eggermont, 1982). The amplitude I/O function for wave V/SN10 demonstrates a similar characteristic shift (Figure 7.26).

The most prevalent middle ear disorder in young children is otitis media, which results from inflammation of the mucoperiosteal lining in the middle ear. The build-up of fluid and thicker glue initially causes an audiometric configuration that increases hearing loss towards lower frequencies but this develops into a flat audiogram across all tone frequencies as the fluid increases and thickens. In many cases of acute and chronic otitis media the threshold of the click-evoked ABR can be raised to 30 dB HL or more because frequencies of 2–4 kHz are often affected to some extent. However, a lower frequency tone-pip stimulus, typically 1 kHz, may provide additional valuable information regarding the degree of slope to the audiogram. A conductive hearing loss at 1 kHz can easily approach levels of 40–50 dB HL.

Complex external and middle ear malformations such as atresia of the auricle (or even simple cases of impacted cerumen in the external auditory meatus) can cause conductive hearing loss. In the majority of these cases the characteristics of the ABR are similar to those already described for otitis media.

Bone-conducted stimuli may be used to evoke an ABR (Schwartz and Berry, 1985), although the characteristics of the stimulus and the

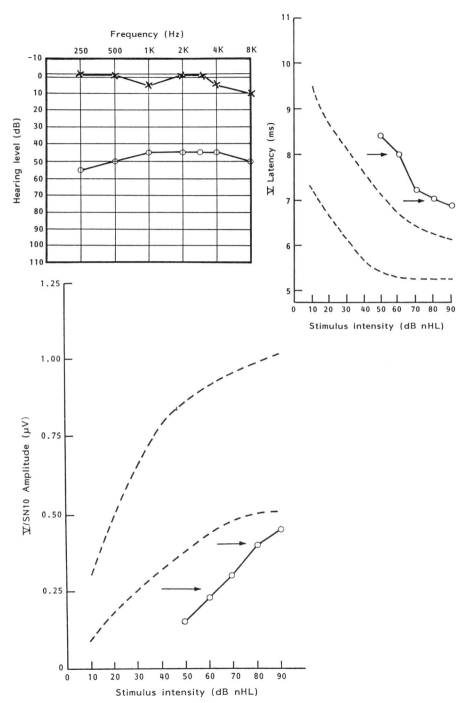

Figure 7.26 An example of the I/O functions of wave V latency and amplitude in conductive hearing loss. The dashed lines indicate the range in normal hearing (± 2 s.d.).

resultant response are slightly different to the air-conduction recording. The technique is useful in the differentiation of conductive and sensorineural loss, particularly in patients with a severe mixed hearing loss. However, some difficulties have been reported regarding the presentation of the stimulus to very young infants (Yang et al., 1991) and the characteristics of the response, particularly latency measurements, are variable (Finitzo-Hieber and Friel-Patti, 1985). The air-conducted ABR therefore remains the first-choice approach for assessment of hearing acuity, with the bone conduction stimulus retained for special cases.

Cochlear hearing loss

Malformation or damage to the delicate hair cells in the cochlea will result in a hearing loss, the characteristics of which will depend on the degree of damage and its position along the cochlear partition. The shape of the audiogram may vary widely. Common configurations are a relatively flat hearing loss across all frequencies or one showing progressively more hearing loss at higher frequencies. The characteristics of the evoked electrical activity from the cochlea will depend on the level and frequency pattern of this hearing loss.

The effect of cochlear hearing loss on the ABR waveform is rather more complex than that of a conductive loss. In many flat cochlear losses the threshold latency of the click-evoked ABR waveform is shorter than that observed in normal hearing (as shown in Figure 7.27), whereas the latencies are similar in a conductive hearing loss (Hyde, 1985). The latency I/O functions often lie within the normal range but do not run parallel with the normal curve at hearing threshold. At high stimulus intensity the latency of wave V is similar to that in normally hearing subjects but may become delayed as threshold is approached (Figure 7.27). A rapid decrease in response amplitude is often associated with these latency changes close to threshold.

These features in the response are consistent with a compression of the range of loudness often observed in cochlear hearing loss (loudness recruitment) that arises predominantly from a selective loss of outer hair cells in the cochlea. The sharp tips of the tuning curves of the auditory nerve fibres at low stimulus levels are lost, causing a rapid increase in the number of fibres activated as the stimulus level increases above the raised threshold of the fibres.

In high-frequency cochlear hearing loss the patterns of the I/O functions to a click stimulus will depend on the active region of the basilar membrane. A severe high-frequency hearing loss arising from damage to both inner and outer hair cells will suppress any contribution to the response from the basal end of the cochlea. This will introduce a general increase in response latency compatible with the time taken for the

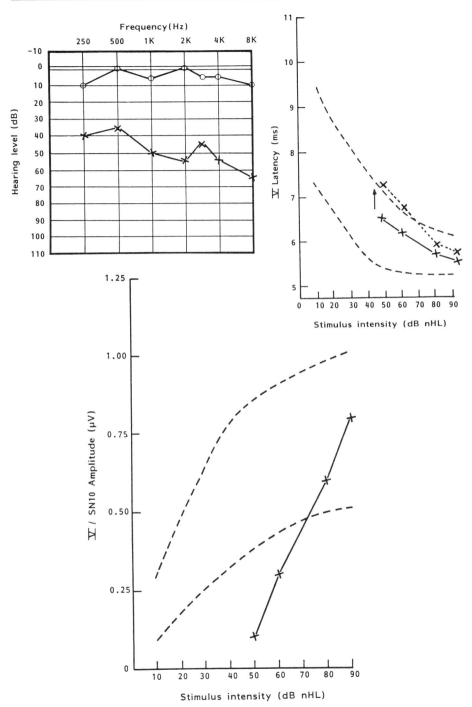

Figure 7.27 An example of the I/O functions of wave V latency and amplitude in flat cochlear hearing loss. The dashed lines indicate the range in normal hearing (± 2 s.d.).

travelling wave to traverse the inactive basal region; the amplitude I/O function is often depressed, as shown in Figure 7.28. If the hearing loss has features of loudness recruitment, due to a predominant loss of outer hair cells at the basal turn of the cochlea, then the latency will tend to shorten towards normal values at high stimulus levels. The slope of the audiogram across 2–4 kHz, where excitation with the click stimulus is maximal, will influence the I/O functions. In a steep, high-frequency loss an increased contribution to the response from the more apical 2 kHz region will occur, with a low-level click stimulus in contrast to a higher intensity stimulus. This tends to enhance the increase in response latency as threshold is approached.

The configuration of the I/O functions can assist in the differential diagnosis of a conductive and cochlear hearing loss. However, caution must be exercised in reporting these findings because of the variation in the shape of I/O functions that can be observed in cochlear hearing losses. Care must be taken to record responses over a wide range of stimulus intensity and to define the threshold of the ABR accurately or the results may be misleading. Tympanometry is a useful additional objective test to assist with this differential diagnosis.

Retrocochlear hearing loss

The most common causes of hearing loss in infants and young children are middle ear disorders or cochlear damage. However, the possibility of retrocochlear pathology at higher levels of the auditory pathway, either the brain stem or the cortex, should not be overlooked. The ABR may be recorded for oto-neurological investigation, recording the interpeak latencies of waves I, III and V, which will help to identify retrocochlear pathology at levels below the generator sites of the wave V and SN10 components (lateral lemniscus and inferior colliculus). An abnormality in the ABR waveform may complicate the assessment of hearing sensitivity, such as described by Kraus et al. (1984) for hydrocephalic patients. Fortunately, retrocochlear pathology is fairly rare in the paediatric population and ABR therefore may be used with confidence for assessment of hearing acuity. Many infants and children with possible brain stem or cortical pathology are likely to have been identified initially from their clinical status by methods including radiological and oto-neurological ABR investigation. The typical I/0 functions observed in a patient with an auditory nerve tumour are shown in Figure 7.29. The wave V component is often delayed and reduced in amplitude.

Configuration of the audiogram

In young children referred for ERA the contour of the audiogram is initially unknown. The click stimulus will provide information regarding

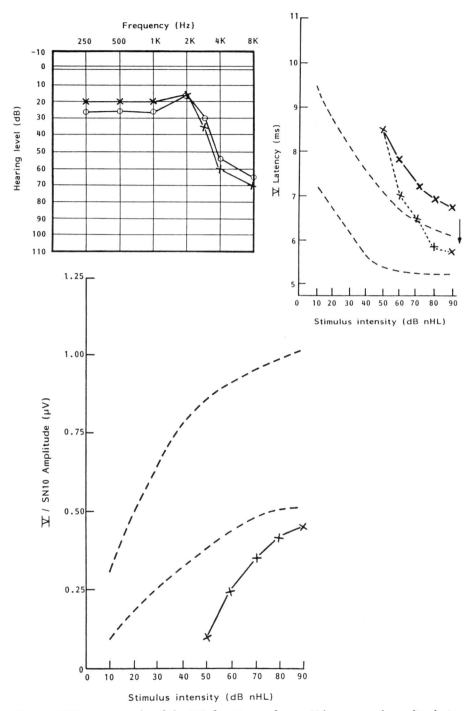

Figure 7.28 An example of the I/O functions of wave V latency and amplitude in high frequency cochlear hearing loss. The dashed lines indicate the range in normal hearing (± 2 s.d).

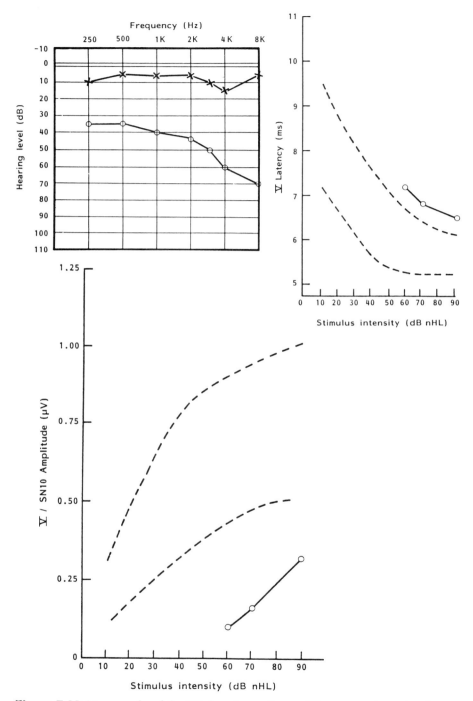

Figure 7.29 An example of the I/O functions of wave V latency and amplitude in a case of retrocochlear hearing loss (auditory nerve tumour). The dashed lines indicate the range in normal hearing (± 2 s.d.).

high-frequency hearing loss across 2–4 kHz and the use of tone pips, particularly those with frequencies below 2 kHz, will provide a valuable supplement to this information. Typical relationships of the click and tone-pip ABR thresholds to the shape of the pure tone audiogram (PTA) are shown in Figure 7.30. The frequency specificity and sensitivity of these ABR thresholds will be limited by aspects of the stimulus and subsequent generation of responses (discussed earlier in this chapter). The audiograms in Figure 7.30 are a representative sample of those reported by Davis et al. (1985), Gorga et al. (1985), Stapells et al. (1985), Keith and Grenville (1987) and from the Nottingham clinic, and are based on recordings of the ABR without the use of ipsilateral high pass or notched noise masking.

The click-evoked ABR thresholds are in reasonable agreement with the PTA at 3 kHz in most cases of flat or only shallow-sloping hearing losses (Figure 7.30 a, b, c). However, when the hearing loss has a steep

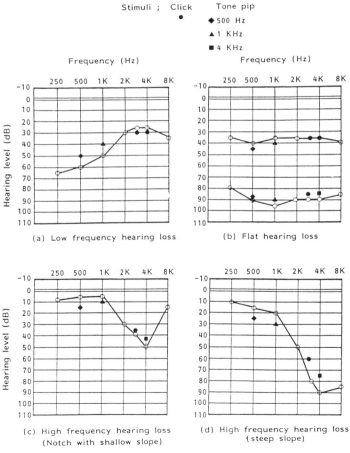

Figure 7.30 The expected accuracy of click and tone-pip ABR thresholds in relation to the shape of the pure tone audiogram.

slope in the region of 2–4 kHz (Figure 7.30d) the click will underestimate the degree of hearing loss present, being biased towards the better hearing at 2 kHz. In some cases of moderate to severe cochlear hearing loss the click may also slightly underestimate the level of hearing loss present (Mason, Field and Coles, 1990) probably because of a relatively faster growth in loudness for wide-band sounds, such as the click, than narrow-band pure tones (Moore, 1989).

The tone-pip ABR will also give reasonably accurate frequency-specific information in situations of a flat or shallow-sloping PTA, particularly with low levels of hearing loss as shown in Figure 7.30b, c. However, with a severe low-frequency hearing loss, as in Figure 7.30a, the degree of loss may be underestimated for the 500 Hz and 1 kHz tone-pips – but up to a limit because, even in subjective PTA, high-intensity low-frequency pure tones may initiate activity in the basal region of the cochlea (Stapells et al., 1985). In steep high-frequency hearing loss (Figure 7.30d) the ABR evoked by a 4 kHz tone-pip may underestimate the degree of hearing loss present, in contrast to a 500 Hz or 1 kHz tone-pip which might have a slight loss in threshold sensitivity depending on the recording conditions. The ABR threshold in profound hearing loss (Figure 7.30b) may underestimate the level of hearing loss slightly due to the effects of distortion and non-linearity of the stimulus at high intensity levels, particularly for the click.

The frequency specificity, and hence the accuracy of threshold information at specific tone frequencies, that can be achieved using the ABR is limited; nevertheless the click and tone-pip stimulus will provide useful information regarding the contour of the audiogram. The click should be the first line of investigation because it gives the best defined response, followed by a tone-pip (typically 1 kHz) provided that appropriate test time and a quiet signal baseline are available. It is important to have good recording conditions, particularly for the tone-pip stimulus, to ensure that significant loss in threshold sensitivity does not occur.

Screening of hearing

The early detection and management of hearing loss in infants is believed to be of paramount importance in alleviating delay in the development of speech, communication and social skills (Ramkalawan and Davis, 1992). In an ideal world a screening programme would identify all infants with a significant hearing loss at a very early age. However, in practice a population in which babies have an increased risk of hearing loss has become targeted. This population includes babies resident in the neonatal intensive care unit, where the risk of severe to profound sensorineural hearing loss is reported as ranging from 0.6% (Davis and Wood, 1992) to 2% (Galambos, Hicks and

Wilson, 1982), compared with 0.1–0.2% for the total new-born population as reviewed by Haggard and Hughes (1991). A more extensive high-risk register could also include factors such as family history of hearing impairment and selected congenital syndromes that are known to be associated with hearing loss (Gerber, 1990).

Several different types of response to sound stimuli have been identified and investigated as a means of assessing the status of hearing in young infants:

- behavioural;
- electrophysiological; and
- oto-acoustic emissions.

Multi-behavioural measurements have been employed in automated screening devices such as the auditory response cradle (Bennett, 1975) and the Crib-O-Gram (Simmons and Russ, 1974). More recently attention has focused on the use of the ABR (Alberti et al., 1983; Mason, 1988) and the evoked oto-acoustic emissions (EOAE) (Lutman 1989; Kemp, Ryan and Bray, 1990; Stevens et al., 1990) as alternatives to behavioural methods of screening. The advent of the ABR and EOAE has cast doubt on the effectiveness of behavioural methods, particularly for screening very young and pre-term babies. The ABR is well-established for the assessment of hearing loss in difficult-to-test young children and babies and its application in screening is a natural extension to the technique.

A screening test may be carried out on a general-purpose piece of commercial ABR equipment using standard methodology and test procedures. However, this is not ideal for implementation in a routine screening programme in which staff relatively inexperienced in ERA measurements (for example nursing staff) may be required to carry out the ABR test. For this reason interest in the development of simple-to-use and highly automated instruments has grown. Machine scoring has been implemented in some of these devices to assist an inexperienced operator to decide whether an ABR is present.

Test protocol

Several aspects of the test methodology, such as electrode placement, signal filtering and averaging, are similar to those of threshold assessment using the ABR and have been described earlier. The click-evoked ABR is widely used in neonatal screening, thereby taking advantage of the well-defined response waveform compared with other types of stimuli. Hyde, Riko and Malizia (1990) reviewed ABR results in infancy with follow-up pure tone audiograms obtained in patients of 3–8 years old. They found that the click-evoked ABR was an excellent predictor of sensorineural hearing loss across 2–4 kHz. Most severe to profound sensorineural hearing losses usually involve impairment across this frequency range.

The optimum test conditions for the ABR are achieved when a baby is settled or asleep and any disturbance during the screening test should be minimized. The response waveform may not be identified when the signal baseline is very noisy; this may result in the baby failing the screening test and being referred for unnecessary follow-up investigations. It is often best to screen a baby soon after it has been fed because this is often a very settled period. Neonates from the neonatal intensive care unit can be tested in their cots. One ear may be immediately accessible and it is advisable to test that ear before moving the baby to test the other. Care should be taken to avoid disturbing the baby when applying the recording electrodes. A pre-amplifier with good performance characteristics will give a reliable signal baseline in most situations with only minimal preparation of the skin.

Machine scoring

Early investigations of machine detection and scoring of evoked potentials in ERA were applied to the auditory cortical response (Schimmel, Rapin and Cohen, 1974; Salomon, 1975) using techniques such as correlation between subsets of a grand average, analysis of the R/N ratio and template methods. The first reports of objective detection of the ABR were by Koizumi (1976) who used measurement of amplitude, and Weber and Fletcher (1980) and Sayers and McClelland (1982), who used correlation techniques. However, these studies presented either few results on patients with hearing loss or a lack of sensitivity of the objective thresholds (20–30 dB) when compared with visual scoring. The reliability and accuracy of machine scoring may be improved by applying a combination of different mathematical techniques (Mason, 1984b). In Mason's study the ABR was detected using a scanning correlation window followed by measurement of the R/N ratio, the final waveform score (++, +, –) being influenced by the absolute amplitude of the response and noise components. Further refinements to this machine scoring algorithm have been reported by Mason (1985).

Instrumentation

Instruments have been developed specifically for screening hearing, incorporating machine analysis of the response waveform, although not all have employed the ABR. These instruments include:

- the Bodyspek 2000;
- the Audit;
- the Algotek (or Algo-1); and
- the Nottingham ABR screener.

The Bodyspek is based on an objective scoring technique for the PAM as described by Fraser et al. (1978). The device screens at a relatively high stimulus intensity of 60 and 80 dB HL. Unfortunately the PAM is not a consistent response in very young infants (who may be asleep for the test) and is therefore not suitable for early screening of the at-risk population.

The second machine, the Audit (Axonics Instruments), objectively detects the 40 Hz steady-state response, which consists of an in-phase overlap of ABR and middle latency response components. It determines the auditory sensitivity as normal, a mild-to-moderate loss, or a severe-to-profound loss. Unfortunately the 40 Hz response is again affected to some extent by sleep, and the in-phase overlapping enhancement of response components at the 40 Hz stimulus rate observed in older children and adults does not occur at the same stimulus rate in infants and neonates.

The Algo-1 records the ABR with a relatively simple and automated test procedure and uses a template method for objective detection of the response waveform (Thornton, Hermann and Berick, 1985; Kileny, 1987). This device has several attractive features for screening hearing in at-risk neonates, although it has two particular drawbacks. First, a very quiet signal baseline is required in order to allow the test to proceed due to the very sensitive level of artefact rejection. Secondly, there is no display of the ABR waveform and interpretation is totally dependent on the objective machine scores. Some workers will not wish to use this technique until they have gained complete confidence in the reliability of the device.

A highly automated ABR screening system, developed in Nottingham (Mason, 1988), provides a display of the on-line signal baseline and all the averaged waveforms as well as incorporating machine scoring. The current system employs an IBM-type personal computer interfaced to a stimulator/amplifier unit. Data collection and analysis are highly automated and, with only minimal training, the device may be used by relatively inexperienced personnel. Typical response waveforms are shown in Figure 7.31.

Evaluation of the ABR

The ABR performs well as a screening test in terms of its sensitivity and specificity. A study of the ABR recorded with a general-purpose ERA system in 600 infants in a neonatal intensive care unit, of which 333 were followed up with pure tone audiometry at 3 years of age, was carried out by Durieux-Smith et al. (1991). A sensitivity of 86% and specificity of 100% were recorded for identification of children with a bilateral sensorineural or mixed hearing loss requiring amplification. Only one child passed the ABR test in infancy and was subsequently

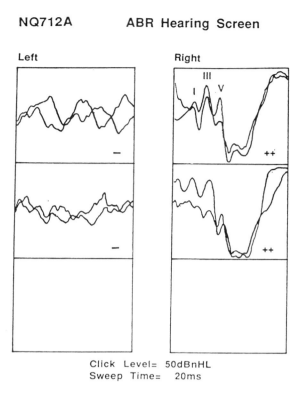

Figure 7.31 Typical ABR waveforms with machine scores recorded in a pre-term neonate who has unilaterally failed the ABR screen at a click level of 50 dB nHL.

given amplification on a trial basis due to delayed speech. The audiogram in this child was rather unusual and exhibited near-normal hearing bilaterally at some frequencies across 1–4 kHz. If the analysis had been carried out according to the classification of a severe to profound hearing loss, rather than children requiring amplification, a sensitivity of 100% for the ABR test would have been recorded. Hyde, Riko and Malizia (1990), in a similar study, found that all the infants studied with bilateral sensorineural loss had been correctly identified with ABR using a 30 dB nHL click stimulus.

Kennedy et al. (1991) compared conventional ABR measurements with those obtained using the Algo-1 device in a group of 370 infants, of whom 75% comprised an at-risk category. The overall failure rate was around 8% in both measurements using a click level of 35 dB nHL. This compares well with results using the Nottingham ABR system, in which typically 7% of at-risk babies fail the screen at 50 dB nHL. Kennedy et al. noted that 2.7% of babies could not be tested with the Algo-1 (compared with only 0.5% with the conventional ABR measurement). This difference was caused primarily by a failure of the baby to settle and the strict requirement of a quiet signal baseline for the Algo-1. Only 1.2% of babies could not be tested with the Nottingham ABR system.

The Nottingham ABR Screener

In this section an analysis of the performance of the Nottingham ABR system for screening an at-risk population of neonates will be presented with respect to machine scoring and the stimulus level of the click. The at-risk group comprised babies resident in the neonatal intensive care unit for longer than 48 h, babies for whom there is significant evidence of a family history of hearing loss and babies with syndromes that are known to be associated with hearing loss. The gestational age at test for most babies was in the range 32–42 (mean 36) weeks. A click level of 40 dB nHL was employed at the start of the study. However, this stimulus level referred too many babies and was changed so that babies younger than 37 weeks' gestational age at the time of the test were allowed to pass the screen at 60 dB nHL (Mason et al., 1986). More recently a screening level of 50 dB nHL was adopted for all the at-risk babies. The protocol was changed because the apparent effects of maturation on the outcome of the screen (which had been observed in earlier results) did not replicate in more recent data. Results of screening 500 babies using the 40–60 dB nHL protocol and a separate group of 500 babies tested at 50 dB nHL have been analysed.

The referral rate of the ABR screen with respect to stimulus level is shown in Figure 7.32: 21% were referred at 40 dB nHL, compared with only 7% at 50 dB nHL (of which 1.8% were bilateral referrals). The number of babies failing the ABR screen is affected by factors such as test conditions and prevalence of middle ear fluid in addition to the stimulus level. The pass or refer result from machine scoring is

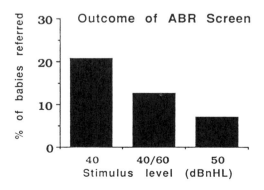

Figure 7.32 Referral rate for the ABR screen with respect to stimulus intensity. There were 7% of the neonates who failed the screen on either ear at 50 dB nHL, of which 1.8% were bilateral referrals.

Table 7.1 Typical agreement between observer and machine scores for screening hearing using the Nottingham ABR system (50 dB nHL, 500 babies, 991 ears tested)

		Machine score	
		Pass	Refer
Observer score	Pass	944 (95.3%)	7 (0.7%)
	Refer	2 (0.2%)	38 (3.8%)

Machine versus observer agreement = 99.1% (observer: marginal pass = pass).

continually assessed with respect to a three-level decision by an experienced observer: pass, marginal pass, or refer. The typical agreement between machine and observer for 500 babies screened at 50 dB nHL is shown in Table 7.1. These data included 23 marginal pass results that were included in the pass category, giving only two false-negative results (0.2%) for the machine, with an overall level of agreement of 99.1%.

All babies that have very little response activity on the ABR screen, and subsequently fail the screening test of hearing, are referred for a full ABR threshold assessment using click and tone-pip stimuli. This follow-up investigation is carried out when the babies are 6 weeks old relative to their expected date of delivery, since many of the babies are born pre-term. The results of this follow up in 33 babies for the 40–60 dB nHL screen and 29 babies for the 50 dB nHL screen are shown in Figure 7.33 (a and b respectively). The outcome for the 50 dB nHL screen compares very favourably with that for 40–60 dB nHL. Eight babies were identified as having a bilateral (five) or unilateral (three) sensorineural hearing loss of greater than 50 dB HL with the 50 dB nHL screen; six for the 40–60 dB nHL screen. A significant number of babies referred the screen but were normal on follow up (44% on the 50 dB nHL screen): transient middle ear pathology in the neonatal period is likely to be the main cause of this discrepancy. The eight babies with severe to profound hearing loss identified by the 50 dB nHL screen represent 1.6% of the total at-risk population screened. Hearing aids were fitted to five of these babies at a very early age. These results agree well with the published findings of a 1–2% incidence of severe to profound hearing losses in the at-risk neonatal population.

The ABR is a popular approach for screening hearing in the at-risk neonatal population. It has good sensitivity and specificity, which compares favourably with the EOAE and behavioural methods. The EOAE has a short test time and has a valuable role to play in screening hearing, particularly in the normal new-born population where it has a good record of sensitivity and specificity. Highly automated and simple-to-use systems for recording the ABR and EOAE should see their wider implementation and evaluation in the future.

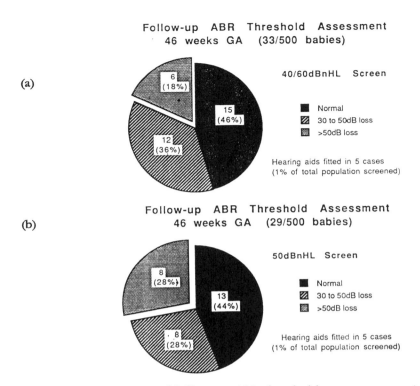

Figure 7.33 Outcome of follow-up ABR threshold measurements in at-risk neonates screened at (a) 40–60 dB nHL; (b) 50 dB nHL.

Electrically evoked ABR

Cochlear implantation is becoming an accepted approach to management of profoundly hearing-impaired children (Staller, 1991) who obtain little or no benefit from conventional amplification. The transfer from acoustic to electrical stimulation of the cochlea has led to the development of techniques for recording electrically evoked potentials (Miyamoto, 1986; Abbas and Brown, 1988). Recent reports (Shallop et al., 1990; Kileny, 1991) have demonstrated use of the electrically evoked auditory brain stem response (EABR), middle latency response (EMLR) and auditory cortical response (EACR). The EABR is appropriate for use in young children and can provide valuable objective assessment of the cochlear implant (Mason et al., 1993).

Methodology

Recording an electrically evoked potential is similar in many ways to that of the acoustic responses, employing well-established recording technology. The main differences are the characteristics and delivery of the stimulus (Shallop et al., 1990; Mason et al., 1993). Electrical stimulation may be a more efficient way of delivering a stimulus to the sensory system, resulting in greater synchronization of evoked neural activity, but the technique does have some drawbacks: there is often a large artefact resulting from the stimulus that the recording system has to handle; current spread arises from the stimulating electrode; the quality of the response may be affected by the level of neuronal survival.

The method of delivery of the stimulus will depend on a number of factors. Pre-implant assessment of electrical stimulation is often carried out using a single stimulating electrode on the promontory or round window in adult subjects and their behavioural response to the stimulus assessed. In young children, however, there are obvious difficulties in implementation of this behavioural technique. Recording an evoked potential from the stimulus (e.g. EABR) while the child is anaesthetized is one way of overcoming the problem of cooperation (Kileny et al., 1992). Electrical stimulation may be extra- or intra-cochlear, using a single or multichannel electrode array. Many reports of electrically evoked potentials involve recordings of the EABR using the Nucleus 22 channel cochlear implant (Allum et al., 1990; Shallop et al,. 1990; Mason et al., 1993). An appropriate stimulus for the EABR consists of a train of individual bipolar electrical pulses presented on a single channel of the electrode array at a repetition rate of typically 31/s. The effective intensity of the stimulus is controlled by the duration and amplitude of the electrical pulse. The signal is recorded from standard EEG-type scalp electrodes with conventional amplification, filtering and averaging being used to recover the response.

Characteristics of the EABR

Responses evoked by electrical stimulation are similar in many ways to those recorded from acoustic stimulation in conventional ERA (Kileny, 1991). Typical characteristics of the EABR are shown in Figure 7.34. Individual components of the EABR are thought to originate from structures in the auditory pathway similar to those for the acoustical ABR and are often identified with a leading 'e' to denote an electrically evoked component (for example, eV). There are, however, minor differences between the electrical and acoustical responses: the absolute latencies of the electrical response components are shorter, with wave eV arising at 4.0–4.5 ms (compared with 5.5–6.0 ms for the acoustical ABR); there is also only a small increase in latency with reduction in stimulus level, as illustrated in the latency I/O functions in Figure 7.35. These findings are consistent with a lack of a cochlear travelling wave as a component of the process that generates the response. The amplitude I/O function for wave eV is very steep (shown in Figure 7.36), often rising from around 50 nV at response threshold up to 500 nV or

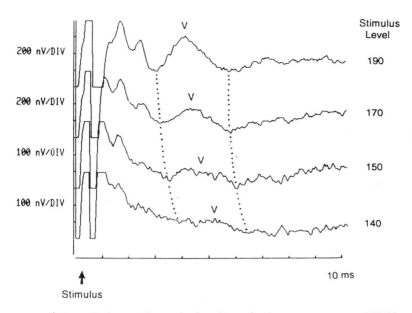

Figure 7.34 Typical electrically evoked auditory brain stem response (EABR) waveforms recorded down to response threshold.

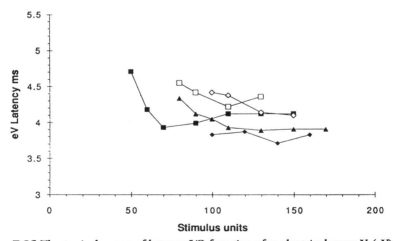

Figure 7.35 The typical range of latency I/O functions for electrical wave V (eV).

more with moderate levels of electrical stimulation. The EABR data in Figures 7.34–7.37 were recorded on Nucleus 22-channel cochlear implants, with stimulus levels from 0 to 239 units.

Clinical application

There is great expectation regarding the clinical application of electrically evoked potentials and in particular the EABR in young children

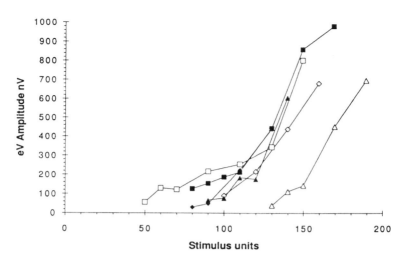

Figure 7.36 The typical range of amplitude I/O functions for electrical wave V (eV).

receiving cochlear implants. The technique is a valuable objective assessment of the cochlear implant and provides information about the levels of electrical stimulation that are required for sensation of the stimulus. There is also interest in assessing the I/O functions of the EABR before surgery as a predictor of the extent and pattern of neuronal survival in both adults and children (Kileny et al., 1992). The EABR evoked by the cochlear implant can be recorded during surgery while the child is still anaesthetized (Mason et al., 1993) and the EABR threshold then used to predict the level of electrical stimulation required for sensation of the stimulus (subjective threshold (T) level) during the initial stimulation period after implantation. The typical relationship between the EABR threshold and T level is shown in Figure 7.37. If a correction factor of –30 stimulus units is applied to the EABR data 82% of thresholds are within 30 stimulus units of T level. This correction factor arises predominantly from the different pulse rates used for measurement of the EABR (31/s) and the subjective T level (250/s).

Intraoperative measurement of the EABR is valuable in young children receiving cochlear implants and should be routinely available in a paediatric cochlear implant programme. Further development of the recording methodology and analysis of data should extend the clinical applications of this technique.

Summary

Electric response audiometry using the ABR is an essential tool for assessing hearing loss in the paediatric population and complements the wide range of behavioural and audiometric tests available. Its con-

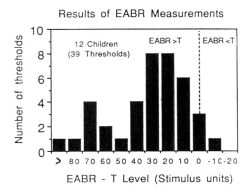

Figure 7.37 The agreement between the intraoperative EABR threshold and the first reliable subjective threshold (T) level. The offset between the two threshold measurements arises to a large extent from the different pulse rates employed for the stimuli – 31 p.p.s. for the EABR and 250 p.p.s. for the T level.

tribution to the early identification of hearing impairment is such that it has become an integral part of screening in populations of infants at high risk.

Electrically evoked potentials, such as the EABR, have been developed to fulfil a need for objective testing in children receiving cochlear implants. This field is likely to experience major growth over the next few years as the number of young children receiving cochlear implants increases.

In the future we can expect advances in the areas of data acquisition, analysis routines and methods of interpretation. Quantification of the recording conditions and the introduction of machine scoring routines should improve the objectivity in the interpretation of ERA results. It is hoped that the time is very close when these objective techniques will be more widely incorporated into clinical ERA equipment.

References

Abbas, P.J. (1988). Electrophysiology of the auditory system. *Clinical Physics and Physiological Measurement* 9, 1–31.

Abbas, P.J. and Brown, C.J. (1988). Electrically evoked brain stem potentials in cochlear implant patients with multi-electrode stimulation. *Hearing Research* 36, 153–162.

Abramovich, S. (1990). *Electric Response Audiometry in Clinical Practice.* Edinburgh: Churchill Livingstone.

Achor, L.J. and Starr, A. (1980). Auditory brain stem responses in the cat. I. Intracranial and extracranial recordings. *Electroencephalography and Clinical Neurophysiology* 48, 154–173.

Alberti, P.W., Hyde, M., Corbin, H., Riko, K. and Abramovich, S. (1983). An evaluation of BERA for hearing screening in high-risk neonates. *Laryngoscope* 93, 1115–1120.

Allum, J.H.J., Shallop, J.K., Hotz, M. and Pfaltz, C.R. (1990). Characteristics of electrically evoked 'auditory' brain stem responses elicited with the Nucleus 22–electrode intracochlear implant. *Scandinavian Audiology* 19, 263–267.

Beagley, H.A. (1972). Progress in objective audiometry. *Journal of Laryngology and Otology* 86, 225–235.

Beagley, H.A. and Kellogg, S.E. (1968). A comparison of evoked response and subjective auditory thresholds. *International Audiology* 7, 420–421.

Békésy, G. von (1947). The variation of phase along the basilar membrane with sinusoidal vibrations. *Journal of the Acoustical Society of America* 19, 452–462.

Bennett, M.J. (1975). The Auditory Response Cradle: A device for the objective assessment of auditory state in the neonate. *Symposium of the Zoological Society* 37, 291–305

Berger, H. (1929) and (1930). *Hans Berger and the Discovery of the Electroencephalogram*, reviewed by Gloor, P. (1969). *Electroencephalography and Clinical Neurophysiology*, Suppl. 28, 1–36

Bickford, R.G., Galbraith, R.F. and Jacobson, J.L. (1963). The nature of average evoked potentials recorded from the human scalp. *Electroencephalography and Clinical Neurophysiology* 15, 720.

Brown, D.D. (1982). The use of Middle Latency Response (MLR) for assessing low-frequency auditory thresholds. *Journal of the Acoustical Society of America* 71, Suppl. 1, S99.

Brownell, W.E. (1986). Outer hair cell motility and cochlear frequency specificity. In: Moore, B.C.J. and Patterson, R.D. (Eds), *Auditory Frequency Selectivity*, pp. 109–120. New York: Plenum Press.

Chiappi, K.H., Gladstone, K.J. and Young, R. R. (1979). Brain stem auditory evoked responses; studies of waveform variations in 50 normal human subjects. *Archives of Audiology* 36, 81–87.

Clark, W.A. Jr. (1958). *Average Response Computer (ARC-1)*. Quarterly Progress Report No. 49 Research Laboratory of Electronics, Massachusetts Institute of Technology, Cambridge, Massachusetts. Cambridge, MA: MIT press.

Coats, A.C. and Martin, J.L. (1977). Human auditory nerve action potentials and brain stem evoked responses. *Archives of Otolaryngology* 103, 605–622.

Davis, A.C. and Wood, S. (1992). The epidemiology of childhood hearing impairment: Factors relevant to the planning of services. *British Journal of Audiology* 26, 77–90.

Davis,. H. (1976). Brainstem and other responses in electrical response audiometry. *Annals of Otology* 85, 3–14.

Davis, H. and Hirsh, S.K. (1976). The audiometric utility of brain stem responses to low-frequency sounds. *Audiology* 15, 181–195.

Davis, H. and Hirsh, S.K. (1979). A slow brainstem response for low-frequency audiometry. *Audiology* 18, 445–461.

Davis, H. and Zerlin, S. (1966). Acoustic relations of the human vertex potential. *Journal of the Acoustical Society of America* 39, 109–116.

Davis, H., Davis, P.A., Loomis, A.L., Harvey, E.N. and Hobart, G. (1939). Electrical reactions of the human brain to auditory stimulation during sleep. *Journal of Neurophysiology* 2, 500–514.

Davis, H., Hirsh, S.K., Shelnutt, J. and Bowers, C. (1967). Further validation of evoked response audiometry (ERA). *Journal of Speech and Hearing Research* 10, 717–732.

Davis, H., Hirsh, S.K., Turpin, L.L. and Peacock, M.E. (1985). Threshold sensitivity and frequency specificity in auditory brainstem response audiometry. *Audiology* 24, 54–70.

Davis, P.A. (1939). Effects of acoustic stimuli on the waking human brain. *Journal of Neurophysiology* 2, 494–499.

Dawson, G.D. (1951). A summation technique for detecting small signals in a large irregular background. *Journal of Physiology* 115, 2–3.

Don, M., Elberling, C. and Waring, M. (1984). Objective detection of averaged auditory brainstem responses. *Scandinavian Audiology* 13, 219–228.

Douek, E.E., Gibson, W.P.R. and Humphries, K.M. (1975). The crossed acoustic response. *Revue de Laryngologie* 96, 121–125.

Drift, van der, J.F.C., Brocaar, M.P. and van Zanten, G.A. (1987). The relation between the pure tone audiogram and the click auditory brain stem response threshold in cochlear hearing loss. *Audiology* 26, 1–10.

Durieux-Smith, A., Picton, T.W., Bernard, P., MacMurray, B. and Goodman, J.T. (1991). Prognostic validity of brainstem electric response audiometry in infants of a neonatal intensive care unit. *Audiology* 30, 249–265.

Eggermont, J. (1982). The inadequacy of click-evoked auditory brainstem responses in audiological applications. *Annals of the New York Academy of Sciences* 388, 707–709.

Finitzo-Hieber, T. and Friel-Patti, S. (1985). Conductive hearing loss and the ABR. In: Jacobson, J.T. (Ed.), *The Auditory Brainstem Response*, pp. 113–132. California: College-Hill Press.

Fjermedal, O. and Laukli, E. (1989). Low-level 0.5 and 1 kHz auditory brain stem responses. *Scandinavian Audiology* 18, 177–183.

Folsom, R.C. (1984). Frequency specificity of human auditory brain stem responses as revealed by pure tone masking profiles. *Journal of the Acoustical Society of America* 75, 919–924.

Fraser, J.G., Conway, M.J., Keene, M.H. and Hazell, J.W.P. (1978). The post-auricular myogenic response: A new instrument which simplifies its detection by machine scoring. *Journal of Laryngology and Otology* 92, 293–303.

Fria, T.J. and Sabo, D.L. (1980). Auditory brain stem responses in children with otitis media and effusion. *Annals of Otology, Rhinology and Laryngology* 68, 200–206.

Galambos, R., Hicks, G. and Wilson, M.J. (1982). Hearing loss in graduates of a tertiary care nursery. *Ear and Hearing* 3, 87–90.

Galambos, R., Makeig, S. and Talamachoff, P.J. (1981). A 40 Hz auditory potential recorded from the human scalp. *Proceedings of the National Academy of Science USA* 78, 2643–2647.

Geisler, C.D., Frishkopf, L.S. and Rosenblith, W.A. (1958). Extracranial responses to acoustic clicks in man. *Science* 128, 1210–1211.

Gerber, S. (1990). Review of a high risk register for congenital or early onset deafness. *British Journal of Audiology* 14, 347–356.

Gibson, W.P.R. (1978). *Essentials of Clinical Electric Response Audiometry*. London: Churchill Livingstone.

Glasscock, M.E., Jackson, C.G. and Josey, A. F. (1987). *The ABR Handbook*. London: Thieme Medical Publishers.

Gorga, M.P., Worthington, D.W., Reiland, J.K., Beuchaine, K.A. and Goldgar, D.E. (1985). Some comparisons between auditory brain stem response thresholds, latencies, and the pure tone audiogram. *Ear and Hearing* 6, 105–112.

Haggard, M.P. and Hughes, E. (1991). *Screening children's hearing: A review of the literature and implications of otitis media*. London: HMSO.

Hashimoto, I. (1982). Auditory evoked potentials from the human midbrain: Slow brainstem responses. *Electroencephalography and Clinical Neurophysiology* **53**, 652–657.

Hawes, M.D. and Greenberg, H.J. (1981). Slow brain stem responses (SN10) to tone pips in normally hearing newborns and adults. *Audiology* **20**, 113–122.

Hecox, K. and Galambos, R. (1974). Brain stem auditory evoked responses in human infants and adults. *Archives of Otolaryngology*, **99**, 30–33.

Hosford-Dunn, H., Runge, C.A., Hillel, A. and Johnson, S.J. (1983). Auditory brain stem response testing in infants with collapsed ear canals. *Ear and Hearing* **4**, 258–260.

Hyde, M.L. (1985). The effect of cochlear lesions on the ABR. In: Jacobson, J.T. (Ed.), *The Auditory Brainstem Response*, pp. 133–146. San Diego, CA: College-Hill Press.

Hyde, M.L., Stephens, S.D.G. and Thornton, A.R.D. (1976). Stimulus repetition rate and the early brainstem responses. *British Journal of Audiology* **10**, 41–46.

Hyde, M.L., Riko, K. and Malizia, K. (1990). Audiometric accuracy of the click ABR in infants at risk for hearing loss. *Journal of the American Academy of Audiology* **1**, 59–66.

Jacobson, J.T. (1983). Effects of rise time and noise masking on tone pip auditory brainstem responses. *Seminars in Hearing* **4**, 363–372.

Jacobson, J.T., Ed. (1985). *The Auditory Brainstem Response*. San Diego, CA: College-Hill Press.

Jewett, D.L. and Williston, J.S. (1971). Auditory-evoked far fields averaged from the scalp of humans. *Brain* **94**, 681–696.

Kavanagh, K.T., Harker, L.A. and Tyler, R.S. (1982). *Auditory brainstem and middle latency responses.* Presented at the Resident's Research Forum, American Academy of Otolaryngology, New Orleans, October 1982.

Keith, W.J. and Grenville, K.A. (1987). Effects of audiometric configuration on the auditory brainstem response. *Ear and Hearing* **8**, 49–55.

Kemp, D.T., Ryan, S. and Bray, P. (1990). A guide to the effective use of otoacoustic emissions. *Ear and Hearing* **11**, 93–105.

Kennedy, C.R., Kimm, L., Cafarelli Dees, D., Evans, P.I.P., Hunter, M., Lenton, S. and Thornton, R.D. (1991). Otoacoustic emissions and auditory brain stem response in the newborn. *Archives of Disease in Childhood* **66**, 1124–1129.

Kiang, N.Y.-S., Christ, A.H., French, M.A. and Edwards, A.G. (1963). Post-auricular electric response to acoustic stimuli in humans. *Quarterly Progress Report of the Laboratory of Electronics, MIT* **68**, 218–225.

Kileny, P. (1982). Auditory brainstem responses as indicators of hearing aid performance. *Annals of Otology* **91**, 61–64.

Kileny, P.R. (1987). ALGO-1 automated infant hearing screener: preliminary results. *Seminars in Hearing* **8**, 125.

Kileny, P.R. (1991). Use of electrophysiologic measures in the management of children with cochlear implants: Brainstem, middle latency, and cognitive (P300) responses. *American Journal of Otology (Supplement)* **12**, 37–42.

Kileny, P.R., Zimmerman-Phillips, S., Zwolan, T., Lougheed, L. and Kemink, J. (1992). *Preoperative EABR in paediatric cochlear implant candidates: classification and follow-up*. Presented at the First European Symposium on Paediatric Cochlear Implantation, Nottingham, September 1992.

Klein, A.J. (1983). Properties of the brain-stem response slow-wave component, I. Latency, amplitude and threshold sensitivity. *Archives of Otolaryngology* **109**, 6–12.

Koizumi, S. (1976). Fundamental studies for automatic scoring of brain stem response. *Journal of Otolaryngology* 79, 591–598.

Kraus, N., Ozdamar, O., Hier, D. and Stein, L. (1982). Auditory middle latency responses (MLRs) in patients with cortical lesions. *Electroencephalography and Clinical Neurophysiology* 54, 275–287.

Kraus, N., Ozdamar, O., Heydemann, P.T., Stein, L. and Reed, N. (1984). Auditory brain stem response in hydrocephalic patients. *Electroencephalography and Clinical Neurophysiology* 59, 310–317.

Lightfoot, G.R. and Mason, S.M. (1992). Electric response audiometry (ERA): principles, techniques and clinical applications. Course notes from the Liverpool ERA Short Course, Institute of Medical and Dental Bioengineering, University of Liverpool and Royal Liverpool Hospital.

Lutman, M.E. (1989). Evoked otoacoustic emissions in adults: implications for screening. *Audiology in Practice* 3, 6–8.

Mahoney, T. M. (1985). Auditory brainstem response hearing aid applications. In: Jacobson, J.T. (Ed.), *The Auditory Brainstem Response*, pp. 349–370. San Diego, CA: College-Hill Press.

Mason, S.M. (1984a). Effects of high-pass filtering on the detection of the auditory brain stem response. *British Journal of Audiology* 18, 155–161.

Mason, S.M. (1984b). On-line computer scoring of the auditory brainstem response for estimation of hearing threshold. *Audiology* 23, 277–296.

Mason, S.M. (1985). *Objective waveform detection in electric response audiometry*. PhD Thesis, University of Nottingham.

Mason, S.M. (1988). Automated system for screening hearing using the auditory brainstem response. *British Journal of Audiology* 22, 211–213.

Mason, S.M., Field, D.L. and Coles, R.A.A. (1990). *Non-linearities of the click evoked ABR threshold in cochlear hearing loss*. Presented at the Fourth International Evoked Potentials Symposium, Toronto, Canada, September 30–October 3, 1990.

Mason, S.M., McCormick, B. and Wood, S. (1988). Auditory brainstem response in paediatric audiology. *Archives of Disease in Childhood* 63, 465–467.

Mason, S.M., Singh, C.B. and Brown, P.M. (1980). Assessment of non-invasive electrocochleography. *Journal of Laryngology and Otology* 94, 707–718.

Mason, S. M., Barber, C., Davis, A.C. and McCormick, B. (1986). Evolution and detectability of the neonatal ABR: Implications for automated screening of hearing. In: Gallai, V. (Ed.) *Maturation of the CNS and Evoked Potentials*, pp. 194–203. Amsterdam: Elsevier Science Publishers.

Mason, S.M., Sheppard, S., Garnham, C.W., Lutman, M.E., O'Donoghue, G.M. and Gibbin, K.P. (1993). Application of intraoperative recordings of electrically evoked ABRs in a paediatric cochlear implant programme. *Advances in Oto-Rhino-Laryngology* 48 (in press).

Miyamoto, R.T. (1986). Electrically evoked potentials in cochlear implants. *Laryngoscope* 96, 178–185.

Mokotoff, B., Schulman-Galambos, C. and Galambos, R. (1977). Brain stem auditory evoked response in children. *Archives of Otolaryngology* 103, 38–43.

Moller, A.R. and Jannetta, P.J. (1984). Neural generators of the brain stem auditory evoked potential. In: Nodar, R.H. and Barber, C. (Eds), *Evoked Potentials II*, pp. 137–144. Boston: Butterworths.

Moore, B.C.J. (1989). Frequency selectivity, masking and the critical band. In: Moore, B.C.J. (Ed.), *An Introduction to the Psychology of Hearing*, pp. 84–136. London: Academic Press.

Musiek, F.E. and Guerkink, N.A. (1981). Auditory brainstem and middle latency evoked response sensitivity near threshold. *Annals of Otology* 90, 236–240.

Okitsu, T. (1984). Middle components of the auditory evoked response in young children. *Scandinavian Audiology* 13, 83–86.

Parker, D.J. and Thornton, A.R.D. (1978). Derived cochlear nerve and brainstem evoked responses of the human auditory system. *Scandinavian Audiology* 7, 1–8.

Parving, A., Salomon, G., Elberling, C., Larsen, B. and Lassen, N.A. (1980). Middle components of the auditory evoked response in bilateral temporal lobe lesions. *Scandinavian Audiology* 9, 161–167.

Pickles, J.A. (1988). *An Introduction to the Physiology of Hearing*. London: Academic Press.

Picton, T.W. and Scherg, M. (1991). Auditory evoked potentials. In: Barber, C. and Taylor, M.J. (Eds), *Evoked Potentials Review No. 4*, pp. 15–28. Nottingham: IEPS Publications.

Picton, T.W., Champagne, S.C. and Kellett, A.J.C. (1992). Human auditory evoked potentials recorded using maximum length sequences. *Electroencephalography and Clinical Neurophysiology* 84, 90–100.

Picton, T.W., Hillyard, S.A., Krausz, H.I. and Galambos, R. (1974). Human auditory evoked potentials. I. Evaluation of components. *Electroencephalography and Clinical Neurophysiology* 36, 179–190.

Picton, T.W., Ouellette, J., Hamel, G. and Smith, A.D. (1979). Brainstem evoked potentials to tone pips in notched noise. *Journal of Otolaryngology* 10, 289–314.

Portmann, M., Lebert, G. and Aran J.-M. (1967). Potentiels cochleares obtenus chez l'homme en dehors de toute intervention chirurgicale. *Revue de Laryngologie* 88, 157–164.

Ramkalawan, T.W. and Davis, A.C. (1992). The effects of hearing loss and age intervention on some language metrics in young hearing-impaired children. *British Journal of Audiology* 26, 97–107.

Reid, A. and Thornton, A.R.D. (1983). The effects of contralateral masking upon the brainstem electric responses. *British Journal of Audiology* 17, 155–162.

Salomon, G. (1975). Automatic evaluation of human auditory evoked potentials from the vertex. *Symposium of the Zoological Society of London* 37, 237–289.

Salamy, A. and McKean, C.M. (1976). Postnatal development of human brain stem potentials during the first year of life. *Electroencephalography and Clinical Neurophysiology* 40, 418–426.

Sanders, J.W. (1978). Masking. In: Katy, J. (Ed.), *Handbook of Clinical Audiology*, pp. 124–140. Baltimore: Williams & Wilkins.

Sayers, B. McA. and McClelland, R.J. (1982). *Evaluation of the cross correlation method for the objective detection of auditory threshold for auditory brain stem potentials*. Presented at the Second International Evoked Potentials Symposium, Cleveland, USA.

Schwartz, D.M. and Berry, G.A. (1985). Normative aspects of the ABR. In: Jacobson, J.T. (Ed.), *The Auditory Brainstem Response*, pp. 65–97. San Diego, CA: College-Hill Press.

Schimmel, H., Rapin, I. and Cohen, M.M. (1974). Improving evoked response audiometry with special reference to machine scoring. *Audiology* 13, 33–65.

Shallop, J.K., Beiter, A.L., Goin, D.W. and Mischke, R.E. (1990). Electrically evoked auditory brain stem response (EABR) and middle latency responses (EMLR) obtained from patients with the Nucleus multichannel cochlear implant. *Ear and Hearing* 11, 5–15.

Simmons, F. B. and Russ, F. N. (1974). Automated newborn hearing screening, The Crib-O-Gram. *Archives of Otolaryngology* 100, 1–7.

Sininger, Y.S. and Masuda, A. (1990). Effect of click polarity on ABR threshold. *Ear and Hearing* 11, 206–209.

Sohmer, H. and Feinmesser, M. (1967). Cochlear action potentials recorded from the external ear in man. *Annals of Otology, Rhinology and Laryngology* 76, 427–435.

Staller, S.J. (1991). Multichannel cochlear implants in children. *Ear and Hearing (Supplement)* 12.

Stapells, D.R., Picton, T.W., Perez-Abalo, M., Read, D. and Smith, A. (1985). Frequency specificity in evoked potential audiometry. In: Jacobson, J.T. (Ed.), *The Auditory Brainstem Response*, pp. 147–180. San Diego, CA: College-Hill Press.

Stapells, D.R., Galambos, R., Costello, J.A. and Makeig, S. (1988). Inconsistency of auditory middle latency and steady-state responses in infants. *Electroencephalography and Clinical Neurophysiology* 71, 289–295.

Stevens, J.C., Webb, H.D., Hutchinson, J., Connell, J., Smith, M.F. and Buffin, J.T. (1990). Click evoked otoacoustic emissions in neonatal screening. *Ear and Hearing* 11, 128–133.

Stockard, J.J. and Rossiter, M.A. (1977). Clinical and pathologic correlates of brain stem auditory response abnormalities. *Neurology* 27, 316–325.

Stockard, J.J., Stockard, J.E. and Sharbrough, F.W. (1977). Detection and localization of occult lesions with Brainstem Auditory Responses. *Proceedings of the Mayo Clinic* 52, 761–769.

Suzuki, T. and Kobayashi, K. (1984). An evaluation of 40–Hz event-related potentials in young children. *Audiology* 23, 599–604.

Teas, D.C., Eldridge, D.H. and Davis, H. (1962). Cochlear responses to acoustic transients: an interpretation of the whole nerve action potentials. *Journal of the Acoustical Society of America* 34, 1438–1459.

Thornton, A.R.D. (1987). Electrophysiological measures of hearing function in hearing disorders. *British Medical Bulletin* 43, 926–939.

Thornton, A.R.D. and Coleman, M.J. (1975). The adaptation of cochlear and brain stem auditory evoked potentials in humans. *Electroencephalography and Clinical Neurophysiology* 39, 399–406.

Thornton, A.R., Hermann, B.S. and Berick, J.M. (1985). *Automated neonatal hearing screening using the auditory brain stem response*. Paper presented at the Ninth Biennial Symposium of the International Electric Response Audiometry Study Group. Erlangen, Germany.

Weber, B.A. and Fletcher, G.L. (1980). A computerised scoring procedure for auditory brainstem responses. *Ear and Hearing* 1, 233–236.

Yamada, O., Ashikawa, H., Kodera K. and Yamane, H. (1983). Frequency-selective auditory brain-stem response in newborns and infants. *Archives of Otolaryngology* 109, 79–82.

Yang, E.Y., Stuart, A., Stenstrom, R. and Hollett, S. (1991). Effect of vibrator to head coupling force on the auditory brain stem response to bone conducted clicks in newborn infants. *Ear and Hearing* 12, 55–60.

Chapter 8
Otoacoustic emissions

YVONNE COPE and MARK E. LUTMAN

Introduction

Low-intensity sound energies generated by the cochlea and measurable within the ear canal are termed otoacoustic emissions (OAEs) and were first demonstrated by Kemp in 1978. Numerous experiments have confirmed Kemp's original findings (for example, Wit and Ritsma, 1979, 1980; Anderson, 1980; Rutten, 1980; Wilson, 1980a; Johnsen and Elberling, 1982 a,b; Grandori, 1985; Probst et al., 1986; Norton and Neely, 1987); Probst, Lonsbury-Martin and Martin (1991) give a comprehensive review of much of the experimental work. The discovery of OAEs has led to significant advances in our understanding of both cochlear mechanisms and mechanics, and over the past 5 years their measurement has developed from being primarily a research tool into a clinical tool being used routinely in many audiology departments.

OAEs may be divided into four distinct but inter-related categories. The first category is *spontaneous*, requiring no external stimulation. The remaining three types all require an external stimulus, their classification depending on the methods used to elicit and measure them. They are termed *delayed, simultaneous* and *distortion product* emissions.

All four types of emission appear to be generated by active processes in the cochlea, more specifically associated with the outer hair cells. Consequently, the cochlea is no longer viewed as functioning solely as a passive organ, receiving acoustic energy, transducing it into electrical signals and transmitting in one direction only. The outer hair cells have been shown to possess a unique electromotility that appears to be responsible for the ability of the cochlea to generate sound. Evidence for this is founded in the existence of spontaneous otoacoustic emissions, and also in the observation that in certain cases stimulated otoacoustic emissions may contain more energy than that of the stimulus (Wilson, 1987). Despite these observations, Allen and Fahey (1992) have proposed a passive model of OAE generation. Arguments against the passive model have been presented by Wit (1992) and Brass and Kemp (1992) – the balance of opinion at present seems to favour an active model.

Of the four types, the delayed OAE has proven to be the most useful clinically, by providing an objective method of assessing the presence of normal or near-normal cochlear function. A number of clinical trials have been undertaken to assess the viability of using delayed OAEs for neonatal screening. Recent experimentation, however, has suggested that the distortion product otoacoustic emission (DPOAE) may also be a practical proposition, particularly as an equivalent test to behavioural pure tone audiometry.

Classification of OAEs

The following classification is widely used.

Spontaneous OAEs

Many individuals spontaneously emit narrow-band acoustic signals from the cochlea without any specific external stimulation. These signals have been termed spontaneous otoacoustic emissions (SOAEs).

Stimulated (or evoked) OAEs

It is possible to evoke otoacoustic emissions by applying an external acoustic stimulus. These are of three types:

- delayed;
- simultaneous; and
- distortion product.

Delayed OAEs

Delayed OAEs arise immediately after a brief stimulus, such as a click or a tone burst. They may last 25 ms or longer.

Simultaneous OAEs

Simultaneous OAEs occur as a synchronous response to a continuous tonal stimulus. They are generally evident as a measurable interaction between the stimulus and the OAE.

Distortion product OAEs

Distortion product OAEs (DPOAEs) arise when two continuous tones closely spaced at frequencies f_1 and f_2 (f_2 greater than f_1) are presented simultaneously to the ear. Emitted distortion products can be measured at intermodulation frequencies such as $f_1 + f_2$ and $2f_1 - f_2$. The largest and most widely measured DPOAE is at the intermodulation frequency $2f_1 - f_2$.

Recording OAEs

The fundamental equipment required to record all types of OAE is an acoustic probe. This is coupled to the external auditory meatus and houses a miniature microphone and, when stimulated OAEs are to be recorded, one or more miniature loudspeakers for delivery of the stimulus. A feature of OAEs is their very low amplitude and because of this a microphone with a low intrinsic noise level and high sensitivity is important to optimally record the OAE signal. Further improvement of signal-to-noise ratio by averaging or frequency-domain filtering is generally required. A method of overload rejection is also desirable to remove interfering signals caused by physiological noise, such as that caused by swallowing or other movement artefacts. A variety of proprietary apparatus is available for recording delayed and DPOAEs, and specialized microphone systems to record SOAEs are also available commercially. Implementation of apparatus required to perform an OAE screening test will be described later.

Characteristics of OAEs

This section presents a brief outline of the features that characterize each type of OAE. Each is described separately, although in a number of instances their characteristics overlap. Table 8.1 summarizes the major properties of spontaneous, delayed and simultaneous evoked OAEs. Readers may wish to refer to this table throughout this section.

Spontaneous otoacoustic emissions

These are narrow-band acoustic signals generated within the cochlea and measurable in the external auditory meatus in the absence of an eliciting stimulus. They are usually evident as a peak in the frequency spectrum of the ear canal microphone signal. A typical recording is illustrated in Figure 8.1. SOAEs have been described by many investigators (e.g. Zurek, 1981; Schloth and Zwicker, 1983; Fritze, 1983; Weir, Norton and Kincaid, 1984; Fritze and Köhler, 1985, 1986; Cianfrone and Mattia, 1986; Wilson, 1986 a,b; Probst et al., 1986, 1987; Bonfils, 1989; Bonfils and Uziel, 1989; Bonfils and Avan, 1990).

Studies of groups of subjects indicate that 30–60% of normal human ears emit at least one SOAE (Table 8.2 summarizes some of the published surveys on the prevalence of SOAEs in people with normal

Table 8.1 Summary of major properties of OAEs (for details see text)

- Spontaneous
    Recordable in a large proportion of normal and a smaller proportion of impaired ears
    Middle and high frequencies most common
    Low SPL (with rare exceptions)
    Can be suppressed by tonal stimuli
    Suppression is sharply 'tuned'
    SOAEs can display frequency locking to tonal stimuli close in frequency
    Frequency can be altered by middle-ear pressure
    Not usually heard by subject under normal circumstances
    Not generally associated with troublesome tinnitus
- Stimulated or evoked
    Recordable in nearly all normal ears
    Abolished by more than mild hearing impairment
    Low SPL
    Can be suppressed by additional sound
    Suppression is sharply 'tuned'
    Little adaptation to rapid stimulation
    Reduced by auditory fatigue
    Frequency shifted by middle-ear mobility changes (or transducer impedance changes)
    Susceptible to cochlear damage (noise, anoxia, drugs)
    Abolished by conductive impairment

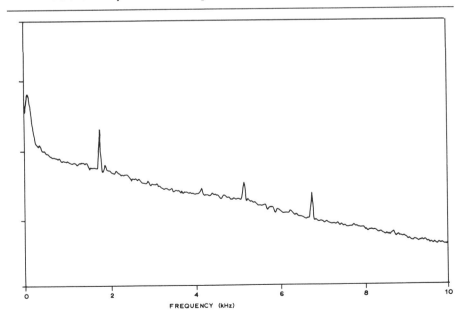

FREQUENCY (kHz)

Figure 8.1 Spectral analysis of SOAEs from an ear with normal hearing. Vertical axis is power spectral density (20 dB/division). The peaks corresponding to SOAEs are at the frequencies 1.775, 5.175 and 6.750 kHz. Their intensities are 13, 1 and −3 dB SPL respectively.

Table 8.2 Incidence of recordable SOAEs in samples of subjects with normal hearing

Study	Number of ears tested	Subject age	Percentage of ears with SOAEs
Zurek (1981)	64	not specified	34
Strickland, Burns and Tubis (1985)	100	mean 9;6 years	31
	38	mean 30 days	26
Probst et al. (1986)	28	Adult	43
Bonfils, Uziel and Narcy (1989)	21	less than 18 months	66
	16	5–10 years	50
Bonfils (1989)	22	less than 18 months	68
	111	10–49 years	35

hearing). There is some variation between studies and age groups, possibly reflecting recording conditions and microphone sensitivity. With the exception of Bonfils (1989) and Bonfils and Uziel (1989), none of the studies shows a particular trend indicating any age-related change in prevalence: these two studies measured SOAEs in subject groups aged from 2 days to over 70 years and found the incidence of SOAEs to decrease with age.

Several studies have demonstrated a relationship between SOAEs and the sex of the subject: it appears that women are about twice as likely to exhibit SOAEs as men (Zurek, 1981; Strickland, Burns and Tubis, 1985; Probst et al., 1986; Burns, Hoberg and Campbell, 1992). This observation is difficult to explain, but may be a consequence of the difference between the average volumes of the external auditory meati of men and women. Women tend to have smaller ears than men, resulting in a possible enhancement of the amplitude of smaller, less easy to detect SOAEs. Contrary to this, Bonfils (1989) found no statistically significant differences between men and women with respect to incidence or spectral content.

Russell and Bilger (1992), in a study of twins with essentially normal hearing, reported SOAEs to be a highly heritable trait. The SOAEs of monozygotic twins were strikingly similar, whereas those of dizygotic twins were not. The genetic determination of SOAE characteristics is underlined by the findings of Whitehead et al. (1993), who demonstrated significant differences between groups of Afro-Caribbean, Caucasian and Asiatic subjects.

SOAEs appear to be fairly stable over time in most subjects. A case investigated by Glanville, Coles and Sullivan (1971) was re-investigated by Wilson and Sutton (1983), who observed that several of the frequency components identified in the original recording were present 13 years later. (At the time of the initial investigation the components were termed 'objective tinnitus'.) Köhler and Fritze (1992) re-examined a sample of 22 ears after a mean lapse of 68 months and reported that the emission spectra were unchanged in 3 ears, no recordable emission was demonstrated in 5 ears and in 14 ears the emission was present but had changed with respect to the number of identifiable components. They presumed this to be a consequence of age-related changes in SOAE generation.

The typical frequency range in which SOAEs are found is 0.5–6 kHz, with the strongest emissions tending to concentrate in the frequency range falling within the octave band 1–2 kHz (Zurek, 1981; Weir, Norton and Kincaid, 1984; Cianfrone and Mattia, 1986). This is likely to be related to the transfer function of the middle ear, which Kemp (1980) calculated to be most efficient in the 1–2 kHz region. Several emissions may be present in one ear, as illustrated in Figure 8.1, in which three narrow spectral peaks corresponding to SOAEs at 1.775 kHz, 5.175 kHz and 6.750 kHz can be seen.

The amplitude of SOAEs generally lies in the range –10 to +20 dB SPL and only very rarely exceeds the upper value. Figure 8.2 illustrates the distribution of intensity levels reported by Zurek (1981) and Weir, Norton and Kincaid (1984). The lower limit may be set by the sensitivity of the instrumentation and recording conditions. A few cases of moderately intense SOAEs have been reported; for example, the case originally investigated by Glanville, Coles and Sullivan (1971) and later

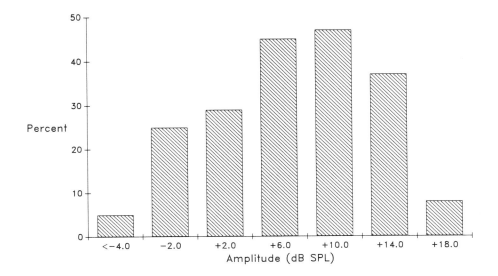

Figure 8.2 Distribution of intensity levels of SOAEs in ears with normal hearing, based on data of Zurek (1981) and Weir, Norton and Kincaid (1984).

by Wilson and Sutton (1983) demonstrated an SOAE with an intensity of approximately 40 dB SPL at a frequency corresponding to a measured hearing threshold level of 60 dB. We have observed a 3-year-old boy who exhibited SOAEs at levels of 44 and 45 dB SPL at 5.168 and 5.591 kHz respectively, associated with hearing threshold levels of 55 dB at 4 and 8 kHz (Figure 8.3).

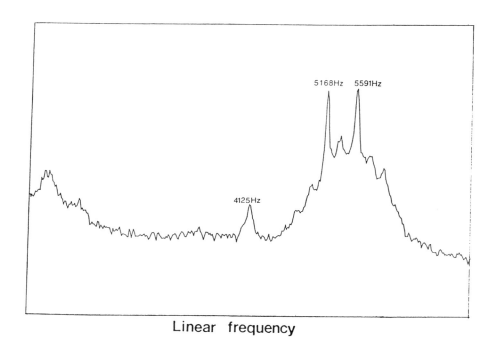

Linear frequency

Figure 8.3 Spectral analysis of intense SOAEs from a 3-year-old boy. The two major peaks at frequencies of 5.168 and 5.591 kHz have intensities of 44 and 45 dB SPL respectively. The smaller peak at 4.125 kHz has an intensity of 12 dB SPL.

Various studies have investigated the influence of a variety of external and physiological factors on the properties of the SOAE: for example, stapedial reflexes and changes in pressure in the external auditory meatus (Wilson and Sutton, 1981; Schloth and Zwicker, 1983; Wilson, 1986a), the effect of suppression and masking by external tones (Zurek, 1981; Wilson and Sutton, 1981; Schloth and Zwicker, 1983; Clark et al., 1984), temporal effects during the menstrual cycle (Wilson, 1986b; Bell, 1992) and shifts in SOAE frequency towards an external tone at an adjacent frequency known as 'frequency locking' (Wilson and Sutton, 1981; Zwicker and Schloth, 1984). Table 8.1 lists several of these properties.

SOAEs are not heard by most subjects: even if a recording of the signal recorded in the external auditory meatus is replayed to them, they usually do not recognize it. This feature is useful in distinguishing SOAEs from other sounds caused by mechanical or hydromechanical events in the middle ear or surrounding tissues, muscles and blood supply: the latter may have narrow-band frequency spectra but are heard by the subject as if presented externally. Thus SOAEs, as defined here, tend to be distinct from the usual form of tinnitus that is heard by the subject but does not have an acoustic representation recordable in the external auditory meatus. This general finding is substantiated by the observations of Zurek (1981), who could find no relationship between SOAEs and tinnitus. Similarly, Tyler and Conrad-Armes (1982) found 3% of their subject population to have sensorineural hearing loss, tinnitus and SOAEs, but found no correlation between the SOAE frequency and the pitch match frequency of the tinnitus. Our own data show no greater prevalence of SOAEs in subjects with tinnitus than those without tinnitus after accounting for hearing threshold level effect, and Penner and Burns (1987) and Bonfils (1989) could not demonstrate any general association between SOAEs and tinnitus. More recently, however, particular cases have been reported in which SOAEs have been demonstrated to be the source of tinnitus. Penner (1988) reported one individual with bilateral tinnitus and bilateral SOAEs in whom suppression of the SOAEs rendered the tinnitus inaudible. The SOAEs were observed to vary in frequency, as did the subject's description of the tinnitus. A tinnitus pitch match to the lowest frequency in the tinnitus corresponded to the lowest frequency in the SOAE. Penner and Coles (1992) reported another case in which tinnitus was thought to arise from an SOAE; the tinnitus disappeared when the SOAE was suppressed by aspirin. A review by Penner (1992) estimated that approximately 4% (confidence interval 1–9 %) of troublesome tinnitus is caused at least in part by SOAEs.

Delayed OAEs

The delayed OAE occurs in response to a brief acoustic stimulus, either a click or a tone burst. Kemp (1978) was the first to demonstrate this type of OAE experimentally, using clicks ranging in intensity from just below the mean normal threshold of audibility to 60 dB above. With the aid of a sensitive miniature microphone sealed into the external auditory meatus and signal averaging techniques, Kemp recorded a brief low-level acoustic response 5–60 ms after the stimulus. The frequency spectrum of delayed OAEs is generally dependent on both the frequency content of the stimulus and the properties of the individual ear. The response in the normal ear corresponds to the intrinsic response of the particular ear convolved with the frequency content of the stimulus (Elberling et al., 1985; Grandori and Ravazzani, 1990). For a click, which has a broad-band spectrum, the response indicates only the intrinsic responses of the individual ear.

It is possible to record delayed OAEs in almost all subjects with normal hearing (Tables 8.3 and 8.4), but Kemp (1978) was unable to record emissions from subjects with immobile middle ears. Two studies have demonstrated an effect of subject age on the incidence of delayed OAEs (Bonfils, Bertrand and Uziel, 1988; Collet et al., 1990), investigating subjects considered to have normal hearing for their age. It was observed that the incidence of OAEs in subjects aged 60 years and over was lower than in younger subjects. However, both studies reported a higher subjective threshold for the stimulus in the subject group aged 60 years and over. Presumably, therefore, the lower incidence is at least partially a consequence of a change in the hearing sensitivity and not a function of age alone.

The occasional failure to record OAEs in younger individuals with normal hearing may be due to poor recording technique or conditions. A consistently absent OAE in the presence of normal hearing sensitivity may be a consequence of the anatomical properties of the individual's middle ear and/or external auditory meatus. However, Martin et al.

Table 8.3 Incidence of delayed stimulated OAEs recordable in samples of subjects with normal hearing (neonates excluded)

Study	Number of ears tested	Percentage of ears with OAEs
Kemp (1978)	35	100
Rutten (1980)	13	92
Probst et al. (1986)	28	96
Stevens and Ip (1988)	36	97
Bonfils and Uziel (1989)	52	100
Dolhen et al. (1991)	71	97
Avan et al. (1991)	44	100

Table 8.4 Incidence of delayed stimulated OAEs recordable in samples of neonates not admitted to a neonatal intensive care unit

Study	Number of ears tested	Percentage of ears with OAEs
Johnsen, Bagi and Elberling (1983)	20	100
Elberling et al. (1985)	199	100
Stevens et al. (1987)	60	96
Dolhen et al. (1991)	39	95
Uziel and Piron (1991)	110	97

(1992) have demonstrated dips in DPOAE audiograms without any corresponding dips in hearing sensitivity, which indicates that parts of the cochlea presumed to be normal may generate abnormally low levels of OAE, or perhaps none at all.

The characteristics of the delayed OAE have been extensively investigated and documented by a number of authors; for example, Kemp (1978), Wit and Ritsma (1979), Wilson (1980a), Rutten (1980), Johnsen and Elberling (1982a,b), Grandori (1985), Probst et al. (1986, 1987), Bray and Kemp (1987), Norton and Neely (1987), Harris and Probst (1991), Hauser, Probst and Löhle (1991), Spektor et al. (1991) and Smurzynski and Kim (1992). The features are summarized below.

Click evoked otoacoustic emissions (CEOAEs)

A typical recording of the averaged sound pressure waveform following click stimulation is shown in Figure 8.4. The response waveform is divisible into two sections:

- the initial component, 0–5 ms after the stimulus onset, is attributable mainly to the impulse response of the transducers but also to that of the outer ear, middle ear and the passive response of the cochlea. This component increases in amplitude linearly with increasing stimulus amplitude;
- the second part of the response waveform is generally smaller in amplitude and is discernible only after the linear impulse response has decayed, usually 3 ms or more after the stimulus depending on the impulse response of the probe. This component is considered

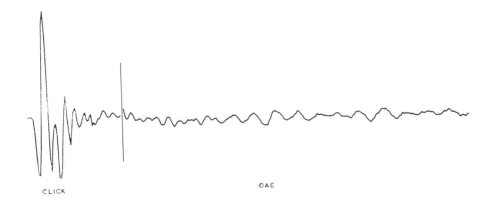

CLICK   OAE

Figure 8.4 Recording of a typical CEOAE. The early part of the trace is the acoustical response of the ear and measurement system to the click stimulus and is mainly due to the ringing of the transducers. The remainder of the trace (amplified by a factor of 32 relative to the earlier part) is the CEOAE.

to be the CEOAE, or 'Kemp Echo'. The duration of CEOAEs can range from a few milliseconds up to several hundred milliseconds (Wit and Ritsma, 1980).

The CEOAE waveform often has the general appearance of bursts of oscillation, each dominated by one frequency (as illustrated in Figure 8.5) but other less periodic waveforms often occur. Each ear has a characteristic pattern of response that is stable over a period of years if no change occurs in the middle ear and/or cochlea. The typical frequency spectrum of the response is 0.5–4 kHz, most emission energy (in adults) falling in the octave band 1–2 kHz, as exemplified in Figure 8.6. The frequency band of the most prominent emissions is thought to correspond to the frequency range of most efficient transmission through the middle ear (in both directions). The CEOAE waveform tends to exhibit frequency dispersion such that the higher frequency components usually occur at the beginning of the waveform and as the latency increases the frequency of the components decreases as a consequence of the tonotopic organization of the cochlea. This effect has been observed by several investigators (Kemp, 1978; Wilson, 1980a; Johnsen and Elberling, 1982b; Grandori, 1985). This frequency dispersion has been assumed to reflect the time taken by the forward travelling wave of the stimulus along the basilar membrane to the site of generation of the OAE, plus the travel time of the reverse travelling wave to the oval window.

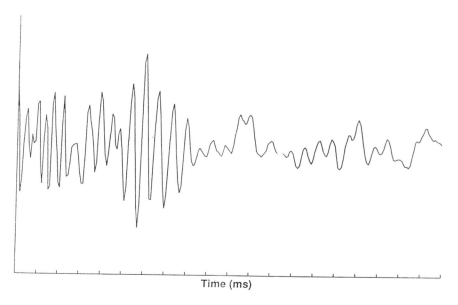

Time (ms)

Figure 8.5 CEOAE recorded in a neonate, showing a burst of oscillation at about 1.5 kHz. The time axis extends from 3 to 23 ms after the onset of the click.

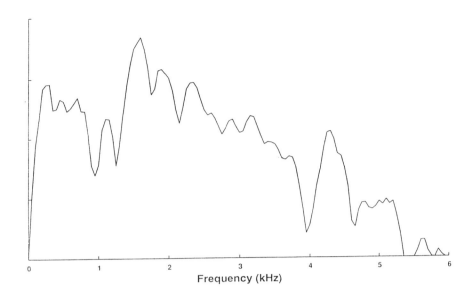

Frequency (kHz)

Figure 8.6 Frequency spectrum of the CEOAE shown in Figure 8.5. Vertical axis is power spectral density (10 dB/division). The main part of the signal energy is in the octave band 1–2 kHz. The energy at frequencies below 1 kHz is mainly due to ambient and physiological noise (movement, breathing etc.).

The sound pressure level of CEOAEs rarely exceeds 20 dB SPL even for high stimulus levels. It is possible to identify a response when using stimuli down to levels slightly below the psychoacoustic threshold. Kemp (1978) reported significant changes in the emission waveform with changing stimulus levels, but at latencies of 5–15 ms prominent features were distinguishable irrespective of the stimulus level used. Kemp observed that the amplitude of the response increased with increasing level of stimulation: at low stimulus levels the increase was linear (1 dB increase in response for each 1 dB increase in stimulus), but the response saturated at more intense stimuli. This compressive non-linearity distinguishes the CEOAE from the passive linear response. Figure 8.7 illustrates responses for stimuli at five different levels in steps of 10 dB.

Grandori (1985) detailed a more complex relationship between the stimulus intensity and latency; he observed non-linearity to be greatest at moderate to high intensities and for the latter part of the response. Deviations from linearity were minimal at the lower levels of excitation and independent of the time after stimulation.

The consistency of CEOAE response waveforms has been demonstrated by Johnsen and Elberling (1982b), who performed retest mea-

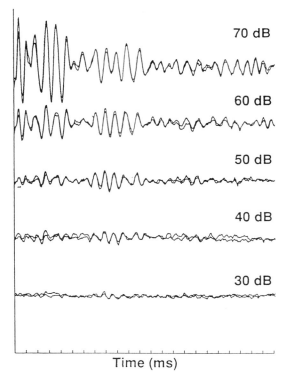

Figure 8.7 Comparison of amplitudes of CEOAEs recorded in an adult ear at stimulus levels of 30, 40, 50, 60 and 70 db peak equivalent SPL (approximately 5, 15, 25, 35 and 45 dB nHL). The vertical scaling is identical for all traces. At each stimulus level two replicate recordings are superimposed, demonstrating the repeatability of the response. The time axis extends from 3 to 26 ms after click onset. Note that the increase in response amplitude is less than 10 dB (x 3.162) for each 10 dB increase in stimulus level, indicating a compressive non-linearity. These waveforms were recorded using the maximum length sequence method (see text) with an inter-click interval of 0.5 ms, allowing 2000 responses to be averaged in 2 s per replication.

surements in the same ear at 4–5-week intervals and found the response pattern to be almost unchanged. Antonelli and Grandori (1986) investigated this property more extensively and demonstrated the temporal stability over almost 4 years. Figure 8.8 shows emissions recorded at intervals in the same individual over a period of 9 years and illustrates the high degree of repeatability. However, the CEOAEs of neonates appear to change with increasing age. The specific details of these changes and differences that have been observed between CEOAEs recorded from adult and infant ears will be discussed later in this chapter.

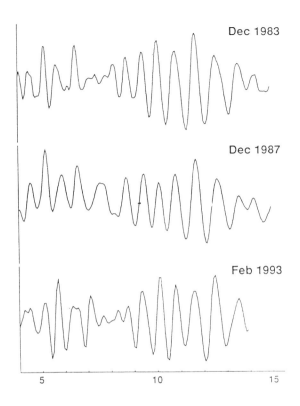

Figure 8.8 Replicate measures of a CEOAE over a period of 9 years. The time scale is from 5 to 15 ms after click onset. Note the high degree of repeatability of waveforms over time. The two earlier waveforms were recorded with the same apparatus. The last recording was made with different apparatus designed along the same principles but with a different probe design and different implementation of other aspects of the recording apparatus.

Differences between individual CEOAE responses occur with regard to the response latency, peak-to-peak amplitude and number of emission bursts but primarily with respect to the waveform morphology and spectral content, as exemplified in Figure 8.9. The incidence of CEOAEs is not dependent on the sex of the subject (Collet et al., 1989).

Tone-burst evoked otoacoustic emissions (TBEOAE)

Several of the features of the CEOAE are also observed when using tone-burst stimuli. Table 8.1 summarizes the common characteristics and Figure 8.10 illustrates a typical response.

The magnitude and the spectral characteristics of the TBEOAE appear primarily to be dependent on the frequency of the evoking

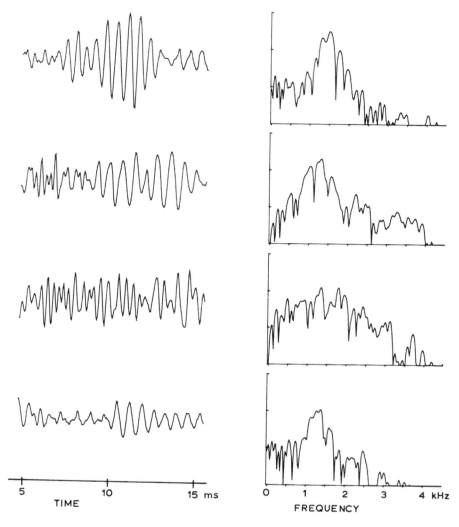

Figure 8.9 CEOAEs and their frequency spectra recorded from adults with normal hearing. Note the inter-subject variation in waveform morphology and frequency content.

stimulus. Wit and Ritsma (1979) documented that the higher the frequency of the stimulus the smaller the response, even when stimuli of different frequency are presented at the same sensation level. Elberling et al. (1985) observed that the energy of the resultant OAE tends to collect about a restricted frequency band, forming specific peaks. They reported that in general the most prominent of these spectral peaks is dependent on the stimulus frequency, such that the largest peaks in the stimulus and the response fall in the same frequency region. Norton and Neely (1987) have reported comparable findings. Elberling et al.

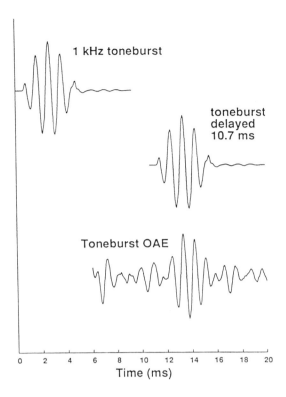

1 kHz toneburst

toneburst
delayed
10.7 ms

Toneburst OAE

0   2   4   6   8   10   12   14   16   18   20
Time (ms)

Figure 8.10 Tone-burst evoked OAE (TBEOAE) recorded in an adult with normal hearing. The upper trace is the 1 kHz tone-burst stimulus as recorded in the ear canal of the subject. The lower trace is the recorded OAE. The middle trace is a copy of the stimulus waveform delayed to match the OAE. Note the similarity of the OAE waveform and the delayed copy of the stimulus waveform. The OAE latency in this subject was 10.7 ms at 1 kHz.

(1985) have indicated that the TBEOAE could be predicted accurately by convolving the CEOAE (impulse response) with the waveform of the stimulus.

The incidence of TBEOAEs appears to be strongly dependent on the frequency of the stimulus. Probst et al. (1986), in their study of individuals with normal hearing, reported a greater percentage of subjects demonstrating emissions in response to 1.5 kHz than to 0.5 kHz tonebursts. Hauser, Probst and Löhle (1991) reported similar observations.

Simultaneous or stimulus frequency evoked OAEs (SFEOAEs)

Less has been published on this mode of generation of OAEs than on delayed OAEs. The SFEOAE is generated during continuous stimulation using a single low-level tone and demonstrates a steady-state response at the same frequency as the stimulus. Kemp and Chum (1980) were the first to demonstrate this technique but it has also been described by Wilson (1980a) and Zwicker and Schloth (1984).

Many of the characteristics of the SFEOAE are similar to those of the delayed OAE. The response adds vectorially to the stimulus in the external auditory meatus and behaves non-linearly with increasing stimulus level (Zwicker and Schloth, 1984). The amplitude tends to be slightly lower than that of the delayed OAE, ranging from −20 to +10 dB SPL (Kemp and Chum, 1980). Prevalence also appears to be slightly lower than for delayed OAEs: 93–94 % according to Probst, Lonsbury-Martin and Martin (1991). This may be, however, a consequence of the greater difficulty in recording this type of OAE.

SFEOAEs are most easily demonstrated by presenting to the ear a tone that is slowly swept across a frequency range. For high stimulus intensities the sound pressure level measured in the auditory meatus is described by a smooth curve representing the overall frequency response of the system. For low stimulus intensities, for example 10 dB SPL, SFEOAEs appear as a series of peaks and valleys as they move in and out of phase with the stimulus. Zwicker and Schloth (1984) observed a trend for the frequency spacing between neighbouring maxima at low frequencies (near 0.5 kHz) to be smaller than at high frequencies (above 2.5 kHz). At present SFEOAEs do not appear to have any practical utility and are generally more difficult to record than the other types

Distortion product OAEs (DPOAEs)

When the ear is stimulated with two tones of closely spaced frequencies (f_1 and f_2 with f_2 greater than f_1) the subject may hear intermodulation distortion products at one or more frequencies such as $f_2 + f_1$ or $2f_1 - f_2$. The presence of distortion in the human auditory system has been demonstrated using several techniques.

- They are recordable electrophysiologically in the cochlear microphonic and subsequent nerve fibre discharge patterns in the auditory pathway.
- They may be detected psychoacoustically.
- It is possible to detect these intermodulation components acoustically within the external auditory meatus. Two-tone stimulation leads to interactions between the two travelling waves, resulting in several distortion products. These can be demonstrated by measuring the frequency spectrum of the sound pressure in the ear canal during stimulation with two tones.

The DPOAE has been the subject of many investigations, for example, Kemp (1979), Kim (1980), Wilson (1980c), Wit, Langevoort and

Ritsma (1981), Kemp et al. (1986), Ohlms, Lonsbury-Martin and Martin (1990), Lonsbury-Martin and Martin (1990), Harris and Probst (1991), Spektor et al. (1991), Smurzynski and Kim (1992), Whitehead, Lonsbury-Martin and Martin (1992). The DPOAE is generally of smaller amplitude than the other types of stimulated OAE, which poses some difficulties as far as measurement is concerned. These may be overcome by using a narrow-band filter tuned to the distortion product frequency or a lock-in amplifier to enhance the signal-to-noise ratio of the measurement system.

The amplitude of the DPOAE is dependent on a number of factors: the levels and frequencies of the primary stimuli, their ratio and the frequency response of the individual ear. A typical DPOAE spectrum is illustrated in Figure 8.11. The $2f_1 - f_2$ distortion product is the most prominent in the human ear. The DPOAE appears to be strongest when it coincides with an SOAE or when it occurs in a frequency region of good TBEOAEs. The presence of a trough in the 2–4 kHz region, which appears to be unrelated to any hearing impairment in this region, has been noted by several authors (Lonsbury-Martin et al., 1990; Spektor

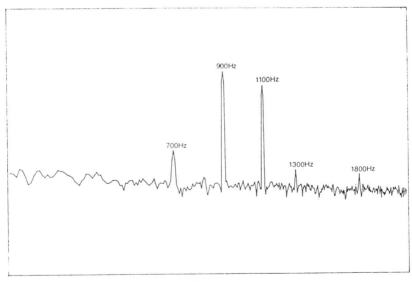

Log frequency

Figure 8.11 Distortion product OAE (DPOAE) recorded in an adult with normal hearing. The logarithmic frequency scale extends from 300 to 2300 Hz. The stimulus primaries at f_1 (900 Hz) and f_2 (1100 Hz) are at intensities of 60 and 50 dB SPL respectively. The most prominent DPOAE is at $2f_1-f_2$ (700 Hz) and at an intensity of 13 dB SPL. There is also a small DPOAE at $2f_2-f_1$ (1300 Hz) with an intensity of 5 dB SPL. The small peak at $2f_1$ (1800 Hz) is harmonic distortion generated in the stimulus delivery system, and is not a DPOAE.

et al., 1991; Smurzynski and Kim, 1992). The cause of this is unclear. Lonsbury-Martin et al. (1990) suggested its presence to be an interaction of the resonances common to a particular individual's ear and cochlea. DPOAEs have a slightly delayed onset, similar to that of the delayed OAE.

DPOAEs share a number of features with the other stimulated OAEs. They are a feature of normal peripheral auditory function. Their frequency response mirrors the subjective pure tone audiogram (Gaskill and Brown, 1990; Lonsbury-Martin et al., 1990; Spektor et al., 1991). They can be detected within the same frequency range as other OAEs and up to higher frequencies, typically over the range 0.5–8 kHz (Smurzynski and Kim, 1992). They demonstrate a high test/retest reliability (Lonsbury-Martin and Martin, 1990). There is a certain degree of variability between subjects but the general pattern of the curve is very consistent (Spektor et al., 1991).

In a study of the physiological vulnerability of DPOAEs in small laboratory mammals, Whitehead, Lonsbury-Martin and Martin (1992) distinguished between the properties of low- and high-level DPOAEs and suggested that two discrete generator mechanisms might be responsible. The two types of DPOAE have been shown to exhibit different physiological vulnerability. Low-level components (those elicited by stimulus levels less than 60–70 dB SPL) appear to be more vulnerable to agents known to cause cochlear insult than the higher level components (those elicited by stimulus levels greater than 60–70 dB SPL). Data from human subjects with sensorineural hearing loss (Lonsbury-Martin and Martin, 1990) have shown that the $2f_1 - f_2$ DPOAE, when elicited by lower-level stimulation, is reduced more by trauma than those elicited by high-level stimulation. However, the properties of OAEs in humans differ from those in laboratory animals and it is difficult to make direct inferences for humans. If DPOAEs are to be used to assess cochlear status, it is important to use stimuli that elicit only the physiologically vulnerable component. Data from humans suggest that stimuli may need to be as low as 50 dB SPL to avoid eliciting the higher level component (Bonfils and Avan, 1992).

Origin and mechanism of production of OAEs

Many properties are common to all types of OAE. It is now generally agreed that OAEs originate from the cochlea and are consistent with the normal, mechanically active, functioning of the outer hair cells. However, conflicting and contrasting opinions exist as to the conditions required within the cochlea for a particular OAE to become manifest and the basic mechanisms for their generation are still not completely known.

At the time of the discovery of OAEs doubts were raised about their physiological origin. They were suspected to be artefactual, resulting from the recording method or some outer or middle ear activity; a neural origin was also proposed. These suggestions were later discounted.

The OAE behaves very differently from a physical artefact: for example, prolonged ringing of the stimulus in CEOAE measurements would demonstrate a linear growth with increasing stimulus amplitude but the OAE displays a clear saturating non-linearity with increasing stimulus amplitude, as described above.

A middle-ear muscle origin may also be ruled out: first, OAEs occur at stimulus levels too low to activate middle ear muscles and, secondly, Evans, Wilson and Borerwe (1981) demonstrated the presence of OAEs after administering a paralysing drug to a laboratory animal, which would inhibit middle ear muscle activity.

Neural origin may also be discounted: OAEs are almost immune to adaptation when using increased rates of stimulation (Kemp, 1978; Grandori, 1985) and secondly, the psychoacoustical detection threshold has commonly been observed to be higher than the CEOAE detection threshold. If the stimulus is not transduced effectively by the cochlea, a neural mechanism cannot operate.

Many of the early investigations supporting a cochlear origin were concerned with demonstrating that the mechanism(s) responsible for OAE generation are susceptible to the same factors that affect the normal functioning of the cochlea. Anoxia, noise exposure and drugs known to be ototoxic all abolish or reduce delayed OAEs and DPOAEs (Anderson and Kemp, 1979; Kim, 1980). Johnsen and Elberling (1982a) demonstrated the temporary reduction of a CEOAE following ingestion of salicylate, which induced a reversible sensorineural hearing loss. McFadden and Plattsmier (1984), Long and Tubis (1988) and Penner and Coles (1992) have shown similar results with SOAEs. Psychoacoustical phenomena, such as the fine structure on a slowly swept Békésy audiogram dependent on a healthy cochlea, and the OAE appear to be interrelated. Wilson (1980a), Horst, Wit and Ritsma (1983), Schloth (1983) and Zwicker and Schloth (1984) demonstrated that subjects with CEOAEs exhibited fine structure in their audiograms, whereas subjects with weak CEOAEs, or no measurable CEOAEs, exhibited audiograms without fine structure. In general agreement with this, Schloth (1983) and Zwicker and Schloth (1984) observed a strong correlation between the frequency of both SOAEs and delayed OAEs and the minima of the fine-structure of the audiogram (i.e. reversals corresponding to acute thresholds). However, it is not clear whether the relationship between fine structure and CEOAE spectrum occurs in subjects without SOAEs, and this property may be a feature particular to SOAEs.

Several researchers, including Kemp (1979), Wit and Ritsma (1979), Wilson and Sutton (1981), Ruggero, Rich and Freyman (1983), Schloth and Zwicker (1983) and Clark et al. (1984) have reported that a suppressor tone reduces the level of the OAE. The frequency specificity of this effect is sharply tuned and is quantitatively and qualitatively very similar to the frequency selectivity of the cochlea measured by psychoacoustical or physiological tuning curves (Kemp, 1979; Zurek, 1981).

Further evidence for a cochlear origin is founded in the numerous investigations involving subjects with known and varying degrees of hearing impairment; this will be discussed in greater detail below. As a general rule, in most cases SOAEs and stimulated OAEs are absent when the hearing loss is in excess of 25–35 dB HL. However, this effect is frequency dependent and, if some frequency regions of normal hearing sensitivity remain, OAEs may be recordable but manifest only at the frequency of normal hearing. An exception to this rule seems to be SOAEs, as discussed above.

Various reasons have been put forward to explain why OAEs are present in certain individuals and absent in others with apparently very similar audiological status. Suggestions that both evoked OAEs and SOAEs are a reflection of a subclinical biomechanical/neuromechanical abnormality or are a product of some pathological phenomenon can probably be discounted for most cases. This is supported by the presence of delayed OAEs in almost all neonates, who are presumed to have normal hearing; also, the proportion of SOAEs in infants is the same as, if not higher than, that in older groups (Strickland, Burns and Tubis, 1985; Bonfils, 1989; Bonfils, Uziel and Narcy, 1989; Burns, Hoberg and Campbell, 1992). Evidence presented by Russell and Bilger (1992) indicated SOAEs to be a highly heritable trait, also suggesting that they are a normal physiological property. It appears, therefore, that the presence of evoked OAEs (and in most cases SOAEs) is a by-product of normal cochlear function.

It is beyond the scope of this chapter to discuss the suggested mechanisms for generation of OAEs in detail. Several models have been proposed: for example Kemp (1980), Wilson (1980b), Guelke and Bunn (1985), Antonelli and Grandori (1986), Zwicker (1986), Furst and Lapid (1988), Allen and Neely (1992), Avan et al. (1991), Whitehead, Lonsbury-Martin and Martin (1992).

Comparison of OAEs in adults, infants and neonates

Several groups have developed recording equipment and have successfully measured delayed OAEs in neonates and infants, mainly using transient stimuli. The incidence of OAEs in neonates and infants is of the same order as adults (Tables 8.3 and 8.4), with the exception of those neonates who have required intensive care during the neonatal period (Table 8.5). A possible explanation for this lower incidence has

Table 8.5 Incidence of delayed stimulated OAEs recordable in samples of neonates and babies admitted to a neonatal intensive care unit

Study	Number of ears tested	Percentage of ears with OAEs
Stevens et al. (1987)	215	81
Stevens et al. (1989)	692	79
Stevens et al. (1990)	74	82
Plinkert et al. (1990)*	95	90
Uziel and Piron (1991)	80	79

*All the babies were neonates except in the study by Plinkert, which included babies up to the age of 7 months.

been given by Stevens et al. (1990), who report that although the absence of OAEs was not related to the age (since birth) when tested, many of the neonates who exhibited negative OAE results were of low gestational age (less than 33 weeks). Such babies tend to have smaller and more flattened heads with distorted external meati, rendering accurate insertion of the probe difficult. Stevens et al. also suggested that this lower incidence is a consequence of middle ear disorder and a relatively high incidence of sensorineural hearing impairment in this particular group of neonates (Galambos, Hicks and Wilson, 1982; Davis and Wood, 1992). Uziel and Piron (1991) report similar observations: they rarely recorded OAEs from neonates with gestational age of less than 35 weeks, although our own experience suggests that CEOAEs may be recorded readily in neonates at much lower gestational ages.

In general, the features of delayed OAEs in adults are also observed in neonates and infants (wide intra-subject variability, saturating non-linearity with increasing stimulus amplitude and comparable latency) (Johnsen, Parbo and Elberling, 1989; Kemp, Ryan and Bray, 1990). Bonfils, Uziel and Narcy (1989) reported a tendency for the incidence of long duration OAEs to decrease with age. The detection threshold has been reported to be comparable to that of adults (Uziel and Piron, 1991). However, neonates and adults do exhibit a few specific differences, particularly with respect to frequency spectrum and amplitude.

Frequency spectra of OAEs in neonates and infants tend to span a wider range of frequencies than in older children or adults, with more power at the high frequencies. Kemp, Ryan and Bray (1990) and Uziel and Piron (1991), in studies on neonates, reported a frequency range of 0.7–5 kHz. Johnsen, Parbo and Elberling (1989), in a study of a group of children examined at birth and again at age 4 years, observed the dominant component of the emission to have shifted to a lower frequency region. Collet et al. (1990) documented a similar lowering of the dominant frequency in the emission spectrum as a function of age in a subject group with ages ranging from 6 weeks to 83 years. Spektor et al. (1991) compared the spectral components of OAEs evoked from adults, children aged 4–10 years and new-borns. A larger number of spectral components in the 4–6 kHz region was reported in the new-born group than the other two groups.

The amplitude of OAEs recorded from neonates is up to 10 dB stronger than those in the adult (Kemp, Ryan and Bray, 1990; Norton and Widen, 1990). Spektor et al. (1991) reported a comparable trend but with a lower magnitude of difference. Contrary to these observations, Johnsen, Bagi and Elberling (1983), Elberling et al. (1985) and Johnsen, Parbo and Elberling (1989) found no such differences; they reported similar orders of magnitude in both adults and neonates.

Studies documenting differences between neonates and adults offer a variety of reasons:

- developmental changes in the cochlea;
- age-associated cochlear changes due to normal wear and tear;
- a consequence of everyday exposure to noise and toxins.

These changes were suggested by Norton and Widen (1990) to cause a decrease in the output of the physiologically vulnerable mechanisms responsible for the production of OAEs.

- Kemp, Ryan and Bray (1990) suggested that OAE activity is intrinsically increased in neonates.
- Another possible explanation is founded in structural differences between the outer and middle ears of neonates and older subjects. The overall shape, size and texture of the neonatal ear tends to result in a much smaller enclosed volume. It is therefore possible that the closer coupling of the transducers of the probe to the cochlea in neonates may influence the OAE generation mechanism itself. Thus, probe characteristics can be a major factor in determining the characteristics of OAEs (Zwicker, 1990).

OAEs and hearing loss

The bulk of work on OAEs and hearing loss has concerned delayed OAEs: therefore this section presents a review mainly of those data. The delayed OAE cannot be used to predict hearing loss directly in terms of a psychoacoustic threshold at each frequency. In subjects with normal hearing the variation of spectrum, amplitude and detection threshold is high for both transient and tone-burst evoked OAEs and it is therefore not possible to identify a reliable predictive formula relating such parameters to the degree of hearing impairment at each frequency. A few authors, however, have attempted to identify certain properties of OAEs that distinguish normal and impaired hearing. The characteristic that has been most widely studied is the degree of hearing threshold elevation above which OAEs are usually absent.

Conductive hearing loss

Several authors have reported the effect of changes in external or middle ear pressure on the OAE (for example, Anderson, Bridgens and Halford, 1989; Kemp, Ryan and Bray, 1990; Robinson and Haughton, 1991). An overall reduction in the amplitude of the emission and a reduction in energy below about 2 kHz generally occurs after a change in pressure from atmospheric. Kemp (1978) and Decreton, Hanssens and Sloovere (1991) were unable to detect OAEs in subjects with immobile middle ears, the emission being obscured by the conductive component causing a heavy loading of the ossicles and tympanic membrane. Hence, screening for middle ear disorder by means of tympanometry is wise before undertaking OAE measurement, as middle ear disease may significantly affect the emission.

Sensorineural hearing loss

Emissions recorded from the ears of subjects with partial cochlear impairment are different from those recorded from ears that are audiometrically normal. Furthermore, a cut-off level, expressed in terms of either the pure tone hearing threshold level or the threshold for the stimulus, is present, above which OAEs are no longer recordable. Kemp (1978) suggested a cut-off level of 30 dB HL, above which OAEs are usually not observed. Rutten (1980) and Kemp et al. (1986) reported that if the hearing loss exceeds 15 dB HL OAEs are usually absent. More specifically, Kemp, Ryan and Bray (1990) reported that OAEs tend not to be recordable in any octave band where the best hearing threshold level is over 15–20 dB. If a pure tone audiogram shows areas of normal hearing, emissions are often, but not always, evoked at these frequencies and are absent at frequencies at which the hearing is abnormal. Slight variations on these cut-off levels have been reported by other researchers: Bonfils et al. (1988) suggested a pure tone hearing threshold level of 35 dB, Stevens and Ip (1988) a mean hearing threshold level of 20 dB and Avan et al. (1991) demonstrated absence of OAEs when the mean hearing threshold level for cochlear impairments was in excess of 20–30 dB HL. Data reported by Lutman (1989) illustrate these general findings, as shown in Table 8.6. In his sample of 514 ears, 81 had hearing threshold levels above 25 dB at the average of the best two hearing frequencies. CEOAEs were only produced in one of those, a marginal case with the best two average equal to 33 dB.

The threshold for the stimulus, rather than for pure tones, has also been used as a criterion to determine the likelihood of recordable

Table 8.6 Cross-tabulation of presence of CEOAE against hearing status. Hearing status was classified according to the average of the best two hearing threshold levels measured among the frequencies 0.25, 0.5, 1, 2, 3, 4, 6, 8 kHz

CEOAE	Best-two average 0.25 Hz–8 kHz	
	<25 dB	>25 dB
Present	318	1
Absent	115	80

OAEs. Stevens and Ip (1988) found that the subjective threshold for a click stimulus must be less than 18 dB nHL for an OAE to be recordable. Probst et al. (1987) were unable to record OAEs when the threshold for the stimulus was in excess of 25 dB nHL: Bonfils et al. (1988) and Bonfils and Uziel (1989) stated a slightly higher cut-off of 35 dB nHL.

Collet et al. (1989) correlated CEOAE threshold with the hearing threshold at 1 kHz and deduced that CEOAEs never occurred when the hearing threshold level at this frequency was above 40 dB or when the mean threshold from the audiogram was over 45 dB. Harris, Probst and Löhle (1991) reported that when CEOAEs are present there is a high probability that the hearing threshold level at one frequency at least is less than 30 dB HL.

It has been stated by many investigators that the occurrence of OAEs tends to decrease progressively with increasing cochlear hearing loss or increasing threshold for the stimulus used. The variation between the values selected as cut-off levels may reflect different recording techniques and identification methods. In general, it can be concluded that the detection of a CEOAE indicates normal or near normal peripheral auditory function at least at one frequency. The absence of an OAE could mean the presence of a conductive element or a cochlear hearing loss, the degree of which can range from mild to profound. However, the consistent failure to record an OAE may not necessarily be associated with the presence of hearing loss. As indicated in Table 8.6, a number of subjects with no recordable CEOAE have hearing threshold levels within normal limits at some frequencies; some of them at all frequencies.

There are, however, some important exceptions to these general findings, although rare. For example:

- Lutman et al. (1989) reported CEOAEs in a case of profound sensorineural hearing impairment. Further diagnostic testing using electrophysiological techniques revealed a predominantly retrocochlear lesion with good cochlear function, although radiological investigation ruled out a space-occupying lesion.

- In all the cases of central deafness studied by Bonfils, Uziel and Pujol (1988), OAE spectra similar to those observed in normally hearing subjects were recorded but only half their group with acoustic neuromas exhibited OAEs; presumably the subjects with no OAE had sustained collateral damage to the cochlea.
- Cane, Lutman and O'Donoghue (1994) recorded OAEs in 47% of ears with confirmed cerebello-pontine angle tumours, the absence of OAEs in the remaining tumour ears being indicative of a cochlear component to the hearing loss.

Correlations between the power spectra of the delayed OAE and audiometric thresholds are difficult to demonstrate due to the wide variation in OAE characteristics in both hearing impaired and normally hearing subjects (Probst et al., 1986, 1987). Collet et al. (1991) showed that the greater the number of spectral components at higher frequencies the better the hearing of the subject at higher frequencies of the audiogram. However, it is not possible to draw any conclusions about the pattern of hearing loss from the spectral content of delayed OAEs. Bonfils and Uziel (1989) demonstrated fewer narrow-band peaks in the spectrum of the OAE recorded from ears with hearing impairment than from unimpaired ears.

The above relationships relate primarily to CEOAEs, although similarities can be expected for DPOAEs. However, because a non-physiologically vulnerable component of DPOAEs is present when higher stimulus levels are used, the exact relationship between DPOAE level and hearing threshold level has yet to be determined. In a recent study Bonfils and Avan (1992) sought to establish the highest stimulus level that would preclude the recording of $2f_1-f_2$ DPOAEs in adult ears with material cochlear impairment (more than 25 dB at the stimulus frequency). This condition was met when the stimuli were at 52 dB SPL, but not at 62 or 72 dB SPL. Hence, studies that report $2f_1-f_2$ DPOAEs for stimuli of 60 dB or greater may be contaminated by the higher level DPOAE component that is not physiologically vulnerable.

More research is required to establish the relationship between DPOAE and hearing threshold level in large groups of subjects with known degrees of cochlear hearing impairment. Current indications suggest that the threshold of the $2f_1-f_2$ DPOAE (i.e. the lowest recordable level of the distortion product), when plotted as a function of the frequency f_2, forms an 'audiogram' that can be compared with the conventional pure tone audiogram. In small groups of subjects the peaks and troughs of the DP 'audiogram' have been shown to mirror the peaks and troughs of the pure tone audiogram, although when the pure tone hearing threshold level exceeds 20–25 dB no DPOAE can be recorded and therefore no further information about the degree of impairment is available. It should be recognized that the peaks and troughs in both types of audiogram are subject to the transfer characteristics of the outer and middle ear and to the coupling characteristics of the probe transducers to the ear, and they may not necessarily reflect variations in cochlear sensitivity with frequency.

With the above caveats, DPOAEs have great promise for assessment of cochlear function. Their major advantage over CEOAEs is frequency specificity and they probably possess the greatest potential as an accurate predictor of hearing threshold level by frequency (Martin, Probst and Lonsbury-Martin, 1990; Ohlms, Lonsbury-Martin and Martin, 1990; Spektor et al., 1991; Smurzynski and Kim, 1992). Further data are required before this potential can be realized.

Clinical application of OAEs

General

OAEs have the potential to provide objective clinical information about the functioning of the cochlea. There is general agreement that the delayed OAE is produced only under the normal working conditions of a healthy, or at least partially healthy, cochlea and middle ear and that its presence indicates mechanically active outer hair cells. If the cochlear mechanisms associated with the micro-mechanical response of the basilar membrane are damaged, then OAEs cease to exist and hearing sensitivity is reduced.

A number of clinical uses have been suggested for the OAE (Bonfils, Uziel and Pujol, 1988; Bonfils and Uziel, 1989; Bonfils et al., 1990; Lutman et al., 1989; Kemp, Ryan and Bray, 1990; Cane, O'Donoghue and Lutman, 1992; Cane, Lutman and O'Donoghue, 1994).

- OAEs have highly individual and repeatable spectra. This feature alone suggests its potential as a monitoring tool to quantify subtle changes in an individual's cochlear status. Such monitoring may be applicable to individuals at risk of cochlear damage, such as those employed in an industry where noise is a hazard, in patients undergoing treatment with ototoxic drugs, to monitor cochlear functioning during acoustic neuroma surgery (Cane, O'Donoghue and Lutman, 1992) or in individuals suffering illnesses known to be potentially damaging to the cochlea, for example meningitis. The DPOAE, because of its frequency specificity, may provide valuable information on individuals with progressive disease, for example some cases of hereditary hearing loss, or when testing response to glycerol for endolymphatic hydrops.
- A second application might be in identifying subtle cochlear pathology in patients complaining of hearing difficulty but with normal

pure tone thresholds, although Lutman and Saunders (1992) failed to show any association of OAEs with obscure auditory dysfunction (hearing difficulty with normal hearing thresholds).

- Another use may be as a diagnostic tool, differentiating between cochlear and retrocochlear lesions or between organic and non-organic hearing loss.
- The most promising application to date is the use of the delayed OAE to screen for normal or near normal cochlear status in neonates, infants and otherwise difficult-to-test individuals.

Neonatal screening

In paediatric audiology it is generally accepted that the early identification of congenital hearing impairment is of great importance and should occur, ideally, in the first few months of life so that appropriate management of the hearing impairment can be initiated. The incidence of severe hearing impairment in childhood in industrialized countries is about 1–2 per 1000 (Peckham, 1986; Sancho et al., 1988; Davis and Wood, 1992), with a higher incidence in neonates who have required special care in the neonatal period (these infants can be up to ten times more likely to have a significant bilateral sensorineural hearing impairment (Davis and Wood, 1992)).

At present in the UK the main hearing screen is administered when a child is 6–8 months old and is mature enough to respond to the distraction test technique. Unfortunately, in the past it has been more of an exception than a rule for hearing loss to be identified in the first year of life: evidence suggests the typical age for the detection of severe and profound hearing impairment used to be of the order of 2;6–3 years of age (Martin and Moore, 1979; National Deaf Children's Society, 1983). The distraction test is potentially an efficient community screen but requires extensive training and continued support to achieve and maintain early identification (McCormick, 1983; McCormick et al., 1984). An objective neonatal hearing screening test, efficient in terms of sensitivity and specificity, could improve screening efficiency, reduce the age at which congenital or neonatally acquired hearing impairment is identified and help to distinguish between cases of congenital and early acquired or progressive hearing loss. Given that nearly all births in the UK are in hospital, screening before mother and baby leave hospital would ensure a high compliance rate. In recent years much effort has been directed towards developing viable screening techniques for hearing applicable to the neonatal population. Examples include:

- the auditory response cradle;
- auditory brain stem response (ABR) audiometry; and
- detection of CEOAEs.

Stevens et al. (1987, 1989, 1990, 1991) compared ABR and CEOAE methods for detecting hearing impairment in neonates at risk (mainly low birthweight), and found both methods to be feasible. However, they considered the CEOAE technique to be a more sensitive indicator of hearing impairment: they report (Stevens et al., 1991) extremely encouraging 'sensitivity' and 'specificity' values (93% and 84% respectively) for a test population of 723 neonates taken largely from a neonatal intensive care unit. 'Sensitivity' and 'specificity' were calculated using ABR as the standard against which the CEOAE test was compared. They proposed that CEOAE should be considered as the initial screening method for hearing impairment in babies in neonatal intensive care units, using the following protocol. The neonate is screened on each ear using the CEOAE method before leaving hospital: if the CEOAE is present in both ears the neonate is deemed to have passed. Neonates that fail (from Stevens' figures these would constitute approximately 20% of the population) would then be assessed using ABR testing. If the same test protocol and management of outcome were applied to babies not treated in the intensive care unit, the follow-up workload would be proportionately lower (although higher in absolute terms) as more babies would pass at the initial stage (Table 8.4). However, a much greater number of babies would require testing.

Requirements of a neonatal screening test

Ideally a screening test should satisfy the following requirements:

1. It must be both sensitive and specific so that few impaired cases are missed and few unimpaired cases are falsely identified.
2. It should have an appropriate cut-off dividing abnormal and normal results (for CEOAEs the intrinsic cut-off appears to be about 25–35 dB HL at the best hearing frequencies).
3. The procedure should be applicable to 100% of the target population (if undertaken shortly after birth and housed in a neonatal unit a high proportion of the target population could be tested).
4. It should be reasonably well tolerated by the subject under test and not put the subject at risk (ideally it should be non-invasive and entail a short test time).
5. It must be affordable in terms of equipment costs, expertise required of the staff and time required to perform each test.

Opinions differ regarding the prevalence of middle ear effusions in the neonatal population. A high incidence would have significant implications for a screening test because OAEs are not measurable in subjects with immobile middle ears (Kemp, 1978; Decreton, Hanssens and Sloovere, 1991). This does not appear to be a material problem if measurements are undertaken shortly after birth in well-baby units, given the data presented in Table 8.4 which indicate a high incidence of measurable OAEs, but the situation is slightly different for babies who have required neonatal intensive care (Table 8.5). Balkany et al. (1978) report middle ear effusions to be present in 30% of infants examined in a neonatal intensive care unit. This should not, however, be considered a contraindication to sceening in this population of neonates, given the data of Galambos, Hicks and Wilson (1982) who state the prevalence of hearing impairment in babies in neonatal intensive care units to be of the order of 1 in 50 and Davis and Wood (1992), who report that as many as 50% of the total number of hearing-impaired children may be detected at birth if a neonatal screen is targeted. Efforts should be made to identify the presence of middle-ear effusions before undertaking OAE measurements. Johnsen et al. (1988) suggest the use of pneumatic otoscopy.

Use of CEOAE in neonatal screening

The CEOAE test appears to be highly appropriate as a neonatal screening test. It is non-invasive, can be undertaken while the subject is asleep and has a short test time. Mean figures for test time range from less than 3 min (Bonfils, Uziel and Pujol, 1988; Plinkert et al., 1990; Kemp and Ryan, 1991; Decreton, Hanssens and Sloovere, 1991) to about 12 min (Kennedy et al., 1991; Stevens et al., 1991). Furthermore, the application of signal-processing techniques that allow an increased rate of click stimulation may substantially reduce test time down to a few seconds* (Thornton, 1993). This, and advances in microelectronic miniaturization, could make the use of a hand-held probe, similar in appearance to an otoscope, a distinct possibility. To administer the test, personnel trained in probe placement and equipment use are required.

A practical OAE screening test

Choice of test

For an OAE screening test to be viable the mode of emission generation selected must show a uniform behaviour in the vast majority of the population with normal hearing. From the foregoing discussion it is clear that the SOAE does not fulfil this requirement, being found in only 30–60% of healthy ears. This leaves a choice between the delayed, simultaneous and distortion product OAEs. Of these, only the delayed

---

*One technique involves the use of a pseudo-random train of clicks, such as a maximum length sequence. Figure 8.7 depicted CEOAEs lasting 26 ms that had, in fact, been obtained using a maximum length sequence that allowed clicks to be presented at intervals as short as 0.5 ms, compared with the theoretical maximum of 26 ms for the conventional method. Averaging of 2000 sweeps was accomplished in 2 s, rather than the 52 s that would have been required for a conventional method.

OAE is sufficiently well described at present in both normal and hearing-impaired subjects to be a practicable screening test.

The DPOAE may provide frequency-specific information and thus be more directly related to the pure tone audiogram, but fewer data are available on its clinical utility. The time required for certain implementations during which the subject must remain quiet is probably too long for screening applications (e.g. 20–45 min per ear; Spektor et al., 1991), although the technique is amenable to optimization, which would substantially improve the speed of testing. Detection of a response also requires more complex equipment, although proprietary systems are now available which should lead to a greater availability of data from which to judge the usefulness of DPOAEs. The simultaneous OAE is probably the most difficult of the OAEs to record, mainly due to the problem of distinguishing emissions from the outer ear sound field. Thus, the clear preference at present is the delayed OAE, although in future the DPOAE may be useful.

Choice of stimulation

The remaining choice for type of test is between click and tone-burst stimulation. The potential for frequency-specific predictive information using tone-burst stimuli has not been fully established as all stimuli appear fundamentally to excite the same emission process, the response simply being the convolution of the impulse response of the intrinsic OAE process and the stimulus. The process can, in principle, be characterized fully from the CEOAE because the click contains components throughout the range of frequencies passed by the stimulation system, although at a lesser amplitude than specific tone bursts.

Therefore, the stimulus of choice appears to be the broad-band click, although Probst et al. (1987) have suggested that a 1.5 kHz tone-burst might slightly improve the specificity of a screening test. Despite this finding and because most existing knowledge of delayed OAEs is based upon click stimulation, the use of clicks is preferable.

Overall design of apparatus

In order to provide a fast, reliable, objective test that can be performed in conditions that are not always ideal and with the minimum of tester skill, special considerations regarding the equipment and analysis used to validate the response are required. The following design principles could be used in the development of bespoke apparatus for a neonatal screening programme and may be of assistance when checking the specification of propriety apparatus purchased for the same purpose.

The basic components comprise

- a stimulus generation system;
- a probe containing a miniature earphone and microphone, pre-amplification and signal conditioning circuitry and a time-domain averager;
- a control system to schedule the test, synchronize the averaging process, display the response and store data for subsequent analysis;
- a method of automatic analysis of the response waveforms to furnish a guide to the presence or absence of an OAE would also give immediate feedback to the operator.

This description will be limited to recording of CEOAEs.

Stimulus characteristics

The exact waveform of the click stimulus is not crucial as the acoustic click arriving at the tympanic membrane is governed primarily by the probe acoustics. Typically, a 0.1 ms unipolar rectangular impulse is applied to the probe earphone. A range of stimulus levels from −10 to +50 dB nHL allows a full range of response levels to be covered. However, if the purpose of the apparatus is simply to establish the presence or absence of a CEOAE, two levels at the upper end of this range, approximately 10 dB apart, will suffice. (Two levels are required to extract the non-linear component of the saturating response – see below.) Clicks may be presented very rapidly, subject to the constraint that a click does not overlap a portion of the response to the previous click that it is required to measure. (Even this constraint may be waived if special analysis is used to deconvolve stimulus and response by, for example, using a maximum length sequence of clicks, as described by Thornton, 1993.) If measurement of the CEOAE extending to 20 ms after the click onset is required, the maximum click repetition rate is the reciprocal of 20 ms (50 clicks/s). In this example, it would be sensible to choose a repetition rate different from the supply line frequency of 50 Hz, for example 47/s. These calculations assume that averaging of the response waveform can occur in parallel with data acquisition and no allowance needs to be made for processing time.

Probe

The probe should be sealed in the ear canal, but have a narrow-bore vent to allow pressure equalization. A very small probe is required for neonates with a port small enough to fit in the ear canal of low birth-weight babies down to a gestational age of approximately 28 weeks. By sealing the probe to the ear canal, the transfer of signal to the microphone is maximized, penetration of external acoustic interference minimized and the waveform of the stimulating click is preserved. The probe is usually connected to the ear canal by a replaceable soft plastic cuff to ensure hygienic conditions and to allow a variety of cuffs to fit ears of different sizes. The probe design must minimize acoustical 'ringing' of the click in the ear canal, which would prevent recording of the earliest (high frequency) components of the CEOAE. This can be achieved by careful optimization of the tubing arrangements within the probe and by introducing acoustic damping into the tube connecting the earphone to the ear canal. Good design will ensure that ringing is controlled in all neonates, even if the fit is not ideal. Our experience of testing several thousands of neonates in intensive care units suggests that a well-designed probe will demonstrate negligible ringing beyond 4 ms in most ears; in approximately 1% of ears ringing will be evident beyond 5 ms but in no cases will ringing extend beyond 6 ms.

Microphone pre-amplifier

The design of the microphone pre-amplifier also requires a great deal of care. It must provide sufficient gain to amplify the low-intensity CEOAE, yet be unperturbed by the relatively high-intensity click stimulus. Typical designs allow the click to overload the pre-amplifier in the knowledge that the analogue-to-digital conversion (ADC) of the microphone signal will not commence until after the click and its subsequent ringing have died away. Thus, the behaviour of the pre-amplifier under conditions of overload is crucial. Experience has shown that small non-linearities in the pre-amplifier performance can occur, lasting several milliseconds after the overload condition has ceased. Because such non-linearities may behave much like CEOAEs, it is of over-riding importance that they do not contaminate the signal passed to the ADC. The pre-amplifier should also provide some signal conditioning to improve signal-to-noise ratio. Filtering the microphone signal with a passband from 0.5 to 5 kHz removes extraneous noise yet allows all material CEOAE components to pass.

The electrical noise output of a low-noise miniature microphone is typically equivalent to approximately 25 dB(A). This is augmented by any physiological or ambient noise that reaches the probe microphone. By comparison, a CEOAE may have an amplitude as low as 0 dB SPL. To improve the signal-to-noise ratio, synchronous time-domain averaging is used, which reduces the relative level of any asynchronous noise progressively as the number of sweeps increases. Typically, 500 sweeps covering a time window from 4 to 20 ms after the onset of each click would give an adequate signal-to-noise ratio. An overload rejection system is essential to reject sweeps containing excessive noise caused, for example, by the subject swallowing, coughing or moving.

Derived waveforms

It has become common practice to consider the non-linear component of the recorded waveform as the CEOAE, because it is unequivocally of physiological origin (barring the pre-amplifier non-linearities described above). This can be accomplished using stimuli at two different intensities, typically 10 dB apart. Because any components that are linearly related to stimulus intensity will be 10 dB larger in the response to the higher intensity stimulus, linear components can be cancelled by reducing the amplitude of the averaged response to the higher intensity stimulus by 10 dB and subtracting it from the averaged response to the lower intensity stimulus, leaving only the non-linear residual. A means to calculate the non-linear residual waveform is required. Ideally, collection of sweeps that contribute to the two raw averages should interleave clicks at the two intensities to minimize any extraneous difference between the averaged waveforms.

Interpretation of waveforms

Interpretation of the CEOAE waveforms is simplified if at least two replicate averages can be compared. If non-linear residuals are obtained, the decision regarding presence of a CEOAE should be based primarily on the similarity of replicate non-linear residual waveforms, although in some cases a CEOAE is evident in the raw averages but becomes buried in noise when the non-linear residuals are calculated. This occurs when the CEOAE displays little saturation. As a rule of thumb, if the non-linear residual waveforms are sufficiently similar that their cross-correlation coefficient calculated over the epoch from 6 to 16 ms after click onset is 0.5 or greater, a CEOAE is present. In a number of cases where a lower correlation coefficient is obtained, a CEOAE may still be visible to the experienced observer. However, the above guideline based on the cross-correlation coefficient is a conservative approach and provides reasonable guidance to the non-expert. The guideline may occasionally give spurious results if the recorded signals are contaminated by low-frequency noise which, by chance, is in-phase in the final averages. This problem is overcome by improved pre-amplifier filtering or by suitable pre-processing of the digitized waveforms.

Attention to the above design considerations has allowed production of apparatus that has been in practical use in 11 neonatal intensive care units in the UK for several years. Although improvements can still be made (to make the test quicker, to produce a smaller probe that will fit more easily into the ears of low birthweight babies, and to give improved feedback to the operator), CEOAE screening apparatus may now be used without great difficulty. Further research will establish the sensitivity and specificity of particular implementations, which should optimize test parameters.

Summary

Of the various types of OAE the bulk of data from humans relates to the CEOAE, which appears to have the main clinical application at present. The presence of a recordable CEOAE indicates normal, or near normal, cochlear function at the level of micromechanical response of the outer hair cells, at least at some frequencies. It also indicates essentially normal transmission of sound through the middle ear. Given the rarity of hearing impairments that involve neither the middle ear nor cochlear micromechanics, the presence of a CEOAE is a reliable general indicator of normal or near normal hearing at least at some frequencies. This has led to its application for neonatal screening and suggests that it may also be useful in the paediatric audiology clinic for testing babies with doubtful hearing ability and who would otherwise be tested by ABR methods. If the baby demonstrates a CEOAE in at least one ear there is no need to consider early fitting of a hearing aid, and detailed assessment can wait until the baby is able to perform the distraction test, or other such behavioural techniques.

Future research concerning the DPOAE may extend the above applications to give frequency-specific predictions of hearing status, improving the sensitivity or specificity of screening programmes. However, important questions regarding DPOAEs, and the possibility of recording DPOAEs in impaired ears, remain unanswered. The use of DPOAEs in paediatric audiology must be considered still to be in the research phase.

References

Allen, J.B. and Fahey, P.F. (1992). Using acoustic distortion products to measure the cochlear amplifier gain on the basilar membrane. *Journal of the Acoustical Society of America* **92**, 178–188.

Allen, J.B. and Neely, S.T. (1992). Micromechanical models of the cochlea. *Physics Today* **45**(7),40–47.

Anderson, S.D. (1980). Some ECMR properties in relation to other signals from the auditory periphery. *Hearing Research* **2**, 273–296.

Anderson, S.D. and Kemp, D.T. (1979). The evoked cochlear mechanical response in laboratory primates. *Archives of Oto-Rhino-Laryngology* **224**, 47–54.

Anderson, S.D., Bridgens, S. and Halford, J. (1989). The effects of middle ear congestion on stimulated oto-acoustic emissions. *British Journal of Audiology* **23**, 356 (Abstract).

Antonelli, A. and Grandori, F. (1986). Long term stability, influence of the head position and modelling considerations for evoked otoacoustic emissions. *Scandinavian Audiology Supplementum* **25**, 97–108.

Avan, P., Bonfils, P., Loth, D., Narcy, Ph. and Trotoux, J. (1991). Quantitative assessment of human cochlear function by evoked otoacoustic emissions. *Hearing Research* **52**, 99–112.

Balkany, T.J., Berman, S.A., Simmons, M.A. and Jafek, B.W. (1978). Middle ear effusions in neonates. *The Laryngoscope* **88**, 398–405.

Bell, A. (1992). Circadian and menstrual rhythms in frequency variations of sponta-neous otoacoustic emissions from human ears. *Hearing Research* **58**, 91–100.

Bonfils, P. (1989). Spontaneous otoacoustic emissions: Clinical interest. *The Laryngoscope* **99**, 752–756.

Bonfils, P. and Avan, P. (1992). *Hearing diagnostic model evaluation using distor-tion-product otoacoustic emissions*. Paper presented to 3rd International Symposium on Cochlear Mechanisms and Otoacoustic Emissions, Rome.

Bonfils, P. and Uziel, A. (1989). Clinical applications of evoked acoustic emissions: Results in normally hearing and hearing-impaired subjects. *Annals of Otology, Rhinology and Laryngology* **98**, 326–331.

Bonfils, P., Bertrand, Y. and Uziel, A. (1988). Evoked otoacoustic emissions: norma-tive data and presbycusis. *Audiology* **27**, 27–35.

Bonfils, P., Uziel, A. and Narcy, P. (1989). The properties of spontaneous and evoked acoustic emissions in neonates and children: a preliminary report. *Archives of Oto-Rhino-Laryngology* **246**, 249–251.

Bonfils, P., Uziel, A. and Pujol, R. (1988). Evoked otoacoustic emissions from adults and infants: Clinical applications. *Acta Oto-Laryngologica* **105**, 445–449.

Bonfils, P., Piron, J.P., Uziel, A. and Pujol, R. (1988). A correlative study of evoked otoacoustic emission properties and audiometric thresholds. *Archives of Oto-Rhino-Laryngology* **245**, 53–56.

Bonfils, P., Avan, P., Francois, M., Marie, P., Totoux, J. and Narcy, P. (1990). Clinical significance of otoacoustic emissions: A perspective. *Ear and Hearing* **11**, 155–158.

Brass, D.N. and Kemp, D.T. (1992). Characteristics of the cochlear amplifier revealed by simplified analysis of macro-mechanical and OAE suppression data. In: Grandori, F., Cianfrone, G. and Kemp, D.T. (Eds) *Proceedings of the 3rd International Symposium on Cochlear Mechanisms and Otoacoustic Emissions, Rome*, p. 3 (abstract). Milan: Centro Ricerche e Studi Amplifon.

Bray, P. and Kemp, D.T. (1987). An advanced cochlear echo technique suitable for infant screening. *British Journal of Audiology* **21**, 191–204.

Burns, E.M., Hoberg, K. and Campbell, S. (1992). Prevalence of spontaneous oto-acoustic emissions in neonates. *Journal of the Acoustical Society of America* **91**, 1571–1575.

Cane, M.A., Lutman, M.E. and O'Donoghue, G.M. (1994). Evoked otoacoustic emis-sions in patients with cerebello-pontine angle tumours. *American Journal of Otology*, **15**, 207–216.

Cane, M.A., O'Donoghue, G.M. and Lutman, M.E. (1992). The feasibility of using oto-acoustic emissions to monitor cochlear function during acoustic neuroma surgery. *Scandinavian Audiology* **21**, 173–176.

Cianfrone, G. and Mattia, M. (1986). Spontaneous otoacoustic emissions from nor-mal human ears. *Scandinavian Audiology Supplementum* **25**, 121–127.

Clark, W.W., Kim, D.O., Zurek, P.M. and Bohne, B.A. (1984). Spontaneous otoa-coustic emissions in chinchilla ear canals: Correlation with histopathology and suppression by external tone. *Hearing Research* **16**, 299–314.

Collet, L., Gartner, M., Moulin, A., Kauffman, I., Disant, F. and Morgon, A. (1989). Evoked otoacoustic emissions and sensorineural hearing loss. *Archives of Otolaryngology, Head and Neck Surgery* **115**, 1060–1062.

Collet, L., Gartner, M., Moulin, A., and Morgon, A. (1990). Age-related changes in evoked otoacoustic emissions. *Annals of Otology, Rhinology and Laryngology* **99**, 993–997.

Collet, L., Veuillet, E., Chanal, J.M. and Morgon, A. (1991). Evoked otoacoustic emissions: Correlations between spectrum analysis and audiogram. *Audiology* 30, 164–172.

Davis, A. and Wood, S. (1992). The epidemiology of childhood hearing impairment: factors relevant to planning services. *British Journal of Audiology* 26, 77–90.

Decreton, S.J.R.C., Hanssens, K. and De Sloovere, M. (1991). Evoked otoacoustic emissions in infant hearing screening. *International Journal of Paediatric Otorhinolaryngology* 21, 235–247.

Dolhen, P., Hennaux, C., Chantry, P. and Hennebert, D. (1991). The occurrence of evoked oto-acoustic emissions in a normal adult population and neonates. *Scandinavian Audiology* 20, 203–204.

Elberling, C., Parbo, J., Johnsen, N.J. and Bagi, P. (1985). Evoked acoustic emission: Clinical application. *Acta Oto-Laryngologica Supplement* 421, 77–85.

Evans, E.F., Wilson, J.P. and Borerwe, T.A. (1981). Animal models in tinnitus. In: Evered, D. and Lawrenson, G. (Eds), *Tinnitus*, pp. 108–138. London: Pitman, Ciba Foundation Symposium 85.

Fritze, W. (1983). On the frequency-distribution of spontaneous cochlear emissions. In: Klinke, R. and Hartmann, R. (Eds), *Hearing, Physiological Bases and Psychophysics*, pp. 77–81. Berlin: Springer-Verlag.

Fritze, W. and Köhler, W. (1985). Frequency composition of spontaneous cochlear emissions. *Archives of Oto-Rhino-Laryngology* 242, 43–48.

Fritze, W. and Köhler, W. (1986). Our experience on spontaneous cochlear emissions. *Scandinavian Audiology Supplementum* 25, 129–137.

Furst, M. and Lapid, M. (1988). A cochlear model for acoustic emissions. *Journal of the Acoustical Society of America* 84, 222–229.

Galambos, R., Hicks, G. and Wilson, M.J. (1982). Hearing loss in graduates of a tertiary care nursery. *Ear and Hearing* 3, 87–90.

Gaskill, S.A. and Brown, A.M. (1990). The behavior of the acoustic distortion product, $2f_1-f_2$, from the human ear and its relation to auditory sensitivity. *Journal of the Acoustical Society of America* 88, 821–839.

Glanville, J.D., Coles, R.R.A. and Sullivan, B.M. (1971). A family with high tonal objective tinnitus. *Journal of Laryngology and Otology* 85, 1–10.

Grandori, F. (1985). Nonlinear phenomena in click and tone-burst evoked otoacoustic emissions from human ears. *Audiology* 24, 71–80.

Grandori, F. and Ravazzani, P. (1990). Deconvolutions of evoked otoacoustic emissions and response nonlinearity. *Advances in Audiology* 7, 99–109.

Guelke, R.W. and Bunn, A.E. (1985). A mechanism for stimulated acoustic emission in the cochlea. *Hearing Research* 19, 185–189.

Harris, F.P. and Probst, M.D. (1991). Reporting click-evoked and distortion product otoacoustic emission results with respect to the pure tone audiogram. *Ear and Hearing* 12, 399–405.

Hauser, R., Probst, R. and Löhle, E. (1991). Click- and tone-burst evoked otoacoustic emissions in normally hearing ears and in ears with high-frequency sensorineural hearing loss. *European Archives of Oto-Rhino-Laryngology* 248, 345–352.

Horst, J.W., Wit, H.P. and Ritsma, R.J. (1983). Psychophysical aspects of cochlear acoustic emissions ('Kemp-Tones'). In: Klinke, R. and Hartmann, R. (Eds), *Hearing, Physiological Bases and Psychophysics*, pp. 89–96. Berlin: Springer-Verlag.

Johnsen, N.J. and Elberling, C. (1982a). Evoked acoustic emissions from the human ear I. Equipment and response parameters. *Scandinavian Audiology* 11, 3–12.

Johnsen, N.J. and Elberling, C. (1982b). Evoked acoustic emissions from the human ear II. Normative data in young adults and influence of posture. *Scandinavian Audiology* 11, 69–77.

Johnsen, N.J., Bagi, P. and Elberling, C. (1983). Evoked acoustic emissions from the human ear III. Findings in neonates. *Scandinavian Audiology* 12, 17–24.

Johnsen, N.J., Parbo, J. and Elberling, C. (1989). Evoked acoustic emissions from the human ear V. Developmental changes. *Scandinavian Audiology* 18, 59–62.

Johnsen, N.J., Bagi, P., Parbo, J. and Elberling, C. (1988). Evoked acoustic emissions from the human ear IV. Final results in 100 neonates. *Scandinavian Audiology* 17, 27–34.

Kemp, D.T. (1978). Stimulated acoustic emissions from within the human auditory system. *Journal of the Acoustical Society of America* 64, 1386–1391.

Kemp, D.T. (1979). Evidence of mechanical nonlinearity and frequency selective wave amplification in the cochlea. *Archives of Oto-Rhino-Laryngology* 224, 37–45.

Kemp, D.T. (1980). Towards a model for the origin of cochlear echoes. *Hearing Research* 2, 533–548.

Kemp, D.T. and Chum, R. (1980). Observations on the generator mechanisms of stimulus frequency acoustic emissions – two tone suppression. In: van den Brink, G. and Bilsen, F. A. (Eds), *Psychophysical, Physiological and Behavioural Studies in Hearing*, pp.34–42. Delft: Delft University Press.

Kemp, D.T. and Ryan, S. (1991). Otoacoustic emission tests in neonatal screening programmes. *Acta Oto-Laryngologica Supplementum* 482, 73–84.

Kemp, D.T., Ryan, S. and Bray, P. (1990). A guide to the effective use of otoacoustic emissions. *Ear and Hearing* 11, 93–105.

Kemp, D.T., Bray, P., Alexander, L. and Brown, A.M. (1986). Acoustic emission cochleography – practical aspects. *Scandinavian Audiology Supplementum* 25, 71–95.

Kennedy, C.R., Kimm, L., Cafarelli-Dees, D., Evans, P.I.P., Hunter, M., Lenton, S. and Thornton, R D. (1991). Otoacoustic emissions and auditory brainstem responses in the newborn. *Archives of Disease in Childhood* 66, 1124–1129.

Kim, D.O. (1980). Cochlear mechanics: implications of electrophysiological and acoustical observations. *Hearing Research* 2, 297–317.

Köhler, W. and Fritze, W. (1992). A long-term observation of spontaneous otoacoustic emissions (SOAEs). *Scandinavian Audiology* 21, 55–58.

Long, G.R. and Tubis, A. (1988). Modification of spontaneous and evoked otoacoustic emissions and associated psychoacoustic microstructure by aspirin consumption. *Journal of the Acoustical Society of America* 84, 1343–1353.

Lonsbury-Martin, B.L. and Martin, G.K. (1990). The clinical utility of distortion-product otoacoustic emissions. *Ear and Hearing* 11, 144–154.

Lonsbury-Martin, B.L., Harris, F.P., Stagner, B.B., Hawkins, M.D. and Martin, G.K. (1990). Distortion-product emissions in humans I. Basic properties in normally hearing subjects. *Annals of Otology, Rhinology and Laryngology* 99, 3–14.

Lutman, M.E. (1989). Evoked otoacoustic emissions in adults: implications for screening. *Audiology in Practice* 6(3), 6–8.

Lutman, M.E. and Saunders, G.H. (1992). Lack of association between otoacoustic emissions and hearing difficulty in subjects with normal hearing thresholds. *Journal of the Acoustical Society of America* 92, 1184–1185.

Lutman, M.E., Mason, S.M., Sheppard, S. and Gibbin, K.P. (1989). Differential diagnostic potential of otoacoustic emissions: A case study. *Audiology* 28, 205–210.

McCormick, B. (1983). Hearing screening by health visitors: A critical appraisal of the distraction test. *Health Visitor* 56, 449–451.

McCormick, B., Wood, S.A., Cope, Y. and Spavens, F.M. (1984). Analysis of records from an open-access audiology service. *British Journal of Audiology* 18, 127–132.

McFadden, D. and Plattsmier, H.S. (1984). Aspirin abolishes spontaneous otoacoustic emissions. *Journal of the Acoustical Society of America* 76, 443–447.

Martin, J.A.M. and Moore, W.J. (1979). *Childhood deafness in the European Community*, EUR 6413. Luxembourg: Commission of the European Communities.

Martin, G.K., Probst, R. and Lonsbury-Martin, B L. (1990). Otoacoustic emissions in human ears: Normative findings. *Ear and Hearing* 11, 106–120.

Martin, G.K., McCoy, M.J., Lonsbury-Martin, B L. and Whitehead, M.L. (1992). Low-level distortion-product otoacoustic emissions in limited frequency regions of normal ears. In: Lim, D.J. (Ed.) *Proceedings of the 15th Midwinter Research Meeting of Association for Research in Otolaryngology, February 2–6 1992*, p.151 (abstract). Des Moines, IA: Association for Research in Otolaryngology.

National Deaf Children's Society (1983). *Discovering Deafness*. A report for the National Deaf Children's Week, 15–21 May 1983.

Norton, S.J. and Neely, S.T. (1987). Tone-burst-evoked otoacoustic emissions from normal-hearing subjects. *Journal of the Acoustical Society of America* 81, 1860–1872.

Norton, S.J. and Widen, J.E. (1990). Evoked otoacoustic emissions in normal-hearing infants and children: Emerging data and issues. *Ear and Hearing* 11, 121–127.

Ohlms, L.A., Lonsbury-Martin, B.L. and Martin, G.K. (1990). The clinical application of acoustic distortion products. *Otolaryngology, Head and Neck Surgery* 103, 52–58.

Peckham, C.S (1986). Hearing impairment in childhood. *British Medical Bulletin* 42, 145–149.

Penner, M.J. (1988). Audible and annoying spontaneous otoacoustic emissions. *Archives of Otolaryngology, Head and Neck Surgery* 114, 150–153.

Penner, M.J. (1992). Linking spontaneous otoacoustic emissions and tinnitus. *British Journal of Audiology* 26, 115–123.

Penner, M.J. and Burns, E.M. (1987). The dissociation of SOAEs and tinnitus. *Journal of Speech and Hearing Research* 30, 396–403.

Penner, M.J. and Coles, R.R.A. (1992). Indications for aspirin as a palliative for tinnitus caused by SOAEs: a case study. *British Journal of Audiology* 26, 91–96.

Plinkert, P.K., Sesterhenn, G., Arold, R. and Zenner, H.P. (1990). Evaluation of otoacoustic emissions in high risk infants using an easy and rapid objective auditory screening method. *European Archives of Otorhinolaryngology* 247, 356–360.

Probst, R., Lonsbury-Martin, B.L. and Martin, G.K. (1991). A review of otoacoustic emissions. *Journal of the Acoustical Society of America* 89, 2027–2067.

Probst, R., Coats, A.C., Martin, G.K. and Lonsbury-Martin, B.L. (1986). Spontaneous, click- and toneburst-evoked otoacoustic emissions from normal ears. *Hearing Research* 21, 261–275.

Probst, R., Lonsbury-Martin, B.L., Martin, G.K. and Coats, A.C. (1987). Otoacoustic emissions in ears with hearing loss. *American Journal of Otolaryngology* 8, 73–81.

Robinson, P.M. and Haughton, P.M. (1991). Modification of evoked oto-acoustic emissions by changes in pressure in the external ear. *British Journal of Audiology* 25, 131–133.

Ruggero, M.A., Rich, N.C. and Freyman, R. (1983). Spontaneous and impulsively evoked otoacoustic emissions: indicators of cochlear pathology? *Hearing Research* 10, 283–300.

Russell, A.F. and Bilger, R.C. (1992). A twin study of spontaneous otoacoustic emissions. *Journal of the Acoustical Society of America* 92, 2409 (abstract).

Rutten, W.L.C. (1980). Evoked acoustic emissions from within normal and abnormal human ears: comparison with audiometric and electrocochleographic findings. *Hearing Research* 2, 263–271.

Sancho, J., Hughes, E., Davis, A. and Haggard, M. (1988). Epidemiological basis for screening hearing. In: McCormick, B. (Ed.) *Paediatric Audiology 0–5 years*, pp. 1–35. London: Taylor and Francis.

Schloth, E. (1983). Relation between spectral composition of spontaneous otoacoustic emissions and fine-structure of threshold in quiet. *Acoustica* 53, 250–256.

Schloth, E. and Zwicker, E. (1983). Mechanical and acoustical influences on spontaneous oto-acoustic emissions. *Hearing Research* 11, 285–293.

Smurzynski, J. and Kim, D.O. (1992). Distortion-product and click-evoked otoacoustic emissions of normally-hearing adults. *Hearing Research* 58, 227–240.

Spektor, Z., Leonard, G., Kim, D.O., Jung, M.D. and Smurzynski, J. (1991). Otoacoustic emissions in normal and hearing impaired children and normal adults. *The Laryngoscope* 101, 965–976.

Stevens, J.C. and Ip, C.B. (1988). Click evoked oto-acoustic emissions in normal and hearing impaired adults. *British Journal of Audiology* 22, 45–49.

Stevens, J.C., Webb, H.D., Smith, M.F., Buffin, J.T. and Ruddy, H. (1987). A comparison of oto-acoustic emissions and brainstem electric response audiometry in the normal newborn and babies admitted to a special care baby unit. *Clinical Physics and Physiological Measurements* 8, 94–104.

Stevens, J.C., Webb, H.D., Hutchinson, J., Connell, J., Smith, M.F. and Buffin, J.T. (1989). Click evoked otoacoustic emissions compared with brainstem electric response. *Archives of Disease in Childhood* 64, 1105–1111.

Stevens, J.C., Webb, H.D., Smith, M.F. and Buffin, J.T. (1990). The effect of stimulus level on click evoked oto-acoustic emissions and brainstem responses in neonates under intensive care. *British Journal of Audiology* 24, 293–300.

Stevens, J.C., Webb, H.D., Hutchinson, J., Connell, J., Smith, M.F. and Buffin, J.T. (1991). Evaluation of click-evoked oto-acoustic emissions in the newborn. *British Journal of Audiology* 25, 11–14.

Strickland, E.A., Burns, E.M. and Tubis, A. (1985). Incidence of spontaneous otoacoustic emissions in children and infants. *Journal of the Acoustical Society of America* 78, 931–935.

Thornton, A.R.D.T. (1993). High rate otoacoustic emissions. *Journal of the Acoustical Society of America* 94, 132–136.

Tyler, R.S. and Conrad-Armes, D. (1982). Spontaneous acoustic cochlear emissions and sensorineural tinnitus. *British Journal of Audiology* 16, 193–194.

Uziel, A. and Piron, J.P. (1991). Evoked otoacoustic emissions from normal newborns and babies admitted to an intensive care baby unit. *Acta Oto-Laryngologica, Supplementum* 482, 85–91.

Weir, C.C., Norton, S.J. and Kincaid, G.E. (1984). Spontaneous narrowband otoacoustic signals emitted by human ears: a replication. *Journal of the Acoustical Society of America* 76, 1248–1250.

Whitehead, M.L., Lonsbury-Martin, B.L. and Martin, G.K. (1992). Evidence for two discrete sources of $2f_1-f_2$ distortion-product otoacoustic emission in rabbit: I.

Differential dependence on stimulus parameter. *Journal of the Acoustical Society of America* 91, 1587–1606.

Whitehead, M.L., Kamal, N., Lonsbury-Martin, B.L. and Martin, G.K. (1993). Spontaneous otoacoustic emissions in different racial groups. *Scandinavian Audiology* 22, 3–10.

Wilson, J.P. (1980a). Evidence for a cochlear origin for acoustic re-emissions, threshold fine-structure and tonal tinnitus. *Hearing Research* 2, 233–252.

Wilson, J.P. (1980b). Model for cochlear echoes and tinnitus based on an observed electrical correlate. *Hearing Research* 2, 527–532.

Wilson, J.P. (1980c). The combination tone $2f_1-f_2$ in psychophysics and ear-canal recording. In: van den Brink, G. and Bilson, F. A. (Eds), *Phychophysical, Physiological and Behavioural Studies in Hearing*, pp. 43–50. Delft: Delft University Press.

Wilson, J.P. (1986a). Otoacoustic emissions and tinnitus. *Scandinavian Audiology Supplementum* 25, 109–119.

Wilson, J.P. (1986b). The influence of temperature on frequency tuning mechanisms. In: Allen, J.B., Hall, J.L., Hubbard, A., Neely, S.T. and Tubis, A. (Eds) *Peripheral Auditory Mechanisms*, pp. 229–236. Berlin: Springer-Verlag.

Wilson, J.P. (1987). Theory of tinnitus generation. In: Hazell, J.W.P. (Ed.), *Tinnitus*, pp. 20–45. Edinburgh: Churchill Livingstone.

Wilson, J.P. and Sutton, G.L. (1981). Acoustic correlates of tonal tinnitus. In: Evered, D. and Lawrenson, G. (Eds), *Tinnitus*, pp. 82–107. London: Pitman, Ciba Foundation Symposium 85.

Wilson, J.P. and Sutton, G.L. (1983). A family with high tonal objective tinnitus – an update. In: Klinke, R. and Hartmann, R. (Eds), *Hearing, Physiological Bases and Psychophysics*, pp. 97–103. Berlin: Springer-Verlag.

Wit, H.P. (1992). Some fundamental aspects of otoacoustic emissions. In: Hazell, J.W.P. (Ed.), *Proceedings of the First European Conference on Audiology, Cambridge* (abstract 85). Reading: British Society of Audiology.

Wit, H.P. and Ritsma, R.J. (1979). Stimulated acoustic emissions from the human ear. *Journal of the Acoustical Society of America* 66, 911–913.

Wit, H.P. and Ritsma, R.J. (1980). Evoked acoustical responses from the human ear: some experimental results. *Hearing Research* 2, 253–261.

Wit, H.P., Langevoort, J.C. and Ritsma, R.J. (1981). Frequency spectra of cochlear acoustic emissions ('Kemp Echoes'). *Journal of the Acoustical Society of America* 70, 437–445.

Zurek, P.M. (1981). Spontaneous narrowband acoustic signals emitted by human ears. *Journal of the Acoustical Society of America* 69, 514–523.

Zwicker, E. (1986). Otoacoustic emissions in a nonlinear cochlear hardware model with feedback. *Journal of the Acoustical Society of America* 80, 154–162.

Zwicker, E. (1990). On the influence of acoustical load on evoked otoacoustic emissions. *Hearing Research* 47, 185–190.

Zwicker, E. and Schloth, E. (1984). Interrelation of different oto-acoustic emissions. *Journal of the Acoustical Society of America* 75, 1148–1154.

Chapter 9
Acoustic measurement of auditory function

DENZIL N. BROOKS

Introduction

The earliest method of assessment of auditory function was use of the human voice, the strength and distance needed for its accurate reception depending on the degree of auditory impairment. Using this seemingly crude method a skilled practitioner could make a reasonable estimate of hearing acuity. From about the beginning of the seventeenth century attempts were made to quantify hearing with more precision.

- Feldmann (1970) reports that Wolke in 1802 produced an instrument consisting of a wooden board to which was hinged a drumstick that could be dropped from measured heights, thereby giving a measure of quantification to the sound produced.
- Itard substituted a copper ring for the wooden board and a pendulum bob for the drumstick: this instrument found widespread acceptance.
- Simple tests such as listening to the tick of a watch or the click of one coin against another were commended by such eminent persons as Hallowell Davis (Davis and Silverman, 1970) as late as 1970.
- John Shore, a trumpeter and lutenist to King James II, is credited with developing the pitch (or tuning) fork around 1711.
- Over a century later Weber described his (now classical) test and a few years later Rinne described his test for differentiating conductive and sensorineural hearing losses.
- More accurate quantification of hearing levels became possible with the development of electrical devices for generating sound – these led up to the modern audiometer.

A second traditional approach to examination of the auditory system is the visual approach: probes for removing earwax are among the oldest medical instruments; available natural light was probably used at first when cleaning the ear canal but later light from an oil lamp or candle was used with a reflector behind the wick to increase the level of illumination. Modern fibreoptics and halogen light sources make illumination of the external ear relatively simple and reliable, and if better vision is required, the optical microscope is invaluable.

Reliability of information

The amount of reliable information provided by tuning fork tests is limited (Browning, Swan and Chew, 1989). Audiometry, even if performed in an adequately sound-treated environment by a skilled individual aware of the need for and the use of appropriate masking using equipment accurately calibrated for both air and bone conduction, is at best inferential in terms of the information provided about middle ear function. The difference between the thresholds for air and bone conduction provides an estimate of the degree of conductive dysfunction, but gives virtually no information about the reasons for that dysfunction. It is generally assumed that the bone conduction threshold reflects the status of the inner ear, but this is not always true: some conductive lesions, and middle ear effusion is a case in point, produce a mass loading on the cochlear windows that inhibits fluid movement in the inner ear giving a semblance of sensorineural hearing loss. Another example of an apparent sensorineural hearing loss that is, in fact, due to a conductive lesion is Carhart's notch in otosclerosis. In a few situations the audiogram may indicate the nature and type of a hearing loss with a reasonable degree of certainty – such as with noise-induced hearing loss – but in many situations audiometry provides little useful pathological information.

Even with all the recent advances in technology the amount of information that can be derived from physical examination of the ear is strictly limited.

- The tympanic membrane is not generally visible over its entire surface, a small segment lying beyond vision in the anterior recess. If the membrane is especially transparent the long process of the incus may be visible, but usually the opacity of the membrane is such that only the malleus is clearly identifiable.
- Disorders such as otosclerosis or ossicular discontinuity, in which the cause of the hearing impairment is located at the medial end of the ossicular chain, provide few if any visual clues as to the nature of the lesion.
- Otitis media with effusion (OME) may be considered as identifiable with certainty by otoscopy, but a number of reports indicate that even experienced otoscopists disagree over its diagnosis (Roeser et al., 1977; Margolis et al., 1979; Renvall and Holmberg, 1981; Karma et al., 1989).

- And, of course, otoscopy will provide very little information about the nature (or even the presence) of sensorineural hearing loss.

Thus, although visual examination and audiometry are undoubtedly of great value in many clinical situations they do, individually and in combination, have manifest limitations. A good history may give additional diagnostic information provided that the patient (or carer of those unable to answer for themselves) is willing and able to furnish such information. In the less than ideal situation that so often faces the clinician, more information about the status of the auditory system would be of inestimable value.

It was probably with these factors in mind that towards the end of the nineteenth century August Lucae decided to explore the potential of sound introduced into the ear canal as a diagnostic tool (Lucae, 1867). His pioneering studies led to the development of acoustic admittance measurement systems such as are in widespread use today (for a historical review see Shallop, 1976).

Principles of measurement of acoustic admittance

Acoustical/physical factors

Sound is propagated through a medium – solid, liquid or gas – by longitudinal waves. Particles of the medium oscillate in the direction of travel of the sound wave, passing their motion on to adjacent particles. If a sudden change is encountered in the propagating medium the efficiency of forward propagation will be affected. For example, if sound moving through air (which is a medium of low density) encounters a water surface only a small part of the incident energy enters the denser medium for onward propagation; most is reflected into the medium of origin because of the different characteristic impedances in the two media.

Characteristic impedance may be defined as the ratio between sound pressure and particle velocity. The velocity of particles in a dense medium such as water will be much lower than in a more tenuous medium such as air for any given sound pressure: water, therefore, has a higher characteristic impedance to sound than air.

The situation in the example above is similar to that which exists in the human auditory system. The medium for sound propagation is air but the acoustic receptors, the hair cells of the cochlea, operate in endolymph, a fluid very similar to water. If airborne sound fell directly on to a window in the cochlea, transfer of energy into the ear would be very inefficient. Wever and Lawrence (1954) calculated that at an air–water boundary less than 0.1% of the incident energy will enter the water: this equates to a loss of around 30 dB.

The middle ear functions as an acoustical transformer or impedance matching device to enhance the transfer of energy from air to endolymph. Two main mechanisms operate to achieve the necessary transformation.

1. The first depends on the difference in area between the tympanic membrane and the footplate of the stapes, the former being some 20 times greater than the latter. The minute variations in ambient pressure that constitute sound are gathered over the relatively large area of the tympanic membrane. This energy enters the cochlea via the small area of the footplate but with increased force or pressure.
2. The second mechanism for increasing the pressure at the footplate is a form of leverage, the malleus being a little longer than the incus (length ratio approximately 4:3).

Together these two factors make the normally functioning middle ear an efficient device for matching air, with its low characteristic impedance, to the endolymph with its relatively high characteristic impedance. Over the last few years the terminology has changed: rather than consider how inefficient an ear may be (i.e. how much sound is impeded), emphasis has moved towards what may be seen as a more positive viewpoint – the efficiency of the system. Modern methods measure the acoustic admittance, this being the inverse of the impedance.

The middle ear can be regarded as being made up of parts or structures having three principal properties: mass, elasticity and resistance (or friction). The malleus and incus with, to some extent, the attached portion of the tympanic membrane constitute a mass that has to be moved by the stimulating sound. This mass is attached to the inner surface of the middle ear by elastic ligaments as well as by the tympanic membrane itself. When the membrane is driven inwards (or outwards) by positive (or negative) changes in pressure, the radial fibres are extended and the air within the middle ear is compressed (or rarefied). As in any system with moving parts the middle ear loses some of the incident energy to friction, or resistance.

Changes in any of the physical properties of the middle ear will affect, usually adversely, the efficiency of the system. Frictional changes reduce the efficiency across the whole auditory spectrum. If the mass elements are altered (a rare occurrence) the transmission of the higher auditory frequencies will be most affected. If the elastic elements change, the effect will be most evident in the lower auditory frequencies.

Physiological aspects

The middle ear also appears, in some circumstances, to have a protective function. The joint between the malleus and incus allows for some disengagement under conditions of excessive stimulation (Mawson, 1967). With sound pressures such as those generated by near speech the malleo-incudal joint is rigid, but if the tympanic membrane is subjected to much greater pressure changes, especially such as to cause the membrane to move outwards, the ossicles subluxate. The movement of the incus is reduced relative to the movement of the malleus, and the cochlea is protected from the large pressure changes.

The function of the muscles of the middle ear is still a matter for conjecture, but it seems likely that a major role is modification of the frequency response of the ear to noise (external, or internally generated by activities such as speaking or chewing) to maximize reception of speech. High levels of noise (above about 80 dB nHL) initiate a contraction of the stapedius muscle, which reduces the transmission efficiency of the middle ear for low-frequency stimuli without impairing performance in the higher auditory frequencies, effectively enhancing the signal:noise ratio for the important consonantal information.

The effective transmission of sound through the middle ear is, therefore, dependent on the whole system – ossicles, ligaments, muscles and eustachian tube – working efficiently.

- If, for example, the footplate of the stapes is fixed in the oval window by otosclerosis, the movement of the stapes will be greatly diminished. As the incudo-stapedial joint has only a small degree of flexibility, the movement of the incus will be severely restricted and movement of the malleus will likewise be inhibited due to the almost rigid coupling between the malleus and incus. The handle of the malleus is embedded in the tympanic membrane, the ability of which to move under the influence of sound pressure changes will be greatly reduced if the malleus is inhibited. The membrane will be stiffer and reflect a higher than normal proportion of the incident energy.
- By contrast, a disruption of the incudo-stapedial joint will allow the malleus–incus system, and hence the tympanic membrane, to move more freely than normal. In such a situation the percentage of the incident energy reflected by the membrane is less than normal.
- If the eustachian tube is functioning poorly a partial vacuum could develop in the middle ear because the tissues will absorb the air contained within the limited space causing the tympanic membrane to become indrawn and stressed. The increased stiffness reduces the ability of the membrane to absorb incident sound and so a greater than normal proportion is reflected.
- Contraction of the stapedius muscle, whether spontaneous or induced, causes the position of the stapes to change and inhibits its movement. This increased stiffness is transmitted to the tympanic membrane and results in increased reflection of incident sound.

Thus the majority of pathological conditions or physical changes in the middle ear change the way in which the tympanic membrane reacts to acoustic energy reaching it down the acoustic meatus. Furthermore, most disorders of the tympanic membrane affect the elasticity of the system; few affect the mass. Tympanosclerosis, retraction of the tympanic membrane, atelectasis, adhesive otitis, disruption of the ossicular system, otosclerosis etc., are predominantly characterized by changes in the mobility of the system. Middle ear effusion also, because of the loading it imposes on the inner surface of the tympanic membrane, greatly stiffens the membrane and loads the whole auditory system. The admittance of the middle ear will reflect the changes in stiffness of the membrane, especially at the lower auditory frequencies (changes in the mass elements of the system mainly affect the higher auditory frequencies). Hence, observation of the acoustic admittance of the ear at low stimulus frequencies should provide valuable diagnostic information about conditions behind the tympanic membrane, information that is frequently unobtainable with conventional examination procedures.

Methods of measurement

The acoustic admittance provides a measure of the efficiency of the middle ear system in receiving and transmitting sound energy. Most measuring instruments employ a probe placed in the external canal or against its entry in such a way that a hermetic seal is obtained while the tests are being performed. The probe contains a small transducer which is energized by an oscillator to produce a low-frequency tone (the frequency recommended in the international standard is 226 Hz) in the cavity bounded by the probe tip, the walls of the external meatus and the tympanic membrane. The probe tip and the walls of the meatus may be regarded as acoustically rigid, i.e. they reflect all the sound energy that falls on them: hence the major determinant of what happens to the sound energy in the cavity is the tympanic membrane. If this is normal and connected to a normally functioning middle ear, most of the incident energy will be absorbed and transmitted to the cochlea; only a small amount of energy will be reflected into the ear canal. If, however, the middle ear is stiff – perhaps due to otosclerosis or effusion in the cavity – then little energy will be transmitted through the tympanic membrane to the cochlea; the largest part will be reflected into the canal.

For the same amount of energy emitted from the probe the first condition will produce a much lower sound pressure level in the ear canal than the second. There is an inverse relationship between the acoustic admittance at the tympanic membrane and the sound pressure in the ear canal. This provides a basis for a system of measurement of the admittance of the ear.

The sound pressure in the ear canal may be measured using a microphone placed in the same probe as the transducer that emits the low tone signal. However, this simple technique has limitations that make it impracticable. The sound produced by the probe is not the only sound in the ear canal: even assuming that the subject being tested is quiet, and that there is no environmental sound, there will still be some normal physiological sounds such as those produced by respiration, swallowing and/or blood pulsation through the arteries adjacent to the middle ear. It is necessary to ensure that in the worst possible situation the sound from the probe can be identified and measured without interference from these adventitious noises. Probably the extreme situation that may be encountered is an extremely flaccid middle ear that absorbs almost all the energy that falls on it. To ensure an adequate signal for the measuring microphone the probe tone sound pressure level must be considerably increased. However, there is a limit to the sound pressure level that can be employed: if it exceeds about 80 dB HL, the stapedius muscles in both ears of an individual with completely normal auditory function will contract, affecting the dynamics of the middle ear. We are then no longer measuring an ear in its normal condition. In other words the probe signal has altered the ear mechanics in such a way that its function cannot truly be assessed.

An alternative technique is to keep the sound pressure level in the ear canal at an optimum level for measurement, high enough to remove the interference of background noise, but low enough to avoid eliciting a stapedius response. In this system the power energizing the output transducer in the probe is varied according to the admittance of the middle ear. More power is needed to drive the transducer and to maintain a given sound pressure level in an absorbent ear than in an ear with a very stiff tympanic membrane. The power required for a given sound pressure level is directly related to the admittance of the ear at the tip of the probe.

Two additional factors need consideration. The first concerns the volume of air between the probe tip and the tympanic membrane. Our interest is in the admittance of the middle ear, but this small amount of air in the ear canal has elastic properties that are interposed between the point of measurement, the probe tip, and the middle ear. The second factor relates to the eustachian tube. If this is functioning normally the pressure in the middle ear will be almost the same as the ambient air pressure, the pressures on the two sides of the tympanic membrane will be equal, and the membrane will be under no tension and operating at maximum efficiency. If the eustachian tube is under-functioning the pressure in the middle ear will probably be below ambient because gases in the middle ear will be absorbed by the membranous lining of the cavity. Under such circumstances the tympanic membrane will be indrawn and stiffened, reducing the admittance of the middle ear. The resolution of both these difficulties is achieved by introducing controlled pressure variation into the external auditory canal.

Tympanometry

The admittance of the normal middle ear is highest when the tympanic membrane is free from stress, i.e. when the air pressure is identical on both sides. If a small pressure differential is created by changing the pressure on either side of the membrane, the radial fibres are stretched and stiffen. This results in a higher than normal proportion of the incident energy being reflected and the admittance falls. A difference in pressure of 0.5% of atmospheric pressure is sufficient to reduce the admittance by around one-half: if the difference rises to 2% the tympanic membrane becomes almost rigid and the admittance falls to almost zero. The process of observing the variation of admittance as a function of the pressure differential across the tympanic membrane is known as *tympanometry*, and the graphical representation of the function is a *tympanogram*.

As a pressure differential between the external canal and the middle ear of more than 2% effectively renders the tympanic membrane rigid and reduces the middle ear's admittance at the membrane to zero, any admittance at the tip of the probe made with such a pressure load on the membrane will be due solely to the elasticity of the air in the ear canal (let us call this A_c). If a second measurement is made when all the stress is removed from the tympanic membrane by exactly equalizing the two pressures, then the admittance at the tip of the probe is the arithmetic sum of the ear canal admittance (for the same volume of air is present between the probe tip and the tympanic membrane as when the membrane is stiffened) and the admittance of the middle ear (A_{me}), i.e. $A_c + A_{me}$. Hence the admittance of the middle ear alone can be derived by subtracting the first measured admittance from the second.

Most commercially available tympanometric instruments express admittance in terms of 'compliance' which, although only one component of the complex acoustic admittance, is a reasonable approximation at the low probe frequencies employed in these instruments. Compliance is expressed in terms of the volume of a cavity that has the same compliance as the ear. The median value of compliance measured at the tympanic membrane is approximately 0.7 ml. The range for normal ears is 0.5–2 times this value (i.e. 0.35–1.4 ml) (Brooks, 1969; Jerger, Jerger and Mauldin, 1972).

The technique of tympanometry transforms a possible disadvantage to a considerable diagnostic asset. It was indicated above that even a small malfunction of the eustachian tube will considerably alter the admittance of the middle ear because of the increased tension induced in the tympanic membrane. If the admittance is observed while the pressure in the external canal is varied in a controlled manner, a maximum will be observed when the external canal pressure is identical with that in the middle ear, thus providing the observer with a measure of that pressure. In an ear with a normally functioning eustachian tube the peak admittance will be at, or very close to, atmospheric pressure and there will be no significant difference between the middle ear pressure and the ambient pressure (Figure 9.1, trace N). The normal range of middle ear pressure spans ± 50 mmH$_2$O.

If the eustachian tube is not functioning normally such that there is some absorption of gas from the middle ear, then the peak admittance will be at some slightly lower (negative) pressure (Figure 9.1, trace A).

If the middle ear is stiffened through some condition such as otosclerosis, then even when there is no pressure differential between the two sides of the tympanic membrane the admittance will be below

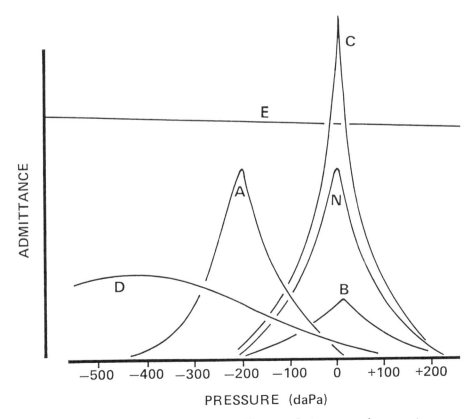

Figure 9.1 Typical tympanometry traces. N, normal; A, retracted tympanic membrane; B, otosclerosis; C, hypermobility; D, middle ear effusion; E, perforation of tympanic membrane.

normal (Figure 9.1, trace B). Typical values of compliance for otosclerosis are about one half to one third of normal.

Limitations of tympanometry

The diagnostic value of such an observation is limited. A number of conditions in addition to otosclerosis can reduce the mobility of the middle ear system, such as fibrosis or tympanosclerosis. The range of admittance values in subjects whose middle ears are classified as normal is very wide (as noted above). In practice there is a considerable overlap between the lower end of the admittance range for normal ears and the upper part of the range for ears with ossicular fixation. As a consequence of this, Browning, Swan and Gatehouse (1985) suggest that tympanometry has little value in the diagnosis of otosclerosis. Similar limitations apply in considering the diagnostic potential of high admittance values (Figure 9.1, trace C). These may occasionally arise from ossicular discontinuity, but are more likely to be caused by thinning of the tympanic membrane, perhaps as a result of long standing middle ear effusion. Again, it is difficult to separate pathological change from the upper range of normality.

Even when a tympanogram indicates admittance near the middle of the normal range, it cannot be assumed that the middle ear is completely normal. It is possible for two (or more) conditions to co-exist in the same ear, one tending to reduce the compliance (such as otosclerosis) and another tending to raise the admittance (for example thin patches on the tympanic membrane). The net result may be a tympanogram that appears to be normal in shape and magnitude.

The flat tympanogram

One type of tympanogram has very considerable diagnostic potential, especially in children. This is the shallow flat curve with an admittance maximum at a markedly reduced middle ear pressure (Figure 9.1, trace D). In adults such a curve may result from a combination of two or more conditions, but in children it is an almost certain indicator of OME. An almost flat tympanogram may result from a middle ear condition that produces extreme stiffness, but more commonly it is seen in ears where the tympanic membrane is perforated. In such a situation it is not possible to create a pressure differential across the membrane; any pressure change produced in the external canal is communicated instantaneously to the middle ear. When the tympanic membrane is perforated the admittance value observed tends to be abnormally high because the probe is looking into a much larger cavity than normal. The ear canal volume is directly coupled to the middle ear and hence the admittance is the sum of the two volumes (Figure 9.1, trace E). The same type of tympanogram will be produced if the perforation is artificial (i.e. a grommet), provided that it is patent.

Measuring effectiveness of grommets

Tympanometry can be of assistance in monitoring the effectiveness of grommets. If the grommet is performing the function for which it was inserted, the tympanogram will be almost flat and the static volume will be high. In some individuals with grommets or perforated tympanic membrane it may be difficult to establish a positive pressure in the ear canal because the eustachian tube opens and vents into the nasopharynx. To obtain a measure of the static volume in such circumstances it may be necessary to change to a negative pressure in the ear canal to 'seal' the eustachian tube. The inability to maintain a positive pressure in the system, assuming this is not due to a poorly sealed probe, provides some information about the functional capacity of the eustachian tube (see later).

If the grommet is not functioning properly a range of different tympanograms may be produced.

- With an occluded grommet the tympanic membrane will function like an intact membrane. If middle ear effusion is present, a flat tympanogram will result, but if the middle ear has largely recovered, a normal or near normal tympanogram will probably be produced.
- If the eustachian tube is still a little sluggish the tympanogram may be of normal shape but displaced towards the side of negative pressure.
- Should the grommet have been extruded and the tympanic membrane healed, then similar patterns will be obtained as with an occluded grommet.
- If the grommet has been extruded but the tympanic membrane has not healed patterns as for a perforated membrane will be obtained.

Several attempts have been made to introduce classification and measurement into tympanometry (Brooks, 1969; Jerger, 1970; Liden, Peterson and Bjorkman, 1970; Beery et al., 1975). Such classifications are particularly valuable in research and in the design of algorithms for screening for specific conditions such as middle ear effusion in children. They are helpful to the enthusiastic clinician who wishes to record the middle ear status and monitor the progression of a condition during or after treatment. However, they are not essential, provided that the individual performing the tympanometry understands the basis of the procedure and the significance of the curve shapes.

Middle ear muscle reflex measurement

Attention was drawn above to the fact that when a normally functioning ear is stimulated with a loud sound, the stapedius muscle contracts,
stiffening the tympanic membrane, with a resultant decrease in the
observed admittance. Observation of the response, or absence of
response, of the stapedius muscle to acoustic stimulation has considerable diagnostic value.

Presence versus absence of response

The stapedius is a tiny, weak muscle. Almost any disorder of consequence in the middle ear results in suppression of the muscular contraction or stiffening of the system so that any elicited change in
admittance is so small as to be undetectable. Hence a detectable
change in admittance when the ear is stimulated by an appropriate
acoustic stimulus strongly suggests that it is free from significant malfunction. In normal ears the stapedius reflex threshold in the frequency
range 250–4000 Hz lies between 80 and 85 dB HL. A mid-frequency
tone of 90–100 dB may thus be regarded as appropriate for determining the normality of the middle ear by elicitation of a stapedius muscle
reflex.

Absence of a stapedius reflex response to acoustic stimulation
should not, however, be regarded as indicative of some dysfunction. A
small percentage of otherwise normal ears do not produce stapedius
muscle contractions to acoustic stimulation. They may have sub-clinical
changes that inhibit the response, or the muscle may be absent.

Acoustic reflex threshold (ART)

The loudness of the stimulus appears to be the primary factor in initiat-
ing the stapedial response. In normally hearing individuals the intensity of the stimulus required to elicit a reflex is about 85 dB re threshold
of hearing. In some individuals with sensorineural hearing loss the ART
lies much closer to hearing threshold: the loudness for triggering the
muscle contraction appears to be attained with a smaller than normal
increase in intensity. This abnormally rapid increase in loudness relative to intensity is, if not identical to, closely akin to recruitment of
loudness. As long ago as 1952 Metz stated that if the difference
between auditory threshold and ART was less than 60 dB this suggested
the presence of recruitment in the ear to which the tonal stimulus was
being applied. The measurement of recruitment is of limited value in
diagnostic terms but may be useful in hearing aid fitting to ensure that
comfort levels are not grossly exceeded.

Acoustic reflex decay (ARD)

If a normal ear is stimulated with a tone 10 dB above the ART, the stapedius muscle contracts and remains contracted as long as the stimulus is present, provided that this period does not exceed a few minutes. With retrocochlear disorders the pattern of response of the muscle is frequently altered. The threshold of stimulus required to produce a contraction may be elevated, possibly beyond the output of the audiometer. In individuals in whom a stapedius response can be obtained, and in whom a stimulus of ART + 10 dB can be employed, the temporal pattern of the response, as monitored by the decrease in admittance, may be abnormal. Instead of the muscle remaining contracted, it relaxes, occasionally within a few seconds. Presumably this relaxation is due to a progressive reduction in the loudness of the tone despite the intensity remaining constant – a form of tone decay. The ARD test is simple to perform and has one of the best correlations with nerve VIII pathology of any of the regularly employed audiological tests (Stach, 1987).

Alerting to possible non-organic hearing loss

Non-organic hearing loss is not uncommon in children, though less so in pre-school children. The acoustic reflex may assist in determining if an apparent hearing loss is genuine. A gap between the given threshold of hearing and ART of 25 dB or less suggests a moderate or severe sensorineural hearing loss (in which situation one would expect confirmatory findings) or, in the absence of such indicators, a non-organic hearing loss.

Assessment of hearing level

Attention has already been drawn to the fact that in normally hearing subjects the ART is about 80–85 dB HL for pure tone stimuli. If instead of using a pure tone as stimulus a broad-band noise is used, the ART is found to be about 60–65 dB HL, a reduction of 20–25 dB. Niemeyer and Sesterhenn (1974) studied the use of different stimuli in subjects with varying degrees of hearing impairment and noted that the gap between ART for pure tones and for broad-band noise decreased as the degree of hearing impairment increased. They suggested that by measuring this difference in threshold between the average ART for pure tones (500, 1000, 2000 and 4000 Hz) and for white noise an estimate of the threshold of hearing could be made. On a test sample of over 200 subjects around three-quarters of the threshold estimates made using this procedure were within 10 dB of the true thresholds. However, this technique provided only an approximation to the average hearing level and no frequency-specific information. Jerger et al. (1974) modified the procedure using high and low pass noise bands as stimuli instead of (or in addition to) the broad-band noise stimulus. They further suggested that a classification of hearing loss according to need and forms of treatment available was needed. The results of their test, the sensitivity prediction from the acoustic reflex (SPAR) test, on 1156 subjects, predominantly adult, indicated that it was reasonably accurate at classifying average hearing loss into the broad groups of normal hearing, mild/moderate, severe or profound hearing loss. Serious classification errors (two categories misplaced) were present in only a small percentage and these tended to over- rather than under-estimate the degree of loss, a less serious type of error. The use of band noise contributed only marginal information about audiogram shape.

A considerably more accurate technique, devised by Sesterhenn and Breuninger (1977), depended on eliciting the acoustic reflex by pure tones either singly or in combination. By this means frequency-specific thresholds could be derived, but to obtain the high level of accuracy required multiple stimulations at each frequency and frequency combination (Brooks and Ghosh, 1982). This made the procedure very lengthy, and hence generally unsuitable for children or those unable to provide behavioural thresholds of hearing.

Eustachian tube function assessment

Tympanometry provides an indication of the functional capability of the eustachian tube. If the pressure in the middle ear, as indicated by the peak of the tympanogram, lies at or near normal, it is reasonable to assume that the tube is functioning within normal limits. If the tympanogram has normal shape and height but is displaced in the direction of reduced middle ear pressure, it can be concluded that the tube is functioning imperfectly, the degree of dysfunction being indicated to some extent by the degree of negativity of the tympanogram peak.

Poorly functioning eustachian tube

A flat tympanogram is highly suggestive of fluid in the middle ear, especially in children. Frequently this indicates a poorly functioning eustachian tube; occasionally the tube is functioning correctly but the fluid is so viscous that the cilia are unable to clear it from the middle ear space.

Further assessment of tubal function is possible if the subject can be persuaded to perform the Valsalva or Toynbee manoeuvres. Tympanograms performed before and immediately after such operations will show a change in the middle ear pressure if the eustachian tube is functioning correctly and the manoeuvre has been successfully completed. An unchanged tympanogram is suggestive of diminished tubal function, but may be due to the inability or unwillingness of the subject to carry through the procedure.

Patent eustachian tube

A patent eustachian tube is rarer than an under-functioning one. It can be consequential on a long period of middle ear effusion. The subject may complain that his or her voice creates an 'echo' as they speak, a phenomenon otherwise known as autophonia. The open eustachian tube is usually very easy to observe with an admittance measuring system. The pressure in the nasopharynx rises and falls with expiration and inspiration, and these pressure changes are transmitted to the middle ear via the open eustachian tube. Thus the inside of the tympanic membrane is now subject to a slowly varying pressure which increases and decreases the tension of the radial fibres and hence produces a cyclical change in the admittance of the tympanic membrane. This is indicated either visually or on a recording by the admittance system. The slow respiration-synchronous admittance change resulting from an open eustachian tube should not be confused with the faster pulse-synchronous admittance change seen in some perfectly normal ears, but more frequently in conditions with an inflamed tympanic membrane, such as in acute otitis media. In extremely rare cases the pulse-synchronous admittance change may indicate a glomus tumour. Confirmation will probably be obtained by direct visualization, a pulsing red 'rising sun' being seen on the tympanic membrane.

Perforated tympanic membrane

The indications of eustachian tube function above are all related to an intact tympanic membrane. If the membrane is perforated tympanometry is of little value, but some useful information may still be obtained about the functioning of the eustachian tube. Physiologically the eustachian tube opens against a slight negative pressure in the middle ear relative to the nasopharynx, this being brought about by gas absorption in the middle ear. The function of the eustachian tube can be tested by establishing a negative pressure of, say, -200 mmH$_2$O in the ear canal and then asking the subject to swallow. Ability to equalize the pressure in a few swallows indicates substantially normal eustachian tube function. If negative pressure cannot be equalized, then a positive pressure may be tried. As noted before, in some ears it is not possible to establish any degree of positive pressure as the eustachian tube opens and equalizes. This is indicative of some degree of function even though it is not as good as in those case in which negative pressure can be equalized. Inability to equalize positive pressures even when swallowing suggests a poorly functioning eustachian tube.

Alternative acoustical techniques for evaluation of auditory function

Acoustic reflectometry

To perform tympanometry it is essential to obtain an airtight seal of the probe in the ear canal. Occasionally this can be difficult, due to the shape of the external meatus or because the child's head cannot be held still for long enough. In an effort to overcome the latter difficulty as well as to produce a simple, low-cost device for evaluating middle ear function, Teele and Teele (1984) devised the Acoustic Otoscope. Although this is described as a new instrument, its principle of operation dates back to the very first attempts at acoustic examination of the ear by August Lucae, being based on quarter wavelength cancellation.

A miniature loudspeaker in the instrument probe (which is placed as close as possible to the entrance to the ear canal) emits a burst of sound that sweeps from 2000 Hz to 5000 Hz in the space of 0.1 s. A microphone in the probe measures the sound pressure level at the mouth of the meatus. This will be a summation of the incident sound wave and the sound wave reflected from the tympanic membrane. If the tympanic membrane is normally absorbent there will be little reflection and the sound pressure level will be around 80 dB SPL. If the membrane is rigid there will be substantial reflection. At the frequency for which the canal length is one-quarter of a wavelength the reflected signal, being one-half wavelength different from the incident signal, will cancel substantially. There will be a nadir in sound pressure.

Two measurements can be made by this means:

- the frequency at which the cancellation occurs can be used to derive the length of the ear canal. If this appears to be abnormally short the canal is probably occluded with wax;
- the degree of cancellation at the quarter wavelength frequency is evaluated, this being low where there is a normally absorbent tympanic membrane and even lower if it is flaccid. By contrast, cancellation is almost complete where the membrane is rigid, as in the presence of middle ear effusion.

Teele and Teele (1984) derived values for sensitivity and specificity with respect to middle ear effusion of 94% and 79% respectively on 190 ears of 160 children aged from 7 days to 13 years. Schwartz and Schwartz (1987) tested 511 ears of 256 children ranging in age from 2 months to 14 years (mean age 4 years) and obtained 88% sensitivity and 83% specificity. Tomlin and Nolan (1989) obtained sensitivities of 91% in children under 5 years of age, falling to 76% in those over 5. Their specificity was 84% in the under fives but rose to 97% in the older group. The accuracy overall in terms of detection of middle ear effusion is not markedly different from that of acoustic admittance measurement, especially in patients under 5 years.

As Teele and Teele suggest, the acoustic reflectometer is a valuable adjunct to the other tools employed in the paediatric diagnostic clinic. It does not provide as much detailed information as admittance measurement (for example it tells little about eustachian tube function), but it may be employed in situations where admittance measurement is impracticable or of dubious accuracy, such as the hyperactive child or the infant under 6/7 months of age where tympanometry may be misleading (Paradise, Smith and Bluestone, 1976)

Tympanic membrane displacement

This technique is a new and interesting development (Marchbanks and Martin, 1984). A probe is hermetically sealed into the ear canal of the subject and is connected to a cavity containing a reference diaphragm which is servo-controlled to keep the pressure in the closed system constant. Any movement of the tympanic membrane is compensated almost instantaneously by the diaphragm, the movement of which is therefore identical to the movement of the membrane. Active eustachian tubal function (such as when swallowing) can be assessed in this way, as can movement of the tympanic membrane brought about by contraction of the stapedius muscle.

The presence of subclinical middle ear conditions may affect the mode of action of the stapes under stapedius muscle contraction, providing an early test for potential disorders of the middle ear. The mode of action of the stapes will also be affected by changes in the inner ear fluid pressures. Tympanic membrane displacement has been used to observe and monitor cerebrospinal fluid pressure in children with hydrocephalus, thereby checking the functioning of the shunt valve mechanism. However, at present this technique is largely a research tool rather than a clinically available option.

Test strategy

Two fundamentally different, clinically practicable, methods of acoustical assessment of auditory function have been considered: acoustic admittance measurement and acoustic reflectometry. For the latter only one instrument is commercially available, but for the former there are many different devices.

Some are, or can be, manually controlled; that is, the pressure in the external ear canal can be adjusted and monitored under the control of the operator, as may the stimuli for eliciting the acoustic reflex. To gather the information desired may, with such instrumentation, take 1 or 2 min. At the other extreme there are instruments where the whole test process is microprocessor controlled, even to self starting the pressure sweep when a hermetic seal has been obtained and testing for stapedius muscle function with one or more tone bursts at predetermined levels. The whole test procedure may be completed in as little as 10 or 15 seconds. However, with automatic tone-burst presentation it may be difficult to be sure that the response indicated by the instrument is a genuine response to the tone and not an adventitious movement response such as a startle. With manual control of the stimulus the length of the tone-burst can be varied so that the observer can check and, if necessary, re-check that there is a definite time-locked 'on' and 'off' response to the stimulus. In other words, there are horses for courses.

If one has the luxury of time (i.e. if the patient is patient and cooperative) use of an instrument which allows the tester personal control over the measurement procedures and stimulus presentations may be preferable. A soft tipped probe inserted into the ear canal leaves the operator both hands free for use. If so desired several measurements can be made. Dubious tympanograms can be repeated to see if the shape is consistently reproduced. Stapedius muscle responses can be assessed with different stimuli and over a range of intensities.

In contrast, if the subject is very active and the time available for testing very limited, then a high-speed response system may be preferable: some results are better than none. Acoustic reflectometry can give useful information in seconds.

Some automatic admittance measurement systems also take only a few seconds to acquire, store and display or print the test results, but such results must be treated with a degree of caution. As noted above, indications of a stapedius muscle reflex response may be spurious, especially if there is only a single positive indication at the highest stimulus level for one frequency. A false flat tympanogram may be obtained in a normal ear due to the tip of the probe sealing against the wall of the ear canal or to collapse of the canal under the pressure of the operator's hand. Ideally the instrument should abort the test under such circumstances, but now and again a misleading tympanogram is produced. A clue to this type of error may be the indication of a very small ear canal volume. Changing the size of the probe tip and using lighter pressure to obtain an acoustic seal can help resolve such problems.

An astute clinician will be suspicious when there is an apparent inconsistency between the audiometric and admittance test results. In any situation where there is doubt as to the accuracy of the instrumental readout a repeat test should help to clarify the situation. Reproducible tympanograms and repeated stapedius muscle responses at the same level suggest that the response is genuine: inconsistency suggests spurious responses.

The three aspects of admittance measurement (tympanometry, reflex measurement and eustachian tube function testing) have, to some extent, been considered in isolation. In practice the first two (and to a lesser extent the third) should be seen as complementary. Each may contribute to the overall picture and the contributions should be harmonious, not contradictory. For example, in an ear with the middle ear filled with effusion the tympanogram will usually be either a very shallow curve or almost flat. Because of the loading effect of the fluid, stapedius reflexes are absent. If, therefore, the test instrument indicates a possible reflex, the findings should be regarded as suspicious: there is a strong probability that the tympanogram is wrong or that the reflex is spurious.

There should similarly be consistency between admittance data and audiometric test results. Better bone than air conduction thresholds are usually regarded as indicative of a conductive loss, although some difference is not unexpected due to the variation in thickness of subcutaneous tissue and headband pressure. Almost any mechanical lesion in the middle ear is sufficient to inhibit detection of the stapedius reflex. Consequently, if an acoustic reflex is observed as a response to either ipsi- or contralateral acoustic stimulation in an ear with a significant air–bone gap, careful thought should be given to how the (possible) contradiction can be resolved. Lutman (1984) investigated the relationship between air–bone gaps and acoustic reflex presence/absence in 1725 ears and stated that: 'clearly, acoustic reflex presence is a more sensitive indicator of middle ear disorder than air–bone gap measurement'. On this basis, the presence of a reflex would suggest that the air–bone gap was not truly representative of a significant conductive lesion, a conclusion that would be reinforced if the tympanogram was of normal shape and indicative of normal middle ear pressure.

In the clinical situation information is obtained primarily from the case history and physical examination. If there is any suspicion at all about the hearing or the status of the middle ear, admittance testing should be carried out, as it may reveal conditions not otherwise evident.

The most prevalent form of auditory dysfunction in infants and young children is OME. A number of studies (e.g. Brownlee et al., 1969; Howie, Ploussard and Sloyer, 1975) indicate that most children have had at least one bout of OME by the age of 2 years. Downs (1975) estimates that the probable net prevalence of middle ear disease in children from birth to 6 years of age is in the range of 20–30%. However, the condition is easily overlooked: it may give little indication on otoscopy and is not usually accompanied by discomfort or pain. Although in most children the condition is transient and appears not to lead to any significantly adverse consequences, in a small percentage it may give rise to educational or behavioural difficulties. Admittance measurement is the most sensitive method for detection of OME.

Summary

The classical methods of evaluating auditory function, otoscopy and tonal assessment by tuning forks or audiometry, even when augmented by a good case history, frequently do not contribute enough information to enable the clinician to make a clear-cut diagnosis. Measurement of the transmission/reflection characteristics of the ear as seen at the tympanic membrane can contribute considerable additional information about conditions within and medial to the middle ear. Observation of changes in the acoustic performance characteristics when the middle ear muscles are stimulated will add further information, not only about the middle ear but also about the mechanics and innervation of the cochlea and auditory pathways.

Current methods of assessing the physico-acoustical properties of the auditory system require only passive participation by the subject and hence are applicable to the very young and to those who either can not or will not cooperate in hearing testing. In combination with the traditional methods for examination of the auditory system these newer techniques enable the swift and accurate diagnosis of most auditory problems.

References

Beery, Q.C., Bluestone, C.D., Andrus, W.S. and Cantekin, E. (1975). Tympanometry pattern classification in relation to middle ear effusions. *Annals of Otology, Rhinology and Laryngology* 84, 56–64.

Brooks, D.N. (1969). The use of the electroacoustic impedance bridge in the assessment of middle ear function. *International Audiology* 8, 563–569.

Brooks, D.N. and Ghosh, A. (1982). Assessment of hearing level by means of the acoustic reflex. *Ear and Hearing* 3, 320–324.

Browning, G.G., Swan, I.R.C. and Chew, K.K. (1989). Clinical role of informal tests of hearing. *Journal of Laryngology and Otology* 103, 7–11.

Browning, G.G., Swan, I.R.C. and Gatehouse, S. (1985). The doubtful value of tympanometry in the diagnosis of otosclerosis. *Journal of Laryngology and Otology* 99, 545–547.

Brownlee, R.C., DeLoache, R.W., Cowan, C.C. and Jackson, H.P. (1969). Otitis media in children: Incidence, treatment and prognosis in pediatric practice. *Journal of Pediatrics* 75, 636–642.

Davis, H and Silverman, S.R. (1970). *Hearing and Deafness*, 3rd edn. New York: Holt, Rinehart and Winston.

Downs, M.P. (1975). Hearing loss: definition, epidemiology and prevention. *Public Health Review* 4, 255–277.

Feldmann, H. (1970). A history of audiology. *Translations of the Beltone Institute for Hearing Research* No.22.

Howie, V.M., Ploussard, J.H. and Sloyer, J. (1975). The 'Otitis-prone' condition. *American Journal of the Disabled Child* 129, 676–678.

Jerger, J. (1970). Clinical experience with impedance audiometry. *Archives of Otolaryngology* 92, 311–324.

Jerger, J., Jerger, S. and Mauldin, L. (1972). Studies in impedance audiometry I: Normal and sensorineural ears. *Archives of Otolaryngology* **96**, 513–523.

Jerger, J., Burney, P., Mauldin, L. and Crump, B. (1974). Predicting hearing loss from the acoustic reflex. *Journal of Speech and Hearing Disorders* **39**, 11–22.

Karma, P.H., Penttilä, M.A., Sipilä, M.M. and Kataja, M.J. (1989). Otoscopic diagnosis of middle ear effusion in acute and non-acute otitis media. 1. The value of different otoscopic findings. *International Journal of Pediatric Otorhinolaryngology* **17**, 37–49.

Liden, G., Peterson, J. and Bjorkman, G. (1970). Tympanometry. *Archives of Otolaryngology* **92**, 248–257.

Lucae, A. (1867). Ueber eine neue Method zur Unterzuchung des Gehoerorgans zu physiologischen und diagnostichen Zwecken mit Hulfe des Interferenz-Otoscopes. *Archiv für Ohren, Nasen und Kehlkopfheilkunde* **3**, 186–200.

Lutman, M.E. (1984). The relationship between acoustic reflex threshold and air–bone gap. *British Journal of Audiology* **18**, 223–229.

Marchbanks, R.J. and Martin, A.M. (1984). Theoretical and experimental evaluation of the diagnostic potential of the TMD measuring system. *Memorandum of the Institute of Sound and Vibration Research* No. 652.

Margolis, C.Z., Porter, B., Barnoon, S. and Pilpel, D. (1979). Reliability of middle ear examination. *Israel Journal of Medical Science* **15**, 23–28.

Mawson, S.R. (1967). *Diseases of the Ear*, 2nd edn. London: Edward Arnold.

Metz, O. (1952). Threshold of reflex contractions of muscles of the middle ear and recruitment of loudness. *Archives of Otolaryngology* **55**, 536–543.

Niemeyer, W. and Sesterhenn, G. (1974). Calculating the hearing threshold from the stapedius reflex threshold for different sound stimuli. *Audiology* **13**, 421–427.

Paradise, J.L., Smith, C.G. and Bluestone, C.D. (1976). Tympanometric detection of middle ear effusion in infants and young children. *Pediatrics* **58**, 198–210.

Renvall, U. and Holmberg, K. (1981). Daignostik av Otosalpingit. *Astra Nytt* **8**, 2–3. Sodertalje, Sweden: Astra Pharmaceuticals.

Roeser, R.J., Soh, J., Dunckel, D.C. and Adams, R. (1977). Comparison of tympanometry and otoscopy in establishing pass/fail referral criteria. *Journal of the American Audiological Society* **3**, 20–25.

Schwartz, D.M. and Schwartz R.H. (1987). Validity of acoustic reflectometry in detecting middle ear effusion. *Journal of Pediatrics* **79**, 739–742.

Sesterhenn, G. and Breuninger, H. (1977). Determination of hearing threshold for single frequencies from the acoustic reflex. *Audiology* **16**, 201–214.

Shallop, J.K. (1976). The historical development of the study of middle ear function. In: Feldman, A.S. and Wilber, L.A. (Eds), *Acoustic Impedance and Admittance – The Measurement of Middle Ear Function*, pp. 8–48. Baltimore: Williams and Wilkins.

Stach, B.A. (1987). The acoustic reflex in diagnostic audiology: from Metz to the present. *Ear and Hearing* **8** (suppl.), 36–42.

Teele, D.W. and Teele, J. (1984). Detection of middle ear effusion by acoustic reflectometry. In: Lim, D.J., Bluestone, C.D., Klein, J.O. and Nelson, J.D. (Eds), *Recent Advances in Otitis Media with Effusion*, pp.237–238. Philadelphia: B.C. Decker.

Tomlin, M.J. and Nolan, M. (1989). The detection of middle ear effusion using acoustic reflectometry. *Journal of the British Association of Teachers of the Deaf* **13**, 7–13.

Wever, E.G. and Lawrence, M. (1954). *Physiological Acoustics*. Princeton, NJ: Princeton University Press.

Chapter 10
Hearing aid systems

PHILIP I. P. EVANS

Introduction

A hearing aid is a device that processes sound in such a way as to make the information it conveys more accessible to the user. It should be seen as an integral part of the receptive communication chain, which includes the signal source and the listener. It should also be regarded as only one important part of a programme aimed at reducing the disability and handicap experienced by the hearing-impaired child. The hearing aid will not restore normal hearing, but optimum communication will be achieved only by the provision of the best available aid. Features of the communication processes that are likely to be most important to the user and the nature of the acoustic environment need to be considered when choosing the most appropriate type of aid. The extent of auditory impairment of the user and the integrity of his or her other sensory modalities will also influence the choice. When the hearing-impaired person is a young child, knowledge of his or her auditory, linguistic, physical and cognitive development and the family environment are important additional factors.

In the form with which most people are familiar, the hearing aid makes ambient sound louder across a limited frequency range. However, signal processing other than uniform linear amplification is necessary for most hearing-impaired children, because of the characteristics of their hearing losses and the conditions under which they will be likely to use their aids. Amplification may vary with frequency, to suit the audiometric configuration of the child or to limit the masking of informative sounds by ambient noise. Output limiting may be used to ensure that the output of the aid always lies within the child's dynamic range of hearing and does not exceed his or her loudness-discomfort level. It may be considered appropriate to amplify sounds preferentially from a particular direction or source (for example, a single speaker), to improve the detection and recognition of important sounds in background noise.

312

However, the signal processing need not be limited to providing the hearing-impaired child with an altered acoustic stimulus. Environmental aids can be chosen to signal specific environmental sounds (e.g. doorbell or telephone) to the child visually. Salient features of the acoustic environment, such as frequency and temporal information, can be presented to the child through vibrotactile stimulation. Direct electrical stimulation of the acoustic nerve can be used to produce auditory perception of important acoustic features. Each of these could be used to fulfil the aim of providing acoustic information to the hearing-impaired child in an optimum way; the last two are available as wearable devices and can accurately be termed 'hearing aids'. It is important that the audiologist should be sufficiently aware of the capabilities, limitations and requirements of the child in selecting the most appropriate device. Vibrotactile aids and electrical stimulating systems will be discussed briefly at the end of the chapter, but most of the subsequent discussion will concentrate on the electroacoustic hearing aid, which is by far the most common device fitted.

At a meeting of the British Society of Audiology in 1979, Poul Lyregaard described two concepts of the term 'hearing aid', each with different implications with regard to design features.

- A hearing aid could be seen as an auditory prosthesis, to help the hearing-impaired person to hear as normally as possible in a wide range of acoustic environments, with a minimum requirement for adjustment of the device by the user. Inevitably, such a device would tend to compromise by producing acceptable, but not optimum auditory perception in most circumstances. It was felt to be most suitable for people whose main requirement is not speech communication, who are generally in relatively quiet auditory environments, or who have physical or mental limitations that make manipulation of controls difficult.

- Lyregaard's alternative concept was of a communication aid, a device that allows the user to manipulate the acoustic environment to provide an optimum input to the disordered auditory system. Such an instrument was envisaged to include several user-accessible controls for altering the performance of the aid to extract the maximum acoustic information from the environment. This concept was seen to be more appropriate for hearing-impaired people with a special need for maximum speech recognition in various situations, often in adverse listening conditions, such as highly reverberant or noisy rooms: school children would be included in this group. Certainly, no observer of a school unit for hearing-impaired children can fail to be impressed by the competence and confidence with which the children manipulate their aids, including complicated radio aid systems, for maximum benefit.

With pre-school children, probably both types of aid will be needed at different times. Indeed, the clear distinction between the two types may not be appropriate. In infancy, auditory learning encompasses all types of acoustic stimuli, in situations that allow the child to develop an understanding of the relationship between sound and everyday events or activities. Speech is only one aspect of the acoustic environment, albeit an important one. The child needs to be provided with as 'natural' an auditory input as possible, without the necessity for (or the possibility of) frequent manipulation of controls. Thus, a prosthetic type of device seems appropriate at this age. The optimization of speech input is rarely an important requirement, as the child is usually spoken to from a close distance, in relatively good acoustic conditions. However, the aid should have an efficient output-limiting or noise-reduction device (preferably functioning automatically) to prevent excessive amplification when the child is in noisy environments such as a busy street. For the older pre-school child, accurate speech recognition becomes increasingly important and the child is more likely to be involved in speech-centred activities in poor acoustic conditions (e.g. listening to stories in a playgroup or nursery). In addition, the child will gradually be able to take more responsibility for manipulating the controls of the aid, including those which optimize its performance. At this stage Lyregaard's 'speech communication aid' may be the more appropriate provision, although the child must still have the opportunity of exposure to the general auditory environment. Again, there is a need for an adaptable aid.

The ideal requirements for pre-school children are rarely available in existing aids. Presumably because of economic considerations, most aids are a compromise between Lyregaard's two concepts. Probably the most satisfactory provision for the pre-school child is a hearing-aid system that provides general amplification of environmental sounds with basic output limitation, but has an optional facility for enhancement of speech recognition in difficult listening conditions. For instance, a child might be provided with a conventional personal hearing aid, with the facility for connecting a FM radio remote microphone system for use in a pre-school educational environment.

With a few notable exceptions, hearing aids are not designed with young children in mind, probably because they represent only a very small proportion of hearing-aid users. Many hearing aids are unacceptably bulky and heavy and are ergonomically unsuitable for young children. Controls are often too accessible and vulnerable to exploratory manipulation by infants, but are difficult for an older pre-school child to adjust accurately. Despite the availability of international standards (e.g. IEC, 1983e) the controls of many hearing aids lack clear markings to indicate their settings. While this may not be a serious problem for the adult user, it can cause considerable difficulties for the parent or teacher of a hearing-impaired child, who needs to ensure that the control settings are consistent. Ad hoc solutions to these inadequacies, such as marking the controls with a felt-tip pen or taping over them to prevent their being moved, are possible, but selection of more appropriate aids, where possible, would place greater pressure on manufacturers to provide better aids for children.

The hearing aid as a system

The instrumental provision that is made for the hearing-impaired child should be regarded as a system, comprising several components. The system as a whole must be effective and efficient, but each of the components should be chosen to be optimal for the child, as well as being well matched one with another. In some cases, components of a system have to be obtained from a single supplier: this has the advantage of ensuring compatibility and so may be preferable even when not essential. However, the selection of components from different suppliers allows updating of the system as technical advances in individual components occur.

The system may be relatively simple or quite complex. Figure 10.1 shows a schematic representation of a simple hearing aid, wholly worn by the user. It consists of:

- a microphone to detect the ambient sound;
- a variable amplifier;
- a receiver to convert the amplified electrical signal back to sound; and
- a battery to provide power to the amplifier.

The layout of the components in a typical post-aural hearing aid is shown in Figure 10.2.

Most hearing aids worn by children are considerably more complex,

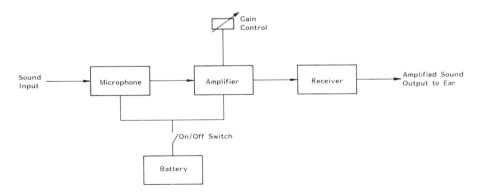

Figure 10.1 Schematic representation of a simple hearing aid.

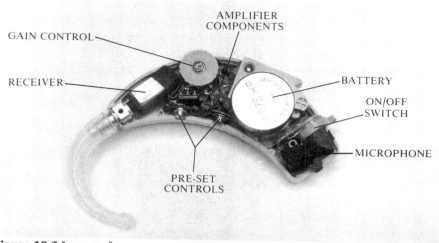

Figure 10.2 Layout of components in a typical post-aural hearing aid.

particularly in the educational context. Figure 10.3 depicts various possible components of a hearing aid system that may be fitted to a child. The enclosed area (b) includes elements that will normally be worn by the hearing aid user. In a post-aural aid the receiver is usually contained in the same case as the rest of the aid and is connected to an earmould by a plastic acoustic tube (Figure 10.4). The functions of the earmould are to retain the tip of the tube at the optimum position in the external meatus, to provide a secure fitting of the aid on the ear and to maintain an effective acoustic seal with the meatal wall. With a body-worn aid fitting, the receiver is external to the body of the aid, being connected directly to the earmould by means of a spring clip and to the main unit by a flexible lead (Figure 10.5).

The controls shown in Figure 10.3 may include some that are accessible to the user (usually an on/off switch, a gain control and, perhaps, a tone control). Others are intended to be pre-set by the clinician and usually take the form of screwdriver-operated switches or potentiometers to alter the frequency gain characteristic and the maximum output of the aid.

The area delineated (a) in Figure 10.3 encompasses components that may be present in a system that uses a remote microphone to provide an optimum signal (usually speech) to the user in adverse listening conditions. The output of the microphone may be relayed to the child's aid by infra-red radiation or by radio-frequency or audio-frequency electromagnetic transmission. In the case of a radio system the child's FM radio receiver may be integral with or separate from the rest of the aid. Infra-red light detectors and audio-frequency electromagnetic coil detectors are almost always fitted into the same case as the rest of the aid. Thus, the concept of the hearing aid system is extended

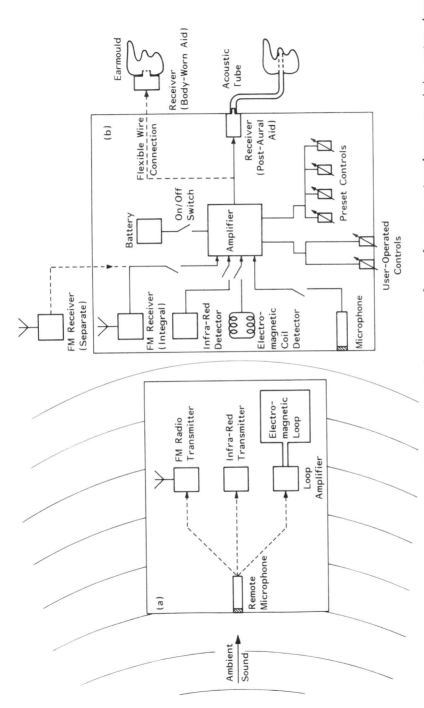

Figure 10.3 Possible components of a hearing aid system. Area (a) shows various forms of a remote microphone-transmission system. Area (b) encloses components which may be included in a single unit worn by the hearing aid user. The FM radio receiver and the audio-frequency receiver of the hearing aid may be worn separately from the main unit.

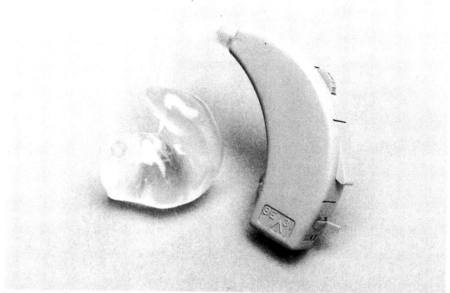

Figure 10.4 A typical post-aural hearing aid and earmould.

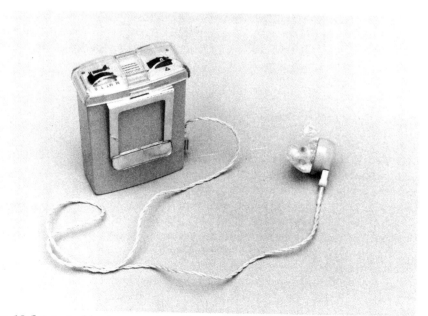

Figure 10.5 A typical body-worn aid with a separate receiver connected directly to the earmould. The retaining clip of the aid and the plastic cover, protecting the upwards-facing microphone and the controls, are both clearly visible.

to all components involved in the processing and transmission of acoustic information to the child. It should also include accessories such as the retaining clip of the body-worn aid and the pocket harness that may be worn by the child to hold the aid, as well as any covers provided to protect the microphone or pre-set controls from interference or damage. A fault in a single component will reduce the efficiency of the system and may impair or break the communication chain to the child. It is therefore imperative that the system is checked frequently and that any faulty component is replaced immediately.

Types of hearing aid systems

A wide range of hearing aid styles exists to meet the needs of most users, each with advantages and limitations when fitted to young children. It is only in recent years that hearing aid manufacturers have started to design aids with children in mind and the choice among these is limited. Many young children are still fitted with aids that are ergonomically unsuitable for them. Audiologists, teachers of deaf and partially hearing children and parents need to take account of the design inadequacies when planning performance monitoring and maintenance schedules for children's aids.

Post-aural aids

The post-aural or behind-the-ear aid is currently the most common style provided for hearing aid users in Britain, young and old alike. Miniaturization of components has produced a device which is relatively inconspicuous and, for adults and older children, convenient to use. The incorporation of all of the electronic components in a single unit makes it reasonably resistant to damage. Its circumaural placement puts the microphone close to the 'natural' position for auditory input. Binaural fitting with post-aural aids provides a close approximation to normal stereophonic stimulation, with its attendant theoretical advantages for directionalization of sound and signal detection in noise. However, the close proximity of the microphone to the receiver requires great care to be taken to ensure sufficient acoustic isolation to prevent feedback, particularly in aids with high levels of amplification. Development of components, in particular the electret microphone, has given the post-aural aid the potential for high gain over a wide frequency range. The performance of the aid can be manipulated by the incorporation of user-operated or preset controls and, in some cases, by substitution of different earhook tubes.

For young children, the fitting of post-aural aids presents difficulties. Despite miniaturization, many post-aural aids are too big and heavy to fit securely on the pinnae of infants. In young babies in particular, the problem is compounded by the 'floppiness' of the pinnae, because the cartilaginous tissue is not fully developed. This difficulty can be alleviated in most cases by selecting aids from the range of small, light models that have recently become available and in difficult cases it may be possible to tape the aid to the child's ear. Alternatively, proprietary retention loops are available to hold the aid in position. Unfortunately, increasing miniaturization has a drawback in making the controls less accessible and more difficult for parents to read and manipulate, particularly while their child is wearing the aid. Although the post-aural aid system is reasonably robust, it is prone to failure in various ways. A frequent problem is condensation, arising from the high humidity of the external meatus, blocking the acoustic tube connecting the aid to the child's earmould. This may be sufficiently controlled by drying the earmould overnight in a warm dry place, such as an airing cupboard (not a hot oven!). When the condensation is excessive, causing blockage of the acoustic tube, the earmould should be detached from the aid and blown through by miniature bellows (available from most hearing-aid suppliers) to clear the drops of moisture. The most common internal faults are likely to be corrosion of the battery terminals or control switches (hastened by the high humidity engendered by perspiration, particularly when the aid is covered by hair) and failure of the microphone suspension, usually caused by impact of the aid on a hard surface. The former will cause increased electrical noise interference or intermittent function. Damage to the microphone suspension will give rise to increased distortion of the amplified sound or internal acoustic feedback.

Body-worn aids

Body-worn aids no longer have any significant acoustic advantages over post-aural aids. However, some very young hearing-impaired children are fitted with body-worn aids, usually because they are considered to be more secure. The aid is placed in pockets in a harness which the child wears on his or her chest. The position, together with the generally larger controls than those on post- aural aids, make them easier for parents to manage in the early stages after the initial fitting. Against this, there are a number of disadvantages to body-worn aids.

- Their placement on the baby's chest makes them susceptible to 'body-baffle', causing a relative low-frequency emphasis due to the absorption of high-frequency energy by the child's clothing and body tissues and the reflection of low-frequency energy back to the microphone.
- Before post-aural aids with extended low-frequency amplification were developed, the relative low-frequency emphasis of body-worn

aids was considered to be an advantage, particularly for severely deaf children, for whom low-frequency voicing components may be the only elements of the speech signal that they can detect, and may still be an advantage for profoundly deaf children, particularly with regard to hearing their own voices. However, the placement of the microphone on the child's chest makes it vulnerable to damage from spilt food, dribble and vomit.

- This problem is enhanced by the tendency for the microphone to be fitted into the top of the aid, rather than the front, in order to pick up the child's voice most effectively. To counteract this problem, manufacturers of body-worn aids usually provide a plastic cover to protect both the microphone aperture and the control switches, which are usually also placed on the top of the aid. This has the additional benefit of preventing the child from playing with or accidentally knocking the control switches. (A similar cover is available for some makes of post-aural aid to prevent controls being altered accidentally.) However, the cover cannot protect the flexible lead, which connects the receiver to the main unit of the body-worn aid and is highly vulnerable to damage.

- The most common cause of failure of this type of aid is loss of electrical continuity of the lead, usually due to a break at the junction with one of the plugs at either end. The most effective way of checking the integrity of the lead is to replace it with a new one. To minimize problems, it is important to use the correct lead as specified by the manufacturer and to ensure that it is properly fitted.

- Another problem with this type of aid is the size of the receiver itself. When fitted to an infant, it may be larger in diameter than the back-plate of the child's earmould and thereby abrade and irritate the pinna.

- Many receivers are too heavy to be supported adequately by the earmould in the flaccid pinna of a baby, with the result that the earmould tends to be pulled partly or wholly out of the meatus. Both this and the previous problem are solved in most cases by fitting a miniature receiver, but even this may be too large for a very young baby.

Bone-conduction aids

It may be difficult or impossible to fit a post-aural or body-worn aid to a child with abnormalities of the external ear:

- an absent or rudimentary pinna will preclude a post-aural fitting;
- the insertion of an earmould may be difficult in an unusually narrow or malformed external meatus;
- earmould insertion will obviously be impossible in a child with meatal atresia (absence of an external ear canal).

In such cases, a bone-conduction aid may be fitted to transmit sound energy to the cochlea by vibration of the skull and, hence, the otic capsule (Figure 10.6). Such an aid may also be useful in a child with a large conductive component in his or her hearing loss, or with persistent suppurative ear infections that prevent consistent use of an aid with a conventional earmould.

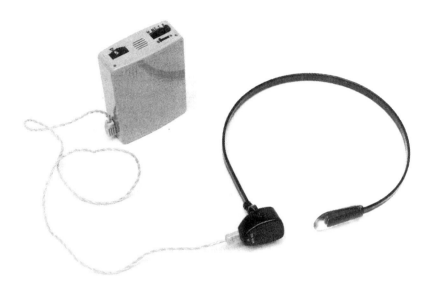

Figure 10.6 A typical bone-conduction aid.

Disadvantages

The interface of the transducer with the soft skin causes considerable distortion in the signal and the relatively large mass of the moving-coil transducer in the bone vibrator limits the output of the system because of the large amount of energy required to drive it. The latter limitation is, however, rarely a problem as the system is most frequently used in children with congenital conductive hearing loss and normal cochlear function. In such cases only minimal gain will be required.

More serious drawbacks are:

- lack of aesthetic appeal of the bone-vibrator fitting;
- physical discomfort;
- lack of firm connection; and
- difficulty in keeping the headband in place.

These lead many clinicians to prefer an air-conduction fitting, if it can be achieved, even with the large amount of gain often necessary for conductive losses. As congenital disorders of the middle and outer ears are often able to be improved by surgical treatment, bone-conduction aids are not often used.

Bone-anchored aids

Where long-term bone-conduction amplification is likely to be necessary, the option of a bone-anchored aid might be considered. In this, the transducer is fixed to the skull by titanium screws and activated by direct connection or by transcutaneous magnetic coupling to the body-worn amplifier. The device provides more reliable sound transmission, higher sound intensities and better sound quality than a conventional bone-conduction aid. Although pre-school children are considered as suitable candidates in some programmes, the need for surgery and the problems that limited skull-bone thickness and increasing skull size pose for the screwed attachment mean that bone-anchored aids are not usually provided for very young children.

Intra-aural aids

Intra-aural (or in-the-ear aids) fit wholly within the concha and ear canal. In the most extreme case, the intra-meatal aid is designed to be placed in the external meatus so that its flat end-plate, in which the microphone and volume control are fitted, lies flush with the meatal entrance. The close proximity of the microphone and receiver limit the available gain of intra-aural aids (because of the increased risk of acoustic feedback), so that they are suitable only for mild–moderate hearing losses. Although these aids are becoming increasingly popular with adult users, they are generally regarded as unsuitable for very young children. The need to replace the earmould for the growing child at intervals of 2–6 months makes the custom-made earmould casing of the intra-aural aid impractical. In addition, the controls of the aid would be difficult to see and inaccessible to parents and teachers when the child was wearing the aid. However, an intra-aural fitting can be useful for a child with a deformed or floppy pinna, which is unable to support a post-aural aid.

Spectacle aids

In these, the aid is incorporated into the spectacle frame and may be provided binaurally. Usually the output of the aid is delivered to the ear in the same way as with the post-aural aid, i.e. through an acoustic tube fitted into an earmould; alternatively a bone vibrator may be fitted into the tip of the spectacle frame, where it lies against the mastoid process, providing a neat solution when a bone-conduction aid is required.

However, neither version is commonly used with young children, because of the permanent linking of the aid to the spectacles, which may frequently need repair or replacement, if only because of the growth of the child.

Contralateral routing of signals (CROS) systems

In CROS systems the microphone and receiver are placed on opposite sides of the head. The basic system consists of two units, similar in appearance to a pair of post-aural aids. One of the units contains a microphone and amplifier, the other only a receiver. The two units may be linked by a flexible lead, or the output from the amplifier may be transmitted to the receiver by electromagnetic induction or FM radio. Such a system is used primarily in cases of unilateral or markedly asymmetrical hearing loss, to overcome the lack of sensitivity to sounds on the side of poorer hearing by amplifying and transmitting them to the better-hearing ear. Many variations of the basic system exist and the reader is referred to Hodgson (1981) for a description.

CROS systems are not often fitted to young children. Those with severe unilateral hearing loss are generally assumed to manage better without an aid, while the more complicated CROS systems are usually thought to be confusing for the child. It could be argued that young children are actually more suitable candidates for CROS aids than adults with acquired losses, as they learn faster and are more adaptable to new stimulus configurations: indeed, the most appropriate candidate may be the very young infant, who is assumed to be in the process of developing an auditory neural representation of the world. It is, perhaps, a fear that an 'incorrect' representation will be developed irreversibly by the child that limits the number of appropriate CROS fittings.

Remote microphone systems

Optimization of signal-to-noise ratio

In order that the child receives maximum benefit from the aid, it is important that the input signal-to-noise ratio should be maintained at the highest possible level, i.e. the intensity of the sound of interest (most commonly speech) should be well above that of the background noise. A hearing aid with a conventional integral microphone will amplify all environmental sounds indiscriminately and equally, within the limits of its frequency response.

Noise interferes with the detection and recognition of sounds that are important or useful to the child. Which sounds are important ('signals') and which are not ('noise') will depend partly upon the circumstances in which the child is using the aid. 'Background' environmental sounds may be important for the child's development of auditory awareness of the world, particularly if he or she is in a position to see or touch the sources of the sounds. The same environmental sounds may disrupt the child's perception of a single sound source of particular interest.

Noise may arise indirectly from the signal itself as well as from other sources. In many everyday environments, reverberation causes delayed 'echoes' by reflection of the signal off walls, ceiling, floor and other hard surfaces. The echoes reach the child's ear an appreciable time after the arrival of the sound along the shortest (direct) path and constitute noise with respect to subsequent elements of the signal. In addition to causing temporal confusion, the echoes have a masking effect upon signal components arriving at the same time by the direct path. Because of the longer travel path of the echoes and the higher absorptive capacity of air for high-frequency sounds, the echoes primarily comprise low-frequency energy, which may mask simultaneous softer sounds, with a tendency to a greater masking effect on high-frequency sounds. Where speech perception is concerned, this may cause weaker high-frequency components to be masked by low-frequency voiced sounds.

The masking effect of background noise is much greater for hearing-impaired people than for those with normal hearing. For example, speech recognition of all children is reduced in background noise, but markedly more so for those who are hearing impaired (Finitzo-Hieber and Tillman, 1978). The fitting of a conventional hearing aid does not improve matters and may cause a further deterioration of speech recognition in noise, especially if the amplification characteristics are not appropriate for the child's hearing loss. In addition, occlusion of the pinna by the earmould may cause a further small deterioration in signal recognition in background noise, because of resultant reduction in directionalization capability.

Several technical approaches to improving the signal-to-noise ratio in hearing aids exist. Their functions depend upon one of two principles:

1. Reducing the sensitivity of the system to sounds which are likely to constitute noise.
2. Selectively increasing the input level of sounds which are regarded as 'signals' (e.g. the voice of a relevant speaker).

One approach is to make use of a *remote microphone system*. The microphone is placed close to the preferred speaker to pick up speech without significant contamination by noise or reverberation effects. Figure 10.7 illustrates the signal-to-noise advantage offered by a remote microphone system. The signal is amplified and transmitted to the child through one of several means.

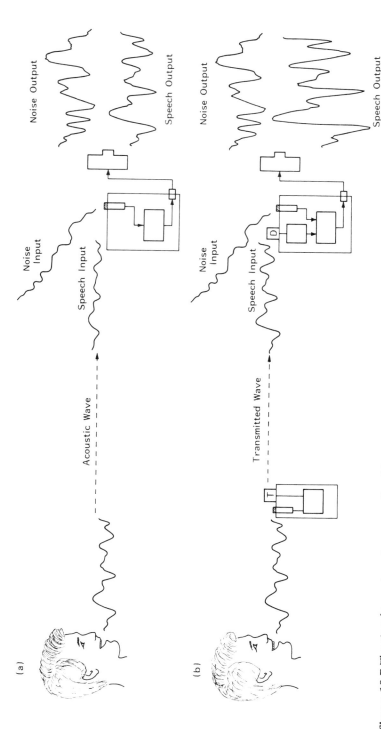

Figure 10.7 The signal-to-noise advantage offered by a remote-microphone system. In (a), the speech acoustic wave reduces in intensity as it travels through the air to the hearing-aid microphone. The amplified speech output is of a similar intensity to the amplified background noise. In (b), the low-gain remote microphone detects the speech with little noise contamination and the signal is passed to the transmitter (T). The transmitted signal is detected (D) and amplified by the child's hearing-aid system. The signal-to-noise ratio is substantially increased and may be further enhanced by switching off the environmental microphone(s) on the child's aid.

Until about 15 years ago, the most common systems were the hard-wired speech-training unit and group aid. The speech training unit is still favoured by some teachers and speech and language therapists when working with individual children, because of its excellent high-fidelity performance. Markides, Huntington and Kettlety (1980) demonstrated the superiority of the speech training unit (and the group aid, which is effectively a group of interconnected speech train-ing units), but pointed out the obvious restriction of movement caused by the physical connection. This disadvantage has led to the increasing use of alternative forms of remote microphone systems.

Electromagnetic induction

In this system the amplified output from the microphone activates a wire loop to create a fluctuating audio-frequency electromagnetic sig-nal within a specified area. Most conventional hearing aids are provid-ed with a switchable integral 'telecoil' (usually labelled 'T' on the function switch) to detect such a signal, sometimes with the optional simultaneous function of the environmental microphone (usually denoted 'MT'). The remote microphone may be connected directly to the loop amplifier, or a body-worn radio-microphone may be used to allow the speaker freedom of movement. British Standard BS 6083 (1981), which is technically equivalent to IEC (1981a), specifies the magnetic field strength required in loops for hearing aids and the Royal National Institute for the Deaf publishes a leaflet giving guidelines for the installation of induction loops (RNID, 1991).

Although the loop system is cheap and can be highly effective in reducing the adverse effects of environmental noise, it has several dis-advantages.

- The electromagnetic field tends to be uneven and can 'spill over' into adjacent areas to be detected by children operating outside the loop.
- The efficiency of the system depends partly on the orientation of the telecoil with respect to the loop, so that the strength of the induced signal may vary as the child's head moves.
- The telecoil will tend to pick up noise from other sources of electro-magnetic radiation, such as control equipment for fluorescent light-ing.
- Finally, the electromagnetic transduction process is sometimes found to cause a relative reduction in amplification at low frequen-cies, compared with its performance with the environmental micro-phone.

For these reasons, the loop system is now rarely used in school classrooms, although it is widely fitted in public halls, churches and theatres for the benefit of hearing-aid users. It offers little advantage for the hearing-impaired child at home, except for connection to the audio output of a television set to provide a low-noise condition for viewing.

Infra-red transmission

Infra-red transmission can be used in remote microphone systems. The output of the microphone is fed into an infra-red transmitter, which may be worn by the speaker. The child wears a unit that detects the infra-red transmission and provides an audio-frequency signal, usually for direct input to the child's hearing aids. The system avoids the spill-over disadvantage of the electromagnetic loop system as the infra-red signal is contained within the walls of the room. It is, however, susceptible to interference from strong sunlight and is therefore not suitable for use outside or in rooms with large windows that allow in a lot of direct sunlight. The body-worn transmitter also requires the speaker and the child to be facing each other for successful reception.

A variation of the system uses a set of transmitters, usually placed at the corners of the room to ensure complete and even coverage. The remote microphone may be free-standing instead of being worn by the speaker. However, this negates the system's advantage by allowing considerable interference from ambient noise and reverberation. Infra-red systems have not gained as much popularity in educational settings in the UK as in continental Europe but are increasingly being used in other applications, such as television listening aids and concert halls.

FM radio transmission

This is the most popular type of remote-microphone hearing-aid system for use with children in the UK. The amplified output of the remote microphone is transmitted to the child by frequency-modulated radio transmission. The radio receiver worn by the child may be integral with a hearing aid in a body-worn unit (Figure 10.8).

The hearing aid frequently has two independent channels, each with its own environmental microphone, in addition to the input from the FM receiver. Usually the environmental microphones and the radio receiver can be selected independently or can be operated together. The aid outputs are connected by wire to button receivers as in a conventional body-worn aid fitting. An alternative arrangement (Figure 10.9) is for the radio receiver to be worn separately, to allow the child to use conventional hearing aids (post-aural or body-worn) independently of the FM system. The connection between the radio receiver and the hearing aid(s) should preferably be made directly by wire (direct audio input).

Various types of plug and socket connections are employed in com-

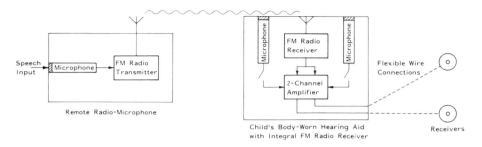

Figure 10.8 A radio/hearing-aid system in which the radio receiver and the hearing aid are in the same unit.

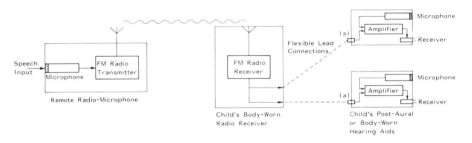

Figure 10.9 A radio/hearing aid system in which the radio receiver and the hearing aid(s) are worn separately by the child. The electrical input socket (a) will usually accept inputs from other electroacoustic devices.

mercial hearing aids. IEC (1984) specifies electrical characteristics for the electrical input circuits in hearing aids, but no mechanical characteristics are specified. Manufacturers have tended to use designs unique to their own systems.

The lead itself is also specific to each aid and it is essential that the correct lead is used or the gain of the system may vary from that specified.

The electrical input circuit of the hearing aid can also be used for direct connection of other devices such as radios, tape recorders or microphones. Some circuits provide a convenient means of incorporating the aid into a CROS system. The standard hearing aid range of the British National Health Service has recently been extended to include a medium-powered model (the BE 36) with direct audio input capability.

For aids that do not have a facility for direct connection to a FM radio system, indirect input is possible. Usually this takes the form of electromagnetic induction, with the aid's telecoil being activated by an electromagnetic field generated by a neck-worn loop connected by wire to the radio receiver. However, the technical problems discussed earlier for electromagnetic loop induction apply to this approach. For a young child, an FM system using direct or indirect connections to separate hearing aids is cumbersome and more liable to damage than one in which the radio receiver and hearing aids are contained in a single unit. Nevertheless, some audiologists and teachers prefer the flexibility of systems with separate components.

Advantages

FM radio transmission offers many advantages for use with young children, particularly in schools.

- It can operate over considerable distances (several hundred yards) with little or no hindrance from solid objects, so that the child is not constrained in a limited area.
- It is rarely subject to interference.
- Spillover or cross-talk between channels used by children engaged in different activities is avoided by the use of different transmission frequencies.

Currently five frequencies are designated for the sole use of FM radio hearing-aid systems in the UK and 15 more are available, though with a slight risk of interference from other types of radio microphone systems (DTI, 1986). In most systems, different frequencies can be selected by a simple change of an oscillator module and some allow the child to switch between the selected module frequency and another fixed frequency. This is useful in an educational environment, where one channel (the fixed frequency) can be common to all children in a group and each child can have his or her own channel for private communication with the teacher. The radio aid is an effective and convenient device for providing the child in school or nursery with high-quality speech input with minimum noise interference. In the UK, it is seen largely as an educational aid and is usually provided by the local education authority. Its advantage for the child at home is less clear, as signal-to-noise ratios are generally good and there are few competing speakers.

Disadvantages

It is important that the limitations and disadvantages of the system are understood, to avoid its abuse by parents and teachers.

- If the young infant is too often distant from the speaker or the source of an environmental sound that is clearly audible through a radio aid system, his or her audio-spatial awareness may be impaired.

- Parents need to be aware that a child using a radio aid cannot be relied upon to recognize warnings and instructions at a distance.
- The convenience of the system may also encourage some parents or teachers to disturb the child at play in an intrusive way that would not be possible if the child was not fitted with the radio aid system.

The system needs to be used thoughtfully and carefully.

Components of hearing aid systems

Microphone

Most hearing aids are fitted with integral microphones, and other forms of input were discussed in the previous section. The progressive miniaturization of hearing aids, together with the demand for high power output, has led to a requirement for a microphone with the following qualities:

- high sensitivity;
- small dimensions and low weight;
- flat frequency response;
- stability and robustness;
- low power requirement.

Such qualities are found in the electret microphone, which is now almost universally fitted to hearing aids. The microphone has a metallized, thin plastic diaphragm, supported on strips of permanently charged dielectric material (electrets), which forms a capacitor in conjunction with a metal backplate in which the electrets are fixed. Incoming sound waves cause the diaphragm to move relative to the backplate, thus changing the capacitance of the device and generating a small fluctuating voltage. A field-effect transistor (FET) amplifies the voltage and generates a current for input to the main amplifier. The response of the electret microphone is relatively flat over a wide frequency range (typically 200–7000 Hz) and the small mass of the diaphragm gives it high sensitivity to acoustic stimuli. At the same time, the device has a low sensitivity to mechanical vibration (e.g. due to movement of the wearer of the aid), is robust against physical damage and is largely unaffected by magnetic fields. This last property makes it particularly suitable for incorporation into miniature hearing aids, in close proximity to receivers.

Directionality

Most hearing-aid microphones are *omnidirectional*, i.e. they are more or less equally sensitive to sound from any direction. In order to improve the signal-to-noise ratio, *directional* microphones have been developed for post-aural aids to provide relatively greater sensitivity to sounds arriving from in front of the wearer than from other directions (Figure 10.10).

The directionality is achieved by providing a second port for entry of sound energy into the microphone behind the diaphragm. Lower sensitivity to sound arriving at the rear port, together with the incorporation of an acoustic delay in the travel time of sounds from the rear port to the diaphragm provides selective reduction in sensitivity to sounds from behind the user, through cancellation of the acoustic energy at

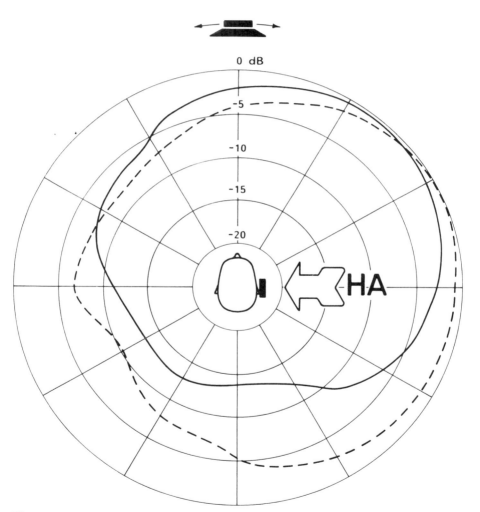

Figure 10.10 Typical relative sensitivity of a hearing aid with a directional microphone (—) compared with the same aid with an omnidirectional microphone (– –). (Redrawn by permission. Courtesy Oticon Ltd.)

the diaphragm. It should be noted that the extent of directionality specified by manufacturers, under laboratory conditions, is not always achieved in everyday use.

Placement

Placement of the microphone inlet is of some importance. In the post-aural aid the inlet may be at the top of the aid (facing forward) or at the bottom. Forward-facing microphones have slight directional advantages and give rise to small improvements in high-frequency amplification. They are all prone to wind noise, but manufacturers usually fit wind-shields to reduce the problem. The placement of the microphone in the body-worn aid has been discussed previously.

Amplifier

To meet the requirements of miniaturization and reduced costs, integrated circuits are increasingly being used for amplifiers in hearing aids. However, circuits using very small discrete components are still fitted in many aids, including the present National Health Service (NHS) standard range. Together, the NHS range and the various commercial aids cover the power requirements of all levels of hearing loss, with the most powerful aids using push–pull amplifiers. These are designed with two transistors in the output stage, operating in such a way as to maximize the current through the receiver. Both post-aural and body-worn aids are available with the capability for maximum output levels in excess of 140 dB SPL, suitable for the most profound hearing losses.

Control components

Most hearing aid amplifying circuits include components to allow the performance of the circuit to be altered.

- A volume (gain) control is nearly always provided to alter the amount of amplification by the amplifier.
- A tone control may be included to change the relative frequency response (the amount of amplification in various frequency regions).
- External controls might be available to allow the user to alter both of these functions.
- Many aids also have internal pre-set controls (usually altered by screwdriver) to allow the clinician or teacher to set limits within which the user may vary the performance of the aid.
- Another function often provided, but nearly always set by an internal control, is a form of output-limiter to prevent the output of the

aid exceeding a specified level (usually at or about the user's loudness discomfort level). Peak-clipping and compression amplification are two forms of output-limiting that are commonly used in hearing aids.

Peak clipping

In many hearing aids the amplification is linear and the amount of gain is independent of the input level. An increase in input level gives rise to a similar increase in output. However, a normal characteristic of amplifiers is that, above a certain input level, the output becomes constant. This non-linearity is called peak clipping, because its effect is to 'clip' the peaks and troughs of the amplified waveform (Figure 10.11).

The level at which peak clipping starts to occur can be designed into the hearing aid and a peak-clipping control allows the level to be varied. This is an effective method of limiting output, but has the disadvantage of introducing marked distortion into the output signal, giving rise to a noticeable 'roughness' in the sound quality.

Compression amplification

Output limiting may also be achieved by compression amplification, more properly termed automatic gain control (AGC). Walker and Dillon (1982) give an excellent review of the use of compression amplification in hearing aids. In a hearing-aid AGC amplifier the gain of the amplifier is varied automatically by a feedback loop which senses the magnitude of the signal at a particular point in the circuit. A generalized input–output curve of an AGC amplifier is shown in Figure 10.12. Above a certain input level (the lower AGC limit) the gain of the amplifier is reduced for increasing input level. The output level rises more slowly, eventually becoming almost constant at high input levels. The

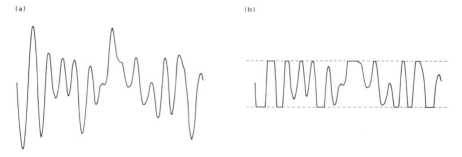

(a)   (b)

Figure 10.11 Peak-clipping of a waveform. When the amplified signal (a) exceeds the maximum amplitude output limits of the amplifier, shown by the dashed line in (b), the peaks and troughs of the waveform are 'clipped'.

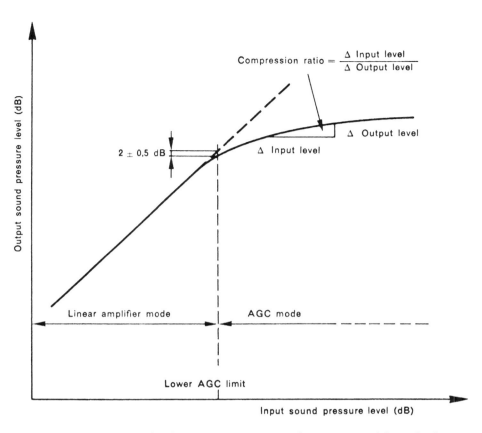

Figure 10.12 A generalized input–output curve of an AGC amplifier. The lower AGC limit is defined as the input sound pressure level which gives a reduction in the amplifier gain of 2 ± 0.5 dB with respect to the gain in the linear mode. (Source BS 6083, 1984.)

lower AGC limit is sometimes adjustable through an internal pre-set control.

The effect of AGC on the performance of the hearing aid depends partly upon the point in the circuit at which the signal level is monitored (Figure 10.13).

Input-controlled compression

In input-controlled compression the amplifier gain is dependent upon the signal level just before the user's gain (volume) control. Thus the maximum output of the aid is dependent on the setting of the volume control (Figure 10.14).

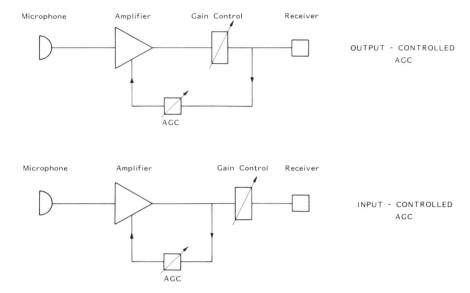

Figure 10.13 Schematic representation of output-controlled and input-controlled AGC circuits.

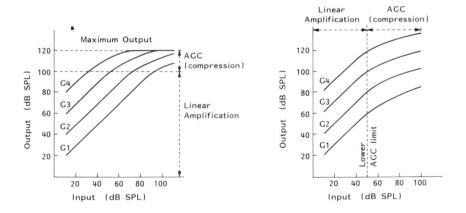

Figure 10.14 Effect of the gain control setting (G_1–G_4) on the maximum output of a hearing aid with output-controlled or input-controlled compression amplification (AGC).

Output-controlled compression

In output-controlled compression the signal level is monitored after the volume control. The setting of the volume control may influence the output indirectly (by modifying the amplifier gain through the feedback network), as well as directly through its attenuating function, but does not alter the pre-set maximum output of the aid.

Uses of compression amplification

Each of the two types of AGC circuit has advantages and disadvantages and is best suited for a particular requirement (Dillon and Walker, 1983).

One aim may be to maintain the output of the aid within a narrow range around the user's most comfortable listening level, in spite of widely varying input levels. This is most likely to be required for patients whose dynamic range of hearing is markedly restricted because of the effect of excessive loudness recruitment. In this case, input-controlled compression is preferable as the input signal to the user's gain control can be made to vary within a pre-determined narrow amplitude range, allowing the user to set the output to a preferred level, which may change with the type of listening task and the ambient conditions.

A second application of AGC can be to restrict the maximum output of the aid to a level which is below the loudness discomfort level of the user. In this case, output-controlled AGC is preferable. Input-controlled compression is probably more appropriate for the responsible older child, who will be able to adjust the aid to suit in various circumstances. Generally, the pre-school hearing-aid user cannot do this and there is a risk that the volume control may inadvertently be knocked by the child, causing the output of the aid to exceed the child's loudness-discomfort threshold when high input sound levels occur. Output-controlled compression is useful in preventing this, but a better alternative would be to fit an aid with both input-controlled compression and a maximum output control (usually a peak clipping device).

Limitations

Although compression amplification distorts the signal less than peak clipping, it is not without its limitations. The attack time and recovery time of the AGC circuit, at the onset and cessation respectively of a sound exceeding the lower AGC limit, must be carefully set. It is important to minimize the risk that the early part of a loud sound will be amplified excessively, while ensuring that transient stimuli do not trigger the AGC unnecessarily.

Similarly, abrupt release of the compression can be disconcerting for the user of the aid, but the reduced gain should not be prolonged to the extent that subsequent quiet sounds are not heard. This is particularly important when listening to speech, to avoid the suppression of soft unvoiced phonemes by the action of the compression circuit in response to louder voiced sounds. If this is a frequent problem, it suggests that the lower AGC limit is set too low. Walker and Dillon (1982) recommend an attack time in the range 0.5–20 ms and a recovery time of 60–150 ms.

Receiver

Electromagnetic receivers (earphones) are almost universally fitted in hearing aids, because of their efficiency and high power-handling capabilities. They are generally designed to have a fairly flat response, but over a narrower frequency range than electret microphones, particularly at high frequencies. For this reason, the receiver tends to be the limiting factor in the overall response of the aid.

The receiver of a body-worn aid is external to the main unit. Both standard and miniature 'button' receivers are available for most models. Although the standard receivers tend to have slightly higher power output, the practical problems in fitting them to young children mean that the miniature receivers are much to be preferred. Some hearing aid manufacturers now fit only miniature receivers to their aids. Whatever their physical size, a range of receivers is usually available for use with each model of body-worn aid, to cater for differing requirements of power output and frequency range. Generally, the higher the output capability of the receiver, the narrower the frequency range and the less smooth the frequency-gain characteristic of the aid. Receivers fitted to aids with push-pull amplifiers have three-hole sockets for the lead plug; others may have only two holes. In some cases, the polarities of the plug and socket are important and the correct alignment is usually ensured by unequal pin size.

Post-aural aids

The user cannot, of course, change the internal receivers of post-aural aids. Different power or frequency-range requirements are met through a much wider range of models than are available in body-worn aids. The construction of the internal receiver differs slightly from that of the button receiver, but the performance characteristics of the two types are not substantially different.

Bone-conduction aids

Bone-conduction receivers work on a similar principle, but the vibrations of the receiver diaphragm are transmitted by direct coupling to the case of the receiver. The flat surface of the case, placed in contact with the head, causes the skull to vibrate, so that the cochlea is stimulated directly through the vibration of the bony otic capsule.

Batteries

Most aids are powered by disposable batteries (more accurately termed primary cells) of various types. Currently, the Department of Health authorizes NHS hearing aid departments to supply most types of disposable batteries free of charge to patients using hearing aids provided by the NHS. These will include nearly all children, whether fitted with standard NHS aids or 'commercial' aids. The Department of Health has published information sheets (B051 and B052) concerning the applications, storage and use of hearing aid batteries. All the batteries are also easily obtainable through retail outlets.

Body-worn aids

Body-worn aids generally use the familiar 'penlite' battery with a nominal voltage of 1.5 V. Two types are available: manganese alkali (IEC type LR6; Department of Health type CP6) and the cheaper carbon–zinc type (IEC R6). The manganese alkali cell is preferable, because of its rather better voltage stability over time and its higher energy density or capacity, measured in milliampère-hours (mAh). It will last up to twice as long as a carbon–zinc cell in service in the same aid. The service life of each type of cell depends greatly on the power demand of the hearing aid and the use made of it by the child. However, the life of a battery can be estimated by dividing its capacity (in mAh) by the nominal current taken by the hearing aid (in mA). The rechargeable nickel–cadmium cell of the same size is not recommended, because of its lower nominal voltage and much smaller capacity.

Post-aural aids

Post-aural aids use the smaller 'button'-type cell used to power many small electronic devices, such as cameras, calculators and watches. This type of cell has a nominal voltage of 1.35 V and is available in several sizes, three of which (IEC types R41, R44 and R48) are commonly used in hearing aids. Both the R44 (often known as the '675' battery) and R48 sizes are generally available through NHS departments. The cells may be of zinc–air (Department of Health types CP44 and CP48) or mercuric oxide (Department of Health type CP1) form.

The electrochemical function of the zinc–air cell depends upon the ingress of air through a number of small holes in the case. The size of the holes limits the current that the cell is capable of providing and the Department of Health recommends the zinc–air cell for use only in low- and medium-powered aids with small current requirements. However, it has several advantages over the mercuric oxide cell, including greater voltage stability, higher energy density and a longer shelf

life. For the pre-school hearing aid user, it also has the significant
advantage of being made of less toxic materials. Reilly (1979) and
Nolan and Tucker (1981) have warned of the risk of young children
swallowing mercuric oxide cells. Should this happen or be suspected,
medical advice should be sought urgently, as there is a possibility of the
case of the cell being corroded in the stomach, with the subsequent
release of its toxic contents. The same action should be taken if a
zinc–air cell is swallowed, even though it is less toxic.

Properties of cells

Table 10.1 lists the properties of the various types of cells and Figure
10.15 shows their typical discharge curves in use and one advantage of
the button battery over the penlite battery. Both mercuric oxide and
zinc–air cells have much flatter discharge curves in use than either of
the penlite cells. The button cell maintains a nearly constant voltage
until the end of its life, when the voltage falls rapidly. Both types of
penlite cell lose voltage steadily in use. As the gain and maximum output of an aid depend partly upon the voltage available from the battery,
a body-worn aid can be expected to show a deterioration in performance over the lifetime of its battery. As the battery nears the end of its
life the sound output of the aid will become increasingly distorted.

For maximum shelf life, batteries should be stored in cool, dry conditions. They should be kept in their packs until use to avoid the possibility of short-circuiting, which will not only rapidly deplete the battery,
but in some types will cause dangerous overheating, with a risk of fire.

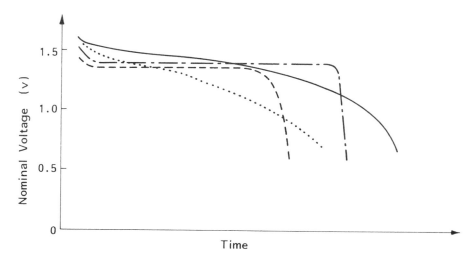

Figure 10.15 Typical discharge curves of various types of primary cells: ...
carbon–zinc; — manganese alkali; – – – mercuric oxide; – . – . zinc–air.

Table 10.1 Properties of common hearing aid batteries

Type	Diameter (mm)	Length/height (mm)	IEC designation	Department of Health code	Nominal voltage (V)	Approximate capacity (mAh)	Electrochemical system
'Penlite'	14.5	50.5	R6	—	1.5	1000	Carbon–zinc
			LR6	CP6	1.45	2200	Manganese alkali
'Button'	7.9	3.6	MR41	—	1.35	36	Mercuric oxide
			AR41	—	1.4	90	Zinc–air
	11.6	5.4	MR44	CP1	1.35	210	Mercuric oxide
			AR44	CP44	1.4	400	Zinc–air
	7.9	5.4	MR48	—	1.35	85	Mercuric oxide
			AR48	CP48	1.4	170	Zinc–air

From BS 397 (1989) and RNID (1990).

All batteries should be stored out of the reach of young children. The air-seal of a zinc–air cell should not be removed until the battery is about to be fitted into a hearing aid.

Problems

The battery compartments of hearing aids tend to be sources of problems, particularly with young children. They are often too easily opened by children, with the risk of loss of the battery or its ingestion by the child. Where possible, children should be fitted with hearing aids with a locking mechanism on the compartment. Where it is not possible, the only solution may be to tape the battery compartment shut. For this reason, hearing aids which incorporate the on/off switch into the battery compartment are unsuitable for young children, unless a locking mechanism is incorporated.

The potential malfunction of the aid due to corrosion of the battery terminals (mentioned for post-aural aids) applies to all other types of aid. If the problem is minor, the terminals can be cleaned by rubbing gently with a rubber eraser.

Rechargeable batteries

Some systems, particularly those employing remote microphones, are fitted with rechargeable batteries and often require special battery chargers provided by the manufacturers. Generally, the batteries require recharging after 6–12 h of continuous aid use, though this depends greatly upon the gain setting. Removable rechargeable battery packs are preferable to permanently wired-in batteries as they offer the convenience of being able to continue using the aid (with a freshly charged pack) while the exhausted battery is being recharged, which may take up to 12 h.

Measurement of performance of the system

Aims

There are two main reasons for checking the performance of a hearing aid electroacoustically.

1. The first is to ensure that the aid meets the performance specifications given for it by the manufacturer. This should be done before the aid is fitted and at regular intervals, not exceeding 1 year. The aid should also be checked whenever a fault is suspected and again when it has been repaired. Listening to the aid is a valuable test and parents and teachers should be encouraged to do this every day,

along with a visual check of the condition of the aid. However, this will identify only the more obvious faults and, in particular, will not detect the slowly progressive deterioration in performance that is inevitable, as a result of wear in the controls and transducers.

2. The other reason for carrying out electroacoustic measurements is to check the effect of any modifications to the aid to achieve more appropriate performance characteristics for the user. This is particularly important for pre-school children, with whom behavioural evaluation can be difficult.

Instrumentation

The equipment required to carry out simple electroacoustic measurements is shown schematically in Figure 10.16. The hearing aid is placed into a sound-attenuating test box with its microphone inlet sited within a target area, in which a pure tone of a specified sound pressure level is generated. The sound pressure level may be maintained by a feedback loop in the stimulation circuit, with a control microphone also within the target area or at a point with a known sound pressure relationship to it. More commonly in modern equipment, the stimulus generator will digitally store information required to ensure that the correct sound pressure is produced. The receiver outlet of the hearing aid is connected to a coupler, which is a cavity of standard design in which a microphone is fitted. The output from the measurement microphone is amplified, filtered and analysed for level or distortion products, as selected. The results are usually displayed on a chart recorder, but occasionally on a meter or an oscilloscope. Integrated measurement

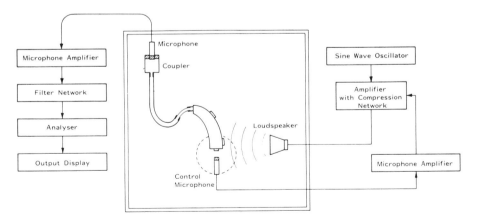

Figure 10.16 Schematic diagram of equipment for electroacoustic measurements of hearing-aid function. The control microphone and feedback loop may be omitted and the stimulation level maintained accurately by digitally stored calibration data.

systems are readily available and are more convenient for routine use in clinical or educational settings than systems built up from separate components. In some systems all the components shown in Figure 10.16 are contained in a single unit, which may be portable, in others the test box is separate from a control unit which usually includes both the stimulation and analysis instrumentation.

The purpose of the coupler is to provide a standard air volume in which to measure the output of the aid for comparison with other data. Two forms of coupler are generally in use.

For comparison of the performance of a hearing aid with the manufacturer's specifications, a 2 cm³ coupler conforming to IEC (1973) is used. Specifications for the measuring equipment, test conditions and the procedures to be used are given in IEC (1983c).

For the purpose of measurement of the electroacoustic characteristics of an aid, particularly for the evaluation of electronic or acoustic modifications to its performance, an occluded ear simulator is used. The ear simulator is a device designed to have the same acoustic impedance as the average normal adult ear. It differs essentially from the 2 cm³ coupler in having side-branch cavities connecting with the main cavity. The sound pressure at the measurement microphone is intended to be similar to that which would be generated by the hearing aid at the eardrum of the average adult ear. Various designs of an occluded ear simulator are available, but all should conform to IEC (1981b). Procedures for measurement of electroacoustic characteristics of hearing aids using the occluded ear simulator are described in IEC (1983a). The ear simulator has the advantage of offering a means for testing the performance of a complete hearing aid system, including the earmould. IEC (1981b) describes arrangements for coupling various types of hearing aids, receivers and ear inserts to the ear simulator.

Hearing-aid gain measured in an ear simulator or a 2 cm³ coupler in a test box is called *transmission gain* and is a measure of the input/output function of the aid. Such measurements do not describe the performance of a hearing aid fitted to a hearing-impaired person, as they do not take account of the diffraction and reflection effects of the head and body of the user on the sound field, nor of the effect of ear-canal resonance on the sound output of the aid. The real gain of a hearing aid in use is referred to as its *insertion gain* and can be defined as the difference between the sound pressure in the external meatus with the hearing aid present and the sound pressure when the hearing aid is absent. To calculate the average insertion gain, it is necessary to make measurements of hearing aid performance in an occluded ear simulator fitted into a manikin, which is placed in a known sound field. IEC (1983d) described the conditions and methods of measurement of simulated in situ hearing aid performance. An international standard for the construction and required properties of a manikin is available (IEC, 1990). The manikin should represent the head and upper torso of the adult human, with dimensions corresponding to the anthropometric medians derived from combined male and female populations. The head should include two pinna simulators with similar shape, dimensions and flexibility to those of the average adult human pinna. One or two occluded ear simulators are mounted in the head of the manikin, each joined by an ear canal simulator to a pinna simulator.

A manikin that meets these requirements is shown in Figure 10.17. Although hearing-aid manufacturers frequently publish in situ performance specifications for their aids, it is important to realize that the performance of an aid in use may be significantly different: for a start, people generally use their aids when wearing clothing and before they lose all their hair, neither of which the manikin has! More importantly,

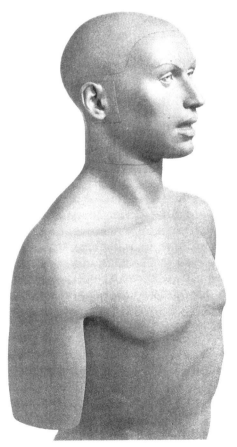

Figure 10.17 A manikin for simulated in situ hearing aid performance measurements. (Courtesy Knowles Electronics.)

most individuals do not conform to the average dimensions represented by the manikin (the differences are likely to be particularly significant for pre-school children). Similarly, the acoustic impedance of the
occluded ear simulator is intended to represent that of the average
adult ear and will be very different from that of the smaller ear of a pre-
school child. The actual output sound pressure of a hearing aid in a
young child's ear is likely to be significantly greater than that measured
in an ear simulator. As there is a risk that the difference may cause the
output to exceed the child's loudness discomfort level, measurement
in a ear simulator (or a 2 cm^3 coupler) should not be relied upon when
setting the maximum output of the aid.

Unfortunately, neither a 'baby manikin' nor a child-sized ear simulator is available. The only satisfactory way of determining the amplification of an aid when fitted to a child is to measure it in use by
measuring the child's aided and unaided performance on various
behavioural or electrophysiological tests, or by means of a probe microphone insertion-gain measurement system. A discussion of the evaluation of real in situ hearing aid performance is not within the scope of
this chapter. However, it should be said that the development of a practical method of measurement of the gain of a hearing aid by placing a
probe microphone into the external meatus behind the user's earmould represents a major advance in the measurement of hearing aid
performances in young children.

Measurement parameters

IEC (1983c) and IEC (1983a) recommend and define performance
measurements which should be made for comparison with manufacturers' specifications, or between different hearing aids or different control settings, respectively. Some manufacturers give specifications in
accordance with the American National Standard (ANSI, 1987). These
differ in some respects from the IEC specifications. When checking an
aid against the manufacturer's specifications, it is important to ensure
that the test conditions (e.g. control settings, input levels and receiver
type) are as shown on the specifications. The main measurements of
interest are likely to be:

- basic frequency response;
- full-on acoustic gain frequency response;
- frequency response for an input sound pressure level of 90 dB;
- effect of control settings on the performance of the aid;
- measurement of amplitude non-linearities (distortion);
- measurement of internal noise of the aid.

Basic frequency response

The frequency response of an aid is the sound pressure level developed in a standard coupler or ear simulator by the hearing aid, expressed as a function of frequency. It gives an indication of the way in which the output sound pressure level of the aid (in dB) varies with frequency, for a specified gain control setting and input sound pressure level. IEC (1983a) defines a basic frequency response measured with an input sound pressure level of 60 dB and with the gain control set to produce a specified output at a reference frequency. If the input level is then varied, a family of curves is produced (the comprehensive frequency response), showing the input–output characteristics of the hearing aid over its full range of operation (dynamic range). Figure 10.18 shows a typical comprehensive frequency response for an aid.

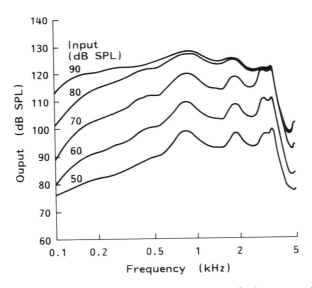

Figure 10.18 A comprehensive frequency response of a hearing aid. The *basic frequency response* is the 60 dB input curve. When the gain control is set to maximum, the 60 dB input curve is the *full-on acoustic gain frequency response* and the 90 dB input curve is the *OSPL90 frequency response*.

Full-on acoustic gain frequency response

This is a frequency response measured with the gain control set to maximum, other controls set as required and with an input sound pressure level of 60 dB. The gain at any frequency is the difference between the input and the measured output sound pressure levels. The maximum gain will be measured when all other controls are set to give the highest output. In some cases 60 dB input sound pressure level will cause the aid to go into saturation, so that the gain measurements will be incorrect. If this happens the input should be set to 50 dB. If the aid is operating in a linear input–output condition, the output for 60 dB input will be (10± 1) dB above the output for 50 dB input at any frequency.

Frequency response for an input sound pressure level of 90 dB

This is the frequency response obtained with the gain control in the maximum setting and with a 90 dB sound pressure level input. It is abbreviated to OSPL90. Usually, any other controls are set for maximum gain and maximum output. In ANSI (1987) this measure is termed 'saturation sound pressure level for 90 dB input sound pressure level' (SSPL90) and is usually taken to be an indication of the maximum output of the aid. However, IEC (1983a) notes that the maximum output may occur at a single frequency with a higher input sound pressure level and is best determined by measurement at discrete frequencies rather than with sweep-frequency measurement.

Effect of control settings on the performance

The effect of changing a control setting may be measured either to determine whether it is appropriate for the user or to check for a suspected fault in the control. The effect of each control should be measured in the mode which best reflects its function. Each control should be assessed separately except when it is specifically desired to measure the change in frequency response with a combination of control settings (perhaps as part of a selection procedure). The effect of the tone control should be measured with respect to the basic frequency response. The function of the user gain control or the preset gain control should be assessed relative to the full-on acoustic gain frequency response, by adjusting the control to give progressively lower gain, while keeping the input sound pressure level constant. The effect of altering a preset maximum output (peak-clipping) control should be measured with respect to the OSPL90 frequency response. Figures 10.19–10.21 illustrate typical effects of these controls. The measurement of the characteristics of a preset AGC is described in IEC (1983b). However, the procedure is time-consuming and cannot be carried out in most automatic hearing aid measurement systems. If a fault is suspected in an AGC circuit, the aid should be returned to the supplier for checking.

The effects of acoustic modifications to the performance of a hearing aid (e.g. venting of the earmould, insertion of acoustic dampers into the tubing, or the creation of a horn-effect tube in the earmould)

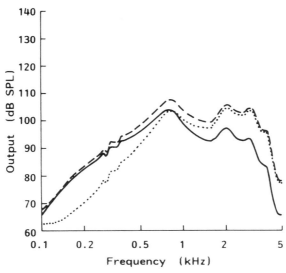

Figure 10.19 Effect of the tone control setting (TC) on the basic frequency response of a hearing aid. — TC-L; – – TC-N; ... TC-H.

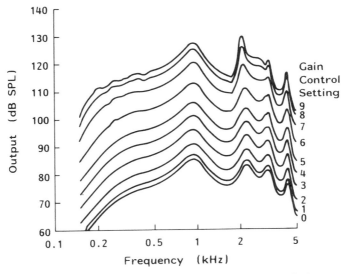

Figure 10.20 Effect of the gain control setting on the output of a hearing aid. The curve with gain control setting 9 is the full-on acoustic gain frequency response of the hearing aid. Note that the function of the gain control is not linear with respect to its nominal setting.

can be measured similarly. The measurements must be made with an ear simulator and the tip of the earmould must be fixed into the inlet of the simulator as specified in IEC (1981b). Figure 10.22 illustrates the effect of insertion of a damper into the tubing of an aid.

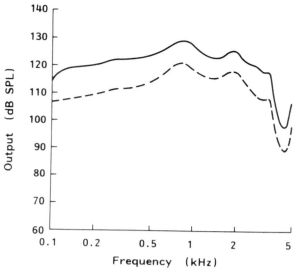

Figure 10.21 Effect of the maximum output control setting (PC) on the OSPL90 frequency response. — PC out; – – PC in.

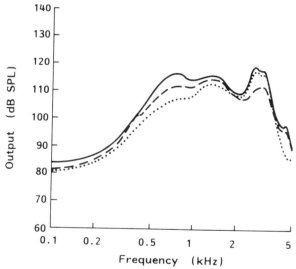

Figure 10.22 Effect of insertion of a 1500Ω damper into the tubing of a hearing aid, measured in an ear simulator conforming to IEC (1981b). Input 60 dBSPL. — no damper; – – with damper (top of tubing); ... with damper (middle of tubing).

Measurement of amplitude non-linearities (distortion)

Distortion arises from limitations in the functions of components of the aid and is present in all systems. Its effect can be seen as the failure of the aid to reproduce faithfully the waveform of the input signal.

Distortion will be present to some extent in any new aid, but is likely to increase over the lifetime of the aid or as a result of damage to individual components. It causes the sound input to have a rough quality and can give rise to loss of clarity.

Frequency distortion occurs largely as a narrowing of the bandwidth of the output. Few hearing aids provide effective amplification outside a frequency range of 200–5000 Hz. Amplitude distortion results from the generation of energy at frequencies which were not present in the input signal. It takes two main forms:

1. *Harmonic distortion* is the generation of frequencies that are integer multiples of frequencies present in the input signal. For a frequency $f_1 = x$ Hz in the input signal, the hearing aid will generate energy at frequencies $2f_1$, $3f_1$, $4f_1$, ... ($2x$ Hz, $3x$ Hz, $4x$ Hz ...) etc. Generally, the amplitude of the harmonics decreases towards the higher harmonics. Many commercial instruments are capable of separately measuring second-order ($2f_1$) and third-order ($3f_1$) harmonics, which are likely to be most troublesome. Some instruments provide a measure of total harmonic distortion (THD), which is largely the combined effect of the second- and third-order harmonics. There are no standards specifying the allowable harmonic distortion in hearing aids, but high-quality aids will usually not exceed a THD value of 5%.

2. *Intermodulation distortion* occurs when two frequencies of similar amplitude are simultaneously present in the input to the aid. Intermodulation distortion products may be of higher or lower frequency than either of the two input frequencies, but only those of lower frequency are likely to be noticeable. Few hearing aid test systems provide facilities for measuring intermodulation distortion and there are no standards specifying allowable limits in aids.

It is important to remember that distortion is markedly increased when a hearing aid amplifier is operating at saturation output, due to the effect of peak-clipping. Distortion measurements must be made under conditions outlined in IEC (1983a) to ensure that the hearing aid is not at saturation output. As an aid will be more likely to reach saturation output if the gain control is set near maximum, it is important to choose an aid which will provide sufficient gain for the child with the gain control set about half way.

Measurement of internal noise

If the internal noise level of the hearing aid is suspected to be unduly high, measurements should be made in accordance with IEC (1983a). It is important to ensure that ambient noise is not sufficiently high to influence the result.

Alternative forms of personal aids to hearing

Vibrotactile aids

These take the form of wearable (usually wrist-worn) devices which present acoustic information to the wearer through vibrotactile stimulation. They are likely to be of particular benefit to profoundly deaf children who may derive little advantage from conventional hearing aids.

Vibrotactile aids generally provide information relating to acoustic energy in one or more limited frequency bands of importance in speech perception. The fundamental frequency of laryngeal vibration is usually cued to give voicing information. Higher frequency bands may be monitored to give cues to sibilant production and first or second formant frequencies. The reader is referred to Summers (1992) for a full description of tactile aids.

Few published data are available for the use of vibrotactile aids by pre-school children, but their neural plasticity and learning capacity may be expected to make them particularly successful as users.

Artificial auditory stimulation

The implantation of devices in profoundly and severely deaf people, to stimulate the acoustic nerve directly, is now available in many centres worldwide. Various systems are available, using one or more stimulating electrodes and one or more channels of acoustic information. The electrodes are activated by a signal processor which either filters the sound input into one or more frequency bands or extracts and codes specific acoustic features in the sound input. The electrode may be implanted in the cochlea or may be extra-cochlear, usually placed on the promontory of the middle-ear cavity.

Several thousand patients have now been implanted worldwide and the results appear promising. Processing strategies, electrode technology and criteria for candidature are all undergoing rapid change as a result of research developments and clinical experience. Previous reluctance to fit children, for practical and ethical reasons, is generally being replaced by a view that severely hearing-impaired children are likely to be the most successful users, if they are fitted in their early pre-school years. Cochlear implantation is covered in detail in Chapter 13 of this book and the reader is referred to Gray (1985) and Cooper (1991) for further information.

References

ANSI (1987). *American national standard: specification of hearing aid characteristics.* ANSI S3.22–1987. New York: American National Standards Institute.

BS397 (1989). *Primary batteries. Part 1: Specification for general requirements.* Milton Keynes: British Standards Institution.

BS6083 (1981). *Hearing Aids. Part 4: Specification for magnetic field strength in audio-frequency induction loops for hearing aid purposes.* Milton Keynes: British Standards Institution.

BS6083 (1984). *Hearing Aids. Part 2: Methods of measurement of electroacoustical characteristics of hearing aids with automatic gain control circuits.* Milton Keynes: British Standards Institution.

Cooper, H. (Ed.) (1991). *Cochlear Implants: A Practical Guide.* London: Whurr.

Dillon, H. and Walker, G. (1983). Compression – input or output control? *Hearing Instruments* 34, 20–21, 42.

DTI (1986). *Performance specifications for radio microphone and radio hearing aid equipment for use in the band 173.35M Hz to 175.02M Hz.* MPT 1345. London: Department of Trade and Industry.

Finitzo-Hieber, T. and Tillman, T. (1978). Room acoustic effects on monosyllabic word discrimination ability for normal and hearing-impaired children. *Journal of Speech and Hearing Research* 21, 440–458.

Gray, R.F., Ed. (1985). *Cochlear Implants.* London: Croom Helm.

Hodgson, W.R. (1981). Special cases of hearing aid assessment: CROS aids. In: Hodgson, W.R. and Skinner, P.H. (Eds),. *Hearing Aid Assessment and Use in Audiologic Habilitation,* 2nd ed., pp. 196–211. Baltimore: Williams and Wilkins.

IEC (1973). *IEC reference coupler for the measurement of hearing aids using earphones coupled to the ear by means of ear inserts.* IEC Publication 126. Geneva: International Electrotechnical Commission.

IEC (1981a). *Magnetic field strength in audio-frequency induction loops for hearing aid purposes.* IEC Publication 118–4. Geneva: International Electrotechnical Commission.

IEC (1981b). *Occluded-ear simulator for the measurement of earphones coupled to the ear by ear inserts.* IEC Publication 711. Geneva: International Electrotechnical Commission.

IEC (1983a). *Measurement of electroacoustic characteristics.* IEC Publication 118–0. Geneva: International Electrotechnical Commission.

IEC (1983b). *Hearing aids with automatic gain control circuits.* IEC Publication 118–2. Geneva: International Electrotechnical Commission.

IEC (1983c). *Measurement of the performance characteristics of hearing aids for quality inspection for delivery purposes.* IEC Publication 118–7. Geneva: International Electrotechnical Commission.

IEC (1983d). *Methods of measurement of performance characteristics of hearing aids under simulated in situ working conditions.* IEC Publication 118–8. Geneva: International Electrotechnical Commission.

IEC (1983e). *Symbols and other markings on hearing aids and related equipment.* IEC Publication 118–11. Geneva: International Electrotechnical Commission.

IEC (1984). *Characteristics of electrical input circuits for hearing aids.* IEC Publication 118–6. Geneva: International Electrotechnical Commission.

IEC (1990). *Provisional head and torso simulator for acoustic measurements on air conduction hearing aids.* IEC Publication 959. Geneva: International Electrotechnical Commission.

Markides, A., Huntington, A. and Kettlety, A. (1980). Comparative speech discrimination abilities of hearing-impaired children achieved through infra-red, radio and conventional hearing aids. *Journal of the British Association of Teachers of the Deaf* 4, 5–14.

Nolan, M. and Tucker, I.G. (1981). Health risks following ingestion of mercury and zinc–air batteries. *Scandinavian Audiology* 10, 189.

Reilly, D.T. (1979). Mercury battery ingestion. *British Medical Journal* i, 859.

RNID (1991). *Installation guidelines for induction loops in public places.* Pamphlet chp 14660. London: Royal National Institute for the Deaf.

RNID (1990). *National Health Service hearing aids.* Pamphlet chp 14211. London: Royal National Institute for the Deaf.

Summers, I., Ed. (1992). *Tactile Aids for the Hearing Impaired.* London: Whurr.

Walker, G. and Dillon, H. (1982). *Compression in hearing aids: An analysis, a review and some recommendations.* NAL Report No. 90. Canberra: Australian Government Publishing Service.

Chapter 11
Hearing aid selection and evaluation for pre-school children

ROGER GREEN

Introduction

The task of fitting a hearing aid to a hearing-impaired child demands a great deal of skill and sensitivity on the part of the clinician. Audiology is a discipline which draws on many areas of knowledge, from physics to psychology, from medicine to management. The clinician needs to combine all of these, along with his clinical experience of what works, if a successful fitting is to be achieved. The subject is a complex one and there is not the space in one chapter to cover in detail all the issues involved. However, by examining some of the central issues it is hoped to give the reader a better understanding of the ideas that underpin the practice of hearing aid selection and evaluation.

To that end this chapter will discuss first the selection of hearing aids, in terms of both ergonomics and electroacoustics and will then proceed to discuss the evaluation of the fitted hearing aid, both in the clinic and in the field.

General points

It is necessary to clarify the difference between selection and evaluation of a hearing aid. When a child presents with a hearing loss which requires amplification, the clinician is faced first with the problem of selection, that is of choosing from an extremely large number of possible hearing aids (and hearing aid settings) the aid which is most likely to provide optimum benefit for that child. This requires an understanding of exactly what amplification is intended to achieve. Do we want to return auditory thresholds to normal or is it sufficient simply to make speech audible? If the latter, how much emphasis do we give to the various frequencies that make up the speech spectrum? Some sort of more or less explicit and more or less precise target for amplification is at the heart of most hearing aid selection strategies. We also require a means of selecting from the range of aids at the clinician's disposal one which is likely to provide the amount of amplification we think the child needs. A good deal of discussion has centred on the problem of selecting an aid that will provide the greatest degree of benefit for each individual hearing loss and we will look at this in the next section.

Once the first choice aid is selected it then requires evaluation. Evaluation is the process by which the actual performance of the aid when fitted to the child is compared with the performance prescribed by the clinician. The child may be tested, wearing the aid, using any of a number of possible test procedures. If, on evaluation, the aid performance is shown to fall short of the required performance, the selected aid may then be modified or replaced, until a satisfactory match is achieved.

In essence then the hearing aid fitting procedure includes the following sequential stages:

1. Measurement of hearing impairment and disability.
2. Specification of the ergonomic and electroacoustic characteristics required to provide optimum benefit for that particular child.
3. Selection of a hearing aid with the required characteristics.
4. Evaluation of the performance of the aid when worn by the child.
5. Modification of the selected aid if necessary to bring the achieved performance in line with the required performance.

Although these stages are usually sequential and rather separate with adults, with pre-schoolers there is often a considerable amount of back and forth movement between the stages. For example, with very young children the initial selection may be based on very limited information, perhaps one or two reliable auditory thresholds. Selection may well need modification as more information about the degree of impairment is obtained in the weeks and months following the initial fitting.

Many of the procedures used in the selection and evaluation of hearing aids for young children are based on work done with adults or older children. Adults can provide two kinds of information which pre-school children usually cannot: first, they provide a (relatively) accurate set of psychoacoustic measurements which can be used to both select and evaluate a hearing aid; secondly, they provide verbal feedback as to their satisfaction with their hearing aid and its benefits. Pre-school children provide audiometric information which is often considerably less precise. This is particularly true for the very young in whom the early audiometric profile, on which the initial aid selection is based, is sometimes very approximate, perhaps including reliable thresholds at only one or two frequencies. Also, of course, such children are not usually sufficiently articulate to tell us what they think of the aids we have given them. We may have to rely on other behavioural indications such as the child refusing to wear the aid, and even then the reasons for rejection may not be clear. For example the aid could be too loud or the mould uncomfortable.

Finally it is not the author's aim to 'sell' one particular set of procedures for selection and evaluation. There are almost as many procedures as there are clinics. The aim is rather to familiarize the reader with some of the principles on which these procedures are based in order to facilitate understanding about what happens when a hearing aid is fitted.

Hearing aid selection

Ergonomic factors

Hearing aids differ not only acoustically (i.e. in the sound they deliver) but also ergonomically (i.e. how easy they are to manage). Selection of ergonomic factors should precede selection of electroacoustic factors. The most carefully adjusted aid is of no use at all if it is too large or cumbersome for the child to wear. Clinicians usually fit hearing aids in the uncluttered confines of their clinic. It is the parent who must manage the aid back in the real world where it is likely to lead a far more boisterous, not to say hazardous, existence. Tales of hearing aids falling into ponds or being chewed by dogs are legion in most clinics.

The main ergonomic choices involved are listed below. They are not entirely independent of each other or of electroacoustic considerations. Thus, for example, a body-worn hearing aid may be selected because of its better low-frequency response rather than its greater convenience in a particular circumstance .

Hearing aid type (body-worn/behind-the-ear/in-the-ear)

Hearing aids worn behind the ear are most commonly fitted in the UK. The increasing sophistication of hearing aid and earmould technology has enabled more severe hearing losses to be reached by powerful behind-the-ear hearing aids, where previously a body-worn aid might have been necessary. Such aids have an obvious cosmetic appeal and they avoid clothes rub noise, which is a major problem with body-worn aids. However, body-worn aids still have some major advantages:

- for some very severe hearing losses, behind-the-ear aids may not be able to provide enough gain, partly because they are not powerful enough and partly because the closeness of the microphone to the receiver in behind-the-ear aids makes them very prone to feedback at high output levels;
- for children with nothing but a small 'island' of low-frequency hearing, a body-worn aid may be preferred;

- the larger receiver on the body-worn aid makes it possible to provide more low-frequency amplification and so to reach such a hearing loss more effectively;
- with some children, for example babies who spend much time in their cots, a behind-the-ear aid may be constantly dislodged by the pillows or clothing worn by the baby: a body-worn hearing aid suffers less from this problem.

In-the-ear hearing aids are becoming increasingly popular in the USA. Generally they are less powerful than behind-the-ear aids and historically they have been less versatile, their small size prohibiting for example the inclusion of adjustable electroacoustic parameters such as frequency response and maximum output or such additions as an induction coil or direct input facility. A greater problem with regard to young children has been that these children require frequent new earmoulds (as much as one every week for some very young children). In the past, in-the-ear aids have been custom built into the earmoulds and the cost of building the circuitry into each new mould is prohibitively expensive. If a behind-the-ear aid requires servicing (not a rare event with children) a loan aid can usually be provided which can be used with the child's own mould. If an in-the-ear aid requires servicing the aid/mould must be sent away and the child is without the aid until it is returned. In-the-ear aid technology has been rapidly expanding and some of these problems are being overcome. Such aids are now available with induction coils and with the facility for direct input. Various 'modular' approaches to their design have advanced to the point where it is possible to remove the circuitry easily from an in-the-ear aid and replace it temporarily with a 'loan' circuit block. With such developments, in-the-ear fittings have become increasingly accessible to this age group. One problem here may be that, while in-the-ear aids have obvious appeal to parents, they cannot always provide the appropriate gain or frequency response. This makes the burden of decision increasingly difficult for the clinician who must strongly resist sacrificing electroacoustic performance for cosmetic appeal. If this is to be achieved against considerable parental pressure for something small and 'invisible', his explanations and demonstrations of the benefits of a correctly fitted aid will need to be clear and convincing.

One possible advantage of an in-the-ear aid is that its microphone is positioned on the concha, enabling sound to be 'focused' from the pinna in a manner similar to that of the normal unaided ear. It has been suggested that this can improve the patient's ability to localize.

Hearing aid size

The great majority of hearing aids fitted to children are small post-aural aids. Again, recent developments in technology have enabled these small aids to provide a similar degree of power to their larger predecessors, as well as providing the necessary range of facilities such as adjustable frequency response and maximum output and direct input. Despite the small size of aids, difficulties are still experienced in keeping them in position on very small ears, though the use of paediatric earhooks and aid retainers (small loops of plastic that fit round the ear and to which the aid may be fastened) can help.

One specific point that should be mentioned is the use of battery locks. Swallowing a battery can be dangerous, sometimes causing stomach burns and even mercury poisoning. If a battery is swallowed it may need to be surgically removed. It is therefore essential to keep prying fingers out of the aid by fitting battery locks. This will not completely solve the problem as little teeth may do what little fingers can not: therefore parents also need careful advice about safety with batteries.

Air conduction/bone conduction hearing aids

While by far the commonest hearing aids fitted transmit their signals by air conduction, there is still occasional need for a bone conduction hearing aid, possibly using a bone-anchored receiver (see Chapter 10). Bilateral atresia with poorly formed pinna and outer canal may mean that the only way to reach the cochlea is by using a bone conduction hearing aid. It may also be necessary with chronically discharging ears, a condition which can be aggravated if the ear canals are closed off by occluding ear moulds.

Monaural/binaural hearing aid fitting

In many clinics there has been some reluctance to fit binaural hearing aids (i.e. an aid for each ear), only doing so when it seems 'necessary'. There seems little doubt that the opposite philosophy should be adopted (but with caution; see Rintelmann and Bess, 1977), in other words that two aids should be fitted unless there is a good reason not to. The well-known comment that you don't go to the optician expecting to be fitted with a monocle still makes the point well. There are some specific advantages of binaural over monaural hearing which can be made accessible with a binaural fitting. These include:

1. Localization – the direction of sound is more easily detected with two ears than with one.
2. Summation – sounds heard with two ears are a little (3 dB) louder, enabling the gain in both hearing aids to be slightly less than with one hearing aid.
3. Fusion – most real life listening conditions are at least partly reverberant and binaural hearing makes us less susceptible to the degrading effects of such reverberation on speech.

4. Unmasking – binaural hearing can make it easier to understand speech in noisy backgrounds, a particular difficulty for the hearing impaired.

In order to develop these auditory abilities two hearing aids should be fitted from the outset. One problem with very young pre-school children can be that it is extremely difficult in a sound field to determine accurately the degree of impairment in each ear. However as Seewald, Ross and Spiro (1985) point out, most hearing losses turn out to be more or less symmetrical and as sound-field test results tend to reflect hearing in the better ear, if we fit as if both ears were the same then we will at worst be underfitting a poorer ear and certainly not overfitting a better one. It is also probably easier for parents to come to terms with two hearing aids at the outset, especially when such fittings are presented as both routine and desirable, rather than when a second hearing aid is introduced at some later stage.

Electroacoustic factors

Matching the electroacoustics of a hearing aid to a patient's individual hearing impairment is a problem which has occupied audiologists over a long period of time and there is not space here to do more than highlight the main issues. The reader is referred to Byrne (1983) for a full review of the topic.

There are three electroacoustic parameters of hearing aids over which we have some control and each of them relates to a particular aspect of the patient's hearing loss.

- First, the overall gain of the hearing aid must be chosen to be appropriate to the degree of hearing loss. Hearing aids tend to be classified in the first instance in terms of their power and more powerful aids are needed for more severe hearing losses.
- Secondly, the configuration of the hearing aid frequency response can be chosen to compensate for the configuration of the hearing loss. Broadly, if a patient hears low frequencies well and high frequencies poorly, the frequency response of the hearing aid can be chosen to give greater emphasis to the high frequencies. (Of course gain and frequency response, while being conceptually distinct, are in reality inseparable in that the 'overall gain' is simply a summary of the gain at each frequency – i.e. the frequency response.)
- Thirdly, the maximum output of the hearing aid should be chosen so that patients will not be exposed to excessively loud sounds. In particular, patients with recruiting hearing losses may be particularly intolerant of even moderately loud sounds.

The main debate in hearing aid selection is not that these parameters need selecting, but on what basis to select them. Let us take as an example the audiogram shown in Figure 11.1. The patient has a severe hearing loss and so needs a powerful hearing aid. But just how much amplification is needed? Should we be trying to improve the thresholds to normal with a hearing aid? Would a more modest amount of gain be sufficient? Hearing is poorer for the high frequencies so some high frequency emphasis seems desirable but just how much? Should we amplify exclusively the high frequencies or only give them a little more emphasis than the low frequencies? At what level should the maximum output be set in order to ensure that normal sounds are loud enough while other sounds are not frequently uncomfortable? These considerations have been addressed in theoretical prescription approaches.

Prescription approaches

Numerous theoretical prescriptive approaches to selection have emerged (e.g. Watson and Knudsen, 1940; Wallenfells, 1967; Byrne and Tonisson, 1976; Berger, Hagberg and Rane, 1977; Seewald, Ross and Spiro, 1985; Byrne and Dillon, 1986; Seewald and Ross, 1988). These have in common the fact that they provide us with a means of selecting a hearing aid for each individual patient based on what is known about the patient's hearing impairment. To be more precise they prescribe a particular gain (and sometimes maximum output) at each frequency based on measurements of the individual hearing loss. Prescription approaches differ both in the measurements they use to derive their prescriptions (e.g. threshold, loudness discomfort, comfortable listening levels, or combinations of these) and in the relative emphasis they give to the measurements (different prescriptions, for example, advocate different degrees of low-frequency emphasis for the same hearing

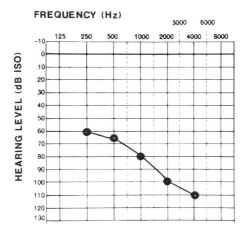

Figure 11.1 Example of a typical audiogram.

loss). Two illustrative examples of the prescription approach to selection will be described.

Byrne and Tonisson (1976) developed a set of tables which enabled the gain and frequency response of a hearing aid to be selected from the patient's audiometric thresholds. There are several steps in the development of their arguments as to why their particular threshold/gain relationships should be used. First, they confirmed a relationship previously reported in the literature, between the degree of hearing loss and the gain at which patients preferred to use their hearing aids. Byrne and Tonisson showed that for each 10 dB increase in hearing loss, the user gain of hearing aids increases by approximately 5 dB.

This relationship between threshold and required gain could be used to predict the required gain for new patients. (It was only applicable to patients with a sensorineural hearing loss and corrections were necessary if a conductive component were present.) However, they were also interested in ensuring that all elements of the speech spectrum were rendered audible. This spectrum is not flat but has most energy in the region around 500 Hz and relatively little at high frequency. The Byrne and Tonisson gain calculations were therefore corrected to take this speech spectrum into account. Further corrections were included for example to allow for the fact that hearing aids are initially selected from their performance measured in a 2 cm³ coupler rather than in real ears and these coupler measurements tend to overpredict the real ear gain (in other words the gain experienced by the patient wearing the aid). The Byrne and Tonisson tables have since been revised (Byrne and Dillon, 1986) resulting in more low-frequency emphasis than the original formula. Examples of the Byrne and Dillon formulae are shown in Table 11.1. The formulae given in that table allow the desired aided thresholds to be calculated. Byrne and Dillon provide other formulae for calculation of real ear gain and various coupler measured desired gains.

The prescriptive approach, attractive though it is, has a number of pitfalls.

- First, it requires hearing aids with almost infinitely variable frequency responses if the prescription is to be matched exactly. In practice hearing aids are not infinitely flexible and in most cases a broad shaping of the frequency response is all that is possible.
- Secondly, aid selection is based on 2 ml coupler measurements. Individual ears will differ considerably from the mean and so the real ear/coupler correction factors built into the prescription may not be appropriate for a particular individual.

Additional problems are encountered when we try to apply such prescriptions to pre-school children. As has been said, the rules from which the prescriptive formulae are derived are based on work with

Table 11.1 Equations for calculating required aided threshold from headphone thresholds, based on the prescriptions of Byrne and Dillon (1986)

1.	Calculate: $X = 0.05*(H(500) + H(1000) + H(2000))$
2.	Calculate aided thresholds (AT) as follows: $AT(250) = 0.69*H(250) - X + 33$ $AT(500) = 0.69*H(500) - X + 18$ $AT(1000) = 0.69*H(1000) - X + 4$ $AT(1500) = 0.69*H(1500) - X + 4$ $AT(2000) = 0.69*H(2000) - X + 4$ $AT(3000) = 0.69*H(3000) - X + 3$ $AT(4000) = 0.69*H(4000) - X + 4$ $AT(6000) = 0.69*H(6000) - X + 10$ Where $H(f)$ is the headphone threshold for frequency

Note that if sound-field unaided thresholds are used as the basis for prediction, then these need to be 'converted' to equivalent headphone thresholds before the formulae can be applied.

adults. We simply do not know to what extent these rules apply to young and often pre-lingually hearing-impaired children. Is it the case, for example, that the frequency response which provides the greatest benefit for the adventitiously hearing-impaired adult who has already developed speech and language will also be the best response for helping the pre-lingually impaired child develop speech and language from residual hearing? Many prescriptions carry corrections for the speech spectrum. This average speech spectrum is based on speech recorded by a number of speakers at a distance of perhaps 1 m from the source. The hearing-impaired infant is probably much closer to the source (mother) for many of the situations in which meaningful communication is taking place. Turner and Holte (1983) have shown that at 20 cm distance from the source the speech level may be increased as much as 20 dB. Furthermore, children listen most frequently not to the average voice but to two particular voices, their own and their mother's. It may therefore be more appropriate to use the mother's speech spectrum in the prescription formula. While we are clinically some way from incorporating such specific information into the hearing aid prescription, the procedure is not complicated, at least in theory. All that is necessary is equipment that is sufficiently inexpensive. To apply prescription formulae requires a set of accurate audiometric measurements. When testing infants, one is usually measuring behavioural thresholds which are less accurate than those obtained with adults and almost certainly at intensities above true threshold.

A systematic approach to selecting hearing aids for pre-verbally hearing impaired children has been put forward by Seewald, Ross and Spiro (1985). They have adapted prescription methods to take into account some of the problems mentioned above. They use a relationship between threshold and the desired sensation level for amplified speech which is:

> ... not strictly based on any specific data set. Rather (it) reflect(s) a general goal to present the range of intensities associated with speech sufficiently above threshold to be useful yet simultaneously considering limitations imposed by the reduced residual hearing associated with increasing degrees of sensorineural loss.

The speech spectrum they adopted, based on work by Cox (1983), is a relatively high-intensity one reflecting the more realistic voice levels of a close proximity parent discussed above.

Seewald and co-workers also include recommendations for maximum output settings. Usually, where such recommendations are included in a prescription, they are based on measures of loudness discomfort level. However, young children cannot respond sensibly to the instruction 'tell me when the sound becomes uncomfortably loud'. It is difficult enough for adults to locate this point with any precision.

Acknowledging that loudness discomfort level measures are simply not obtainable on infants, Seewald et al. base their maximum output values on ensuring that the maximum output is sufficiently elevated above the amplified speech signal to prevent speech reaching saturation more than necessary while, at the same time, using guidelines established by other workers (Rintelmann and Bess, 1977; Kamm, Dirks and Mickey, 1978) to ensure that maximum output is not excessive, from the point of view both of causing discomfort, and of damaging residual hearing. Figure 11.2 illustrates their approach.

This approach is similar to others such as Byrne and Tonisson in that only threshold data are needed from the patient, though with the Seewald et al. approach these thresholds then yield both required gain and maximum output. We have already stated, however, that accurate threshold data at all frequencies may not always be available. As a consequence the aid may initially be selected based on limited information. Once the initial assessment has given a broad picture of the degree of loss, it is better to work at obtaining one or two reliable thresholds in each session and then select the aid on the basis of these results. A fuller (across frequency) audiometric profile can gradually be built up in subsequent sessions and modifications made to the aid as more information comes to light. The relationship between measured and true thresholds will depend to some extent on age. Table 11.2 (taken from Northern and Downs, 1984) gives an indication of both the type of response and the level above audiometric zero at which it is likely to be elicited in normal hearing children of different ages. When the hearing aid is selected these levels need to be borne in mind.

The aim of this section has been to introduce the reader to the idea of hearing aid prescription. It is strongly recommended that the origi-

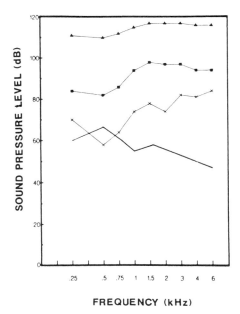

FREQUENCY (kHz)

Figure 11.2 Prescription of gain and maximum output for the hearing loss shown: X—X unaided thresholds (converted to dB SPL); ———— idealized speech spectrum; ■—■ required levels for aided speech. The difference between the idealized speech spectrum and the required aided speech levels represents the amount of gain which the hearing aid must deliver. ▲—▲ required maximum output.

nal references are referred to before any such procedures are incorporated into clinical practice.

In practice, hearing aid selection is greatly simplified by the use of a microcomputer. In the author's clinic a software package is used that was developed to generate required hearing aid performance from measures of unaided thresholds, based on prescriptions such as that of Seewald et al. Unaided thresholds from either sound-field or headphone testing are entered. These are appropriately converted and the prescription then used to generate required aided thresholds, and required hearing aid frequency response and maximum output of the aid into a coupler (using coupler/real ear correction factors, based on age if required). These prescriptions can then be compared with the measured frequency response and maximum output and the aid modified until a good approximation is obtained.

Frequency response modification can be achieved by changing high and low-frequency tone control settings, by earmould plumbing and if necessary by using a different aid from that initially selected.

Output control can be achieved in a variety of ways. A simple peak clipping circuit enables us to prevent the output of the aid reaching levels greater than a preset amount (as measured in a coupler). This

Table 11.2 Index of auditory behaviour for infants

Age	Noisemakers (Approx. SPL)(dB)	Warbled pure tones (re:audiometric zero)(dB)	Speech (re: audiometric zero)(dB)	Expected response
0–6 weeks	50–70	78 (6)	40–60	Eye-widening, eye-blink, stirring or arousal from sleep, startle
6 weeks–4 months	50–60	70 (10)	47 (2)	Eye-widening, eye-shift, eye blinking, quieting; beginning rudimentary head turn by 4 months
4–7 months	40–50	51 (9)	21 (8)	Head-turn on lateral plane toward sound; listening attitude
7–9 months	30–40	45 (15)	15 (7)	Direct localization of sound to side, indirectly below ear level
9–13 months	25–35	38 (8)	8 (7)	Direct localization of sounds to side, directly below ear level, indirectly above ear level
13–16 months	25–30	32 (10)	5 (5)	Direct localization of sound on side, above and below
16–21 months	25	25 (10)	5 (1)	Direct localization of sound on side, above and below
21–24 months	25	26 (10)	3 (10)	Direct localization of sound on side, above and below

The three middle columns show the levels above audiometric zero at which infants of different ages will respond to different types of stimulus (if they have normal hearing). Aided and unaided thresholds need to be corrected by these amounts, though the figures should be treated as 'orders of magnitude' rather than exact amounts. Values in parentheses are the standard deviations.

Reproduced from Northern and Downs (1984) with permission.

can be combined with or replaced by a compression circuit. If the compression circuit acts on the output it serves to provide a more distortion-free, fixed-maximum output. If the compression circuit acts on the input it enables the user to effectively select the maximum output for different situations. Unfortunately, control of maximum output is one of the least researched areas of paediatric audiology. Even if LDLs are known, the relationship between the discomfort levels and the output control settings on the aid is unclear. For example, an aid may have an output limit which can be preset to 105 dB SPL. This means that, in a coupler, the greatest output at any frequency is 105 dB SPL. The output in the individual ear may be very different. In particular, ear canals of young children are smaller than those of adults, resulting in hearing aid output being both shifted to higher frequencies and increased overall. Figure 11.3, taken from a study carried out by the author, shows this effect. It compares the output of a hearing aid measured in the ear canals of adults and children. The measurements are averaged for seven adults and four children (all under 2 years old). Also included is one individual trace. The figure demonstrates the difference between adult and child ears described above. The output in the child ear canals is shifted in frequency and reaches a maximum level of some 7 dB higher than in the adult ear canals. The figure also demonstrates the considerable individual differences which can arise.

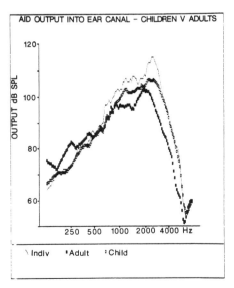

Figure 11.3 Plot of the output of a hearing aid into the ear canal, averaged for a group of adults (n = 7) and a group of children (n = 4). Also shown is the output for one individual child. The measurements were taken by inserting the tube of the probe microphone into the ear canal around the earmould and measuring the output levels in the canal for a constant (across frequency) 60 dB input to the aid microphone.

Hearing aid evaluation

Clinical evaluation

Having selected an appropriate first-choice hearing aid, we cannot then simply slip it on the pre-school child's ear and ask them what they think of it. (In a sense this is not a major disadvantage. Even using such an approach with adults is fraught with pitfalls. Hearing impaired people are not always good judges as to what is best for them, particularly if they have not had previous experience of hearing aids. (See, for example, Green, 1986.) Real ear evaluation is necessary both to check the aid's actual performance against its expected performance and to get some feel for how well the child performs when aided. An important side effect of the hearing aid evaluation is that it serves to demonstrate to parents the difference the aid makes to their child and, where parental resistance is met, to convince them of the need for amplification.

In fact very little evaluation is carried out at the first fitting visit. If the initial selection of the aid is to be tried has been done carefully (and it is worth noting that this process of selecting the initial aid can be quite time consuming and needs to be done before the patient arrives) then much of the session itself can concentrate on the process of introducing the family to the aid. Evaluation begins in earnest usually at the first follow-up visit.

Evaluation includes measuring the aided thresholds to check that they are at, or close to, the required aided thresholds. The techniques used are exactly the same as those used for measuring unaided thresholds (see Chapters 4 and 5).

Some clinics use a less rigorous approach to aid selection, simply requiring that the hearing aid render all speech sounds audible. In this case evaluation consists of checking from the aided thresholds that all sounds of the speech spectrum are amplified above threshold. In practice this is best achieved by recording the aided thresholds on a pre-printed chart showing the speech spectrum. Calibration of the room (and so the sound level axis of the chart) should of course be in sound pressure level. A number of speech spectra have been reported. The Seewald et al. spectrum discussed above is shown in Figure 11.2. Byrne and Dillon give the following figures for their speech spectrum:

250 Hz = 62 dB SPL, 500 Hz = 61 dB SPL, 1000 Hz = 50 dB SPL,
1600 Hz = 51 dB SPL, 2000 Hz = 49 dB SPL, 3150 Hz = 47 dB SPL,
4000 Hz = 48 dB SPL, 6000 Hz = 46 dB SPL.

If aided thresholds above the speech spectrum have been achieved and further modification of the aid still seems necessary (e.g. because of 'too much' low-frequency emphasis) this can be carried out.

While this approach is perhaps theoretically less satisfactory than the more exacting prescriptive approach, it is often at least realistic. This is partly because hearing aids are not infinitely flexible and simply to find an aid which puts the speech spectrum above threshold across frequency can be a considerable achievement. It must also be remembered that precise use of prescriptive procedures involves finding a hearing aid that delivers precise gains based on a set of rules whose validity is not entirely proven (particularly for this age group) and on a set of audiometric measurements which are usually less accurate and less reliable than those of adults. Prescriptions can provide broad guidelines but each individual is unique and not always well described by such rules.

In an evaluation session, time allocation should be geared carefully to obtaining the important information first. Thus, aided thresholds across frequency should be measured until reliable results across frequency have been established or until the child's cooperation is lost. The next stage will depend on the situation. Two particular problems may arise.

- First, it may be that the child has not provided very accurate thresholds (due to age, or disposition or whatever). In this case the next step may be to use some form of speech test to establish voice detection threshold or, for older children, speech reception threshold (using some form of toy test – see Chapter 4). The relationship between these speech measures and audiometric thresholds has been shown (e.g. Bamford et al., 1980) to be close enough for the speech result to be used to back up the threshold findings.
- Secondly, it may be that, while aided thresholds are satisfactory, parents might still remain unconvinced of the need for an aid. In this circumstance it may be worth performing some unaided testing in order that the immediate aided/unaided comparison can demonstrate the benefit of the hearing aid. If this kind of demonstration is required it can be more effective if speech testing is used because the speech signal is more meaningful to parents than the warble tones or narrow-band noises used for threshold testing.

An example of an evaluation session is shown in Figure 11.4. It does show a rather full complement of data, in other words a very cooperative child. It shows a situation in which the aid is providing rather too much mid-frequency gain, and would require some modification.

The correctness of the maximum output setting can be broadly checked by presenting the child with loud inputs and observing carefully for signs of distress. Different clinicians suggest different techniques. Tucker and Nolan (1984) for example use a voice stimulus such as 'go' or 'ba' and look for any signs of distress in the child as the level of the stimulus is raised from conversational (65 dB SPL) to very loud

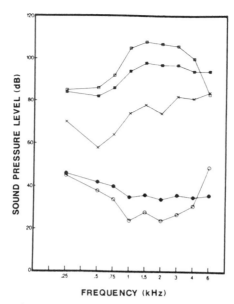

FREQUENCY (kHz)

Figure 11.4 Required and achieved hearing aid gain for the example shown in Figure 11.2. X—X unaided thresholds; ■—■ required levels for aided speech; •—• required aided thresholds; O—O achieved aided thresholds; □—□ achieved levels for aided speech (calculated by adding the difference between required and achieved aided thresholds to the required levels for aided speech). It is clear in this example that the patient is receiving relatively too much mid-frequency gain.

speech (90 dB SPL). A similar procedure can be carried out using more frequency-specific stimuli (such as narrow band or warble tones).

Field evaluation

The nature and number of unknowns previously discussed mean that a satisfactory fitting at an early stage, backed up by a comprehensive set of evaluative measures, is perhaps the exception more than the rule. An extremely important aspect of evaluation comes from observation of the child in the real world outside the clinic. The family will need to make frequent visits to the clinic in the early stages so that a picture of the child's aided performance can be gradually built up. At these sessions parents can be questioned in detail about the success of the fitting. In most places the family will also be visited regularly by a teacher/counsellor. Such professionals are more used to the effects of a hearing aid and comment from them is also valuable here. Essentially we need to know two things. First, is the hearing aid doing any good? As Tucker and Nolan point out this may not show up early in the fitting in terms of speech and language development. Rather it will be apparent from less specific behaviour such as the child being generally more responsive to sounds, being reluctant to take their hearing aids out, having their attention caught more easily and so on. The second question is whether reasons can be found for any tendency to reject the aids? Is the child easily upset or startled by loud noises? Does he or she reject the hearing aids in certain situations (e.g. noisy playgroup)? Is he or she reluctant to wear them at all (a possible sign of poorly fitting earmoulds)?

Information from observation both in the field and the clinic needs to be pieced together to decide on the adequacy of the fit. Sometimes the two sets of information are complementary (e.g. not enough gain achievable according to clinical measurements, and parents reporting little improvement in response to sound). In such situations steps must be taken to try to bring about a more satisfactory fitting. Sometimes the two sets of information are contradictory (e.g. the parents report no tolerance problems but the child reacts vigorously to modestly raised speech and narrow-band noise in the clinic). In such situations it may be necessary to ensure first that the parents have understood exactly what is being asked; that they are not answering one question where the clinician is asking another. Audiologists are used to using a wide range of terms to talk about sound. Some of these terms have been taken from general parlance, but have come to mean quite specific things. Words such as 'low' and 'high', 'comfortable' and 'uncomfortable' may mean something different to the non-expert who usually has a much less sophisticated set of terms to deal with sound (at least in the early stages of assessment and rehabilitation). Because of this, misunderstandings can arise. If contradiction remains then it is probably better to rely cautiously on the real-world performance of the child than on the less representative clinical results, until such a time as the contradiction can be resolved.

The fitting of a hearing aid to a young child affects both the child and their family in many complex and sometimes subtle ways. In the early stages parents must come to understand both the benefits and limitations that aids provide. They must cope with the new image of their child and learn how to develop ways of communication with the child that bring out the best in them. The role of the visiting teacher is vital in leading the family to a better understanding of what is happening, and facilitating the development of their child's potential. Liaison between the audiology services and the teaching services is therefore essential. The teachers provide important information which can help assess the success of a particular aid fitting.

In practice, field evaluation usually takes place during some form of 'hearing aid review' clinic. Such clinics are used to obtain the following information.

1. General comments from the parents, the visiting teacher and, if he or she is old enough, the child. Comments are sought on wearing time, apparent comfort, responses to sound when aided, changes in speech or language and signs of tolerance problems.
2. The ears are checked for occlusion by wax etc. The moulds are checked for damage or obstruction and fit. The aids are checked (on a hearing aid test box) for frequency response, gain, maximum output and distortion. Tympanometry can be useful to check for the presence of middle ear problems.
3. Various aided and unaided tests can be performed to:
   (a) obtain a clearer picture of unaided hearing;
   (b) confirm the adequacy of the aided thresholds;
   (c) check the child's tolerance of loud sounds;
   (d) check on the stability of the hearing and in particular that it shows no deterioration as a result of wearing the aid.

Speech tests of hearing can be performed here, though these are more useful as a demonstration to parents of aided benefit than as a means of confirming the adequacy of the aid or of choosing between different aids (see e.g. Green, 1988) .

Modification

If the field performance of the aid does not meet the required specifications then modification may be necessary. As before, various forms of modification are possible, involving re-setting the aid, changing it or altering the earmould. If the aided thresholds are not correct, the frequency response can be re-shaped with a combination of tone and volume control settings, or earhooks and earmoulds specially plumbed or filtered. If maximum output is not correct the hearing aid output control can be adjusted (though this usually produces a rather broad change across frequency). For children with very reduced dynamic ranges, carefully set compression limiting may be necessary. Earmould plumbing with sintered filters can also be used to control maximum output and this can provide an effective form of 'quasi-compression' limiting. However, the management of such filters with frequently changing earmoulds can be a problem.

If feedback is a problem it may indicate an occluded ear (e.g. wax) or a poorly fitting mould. If these possibilities have been ruled out then the fitting of a more powerful aid worn on a lower volume setting, or an aid with less high-frequency emphasis may solve the problem.

If exact modifications are required, say to bring aided thresholds in line with a prescription, these modifications can be monitored in a test box rather than on the patient. This is done by noting the difference between required and achieved aided thresholds, measuring the hearing aid frequency response in a test box at the initial setting and then resetting the aid until the difference between the final and initial setting matches the difference between required and achieved aided thresholds. Two cautionary comments are appropriate here: first, the limited flexibility of both the frequency response and maximum output adjustments of a hearing aid mean that an exact match may not be possible (or indeed strictly necessary); secondly, if the impedance of the hearing aid/earmould is changed, either by earmould plumbing or by trying a new hearing aid, the relationship between the differences of the initial and final settings in the test box and the same settings in the ear may change.

Objective evaluation

All of the above discussion has assumed at least some behavioural cooperation of the child at the centre of things. Various test procedures are being developed to enable us to obtain useful information from procedures which do not require such cooperation (other than that the child sit still). While there is not the space here to discuss these in any detail, it is at least worth while mentioning and referencing them so that the interested reader can explore them further.

Stapedius reflex testing

The stapedius reflex has been used for some time in paediatric work. Apart from being a useful diagnostic tool, its effectiveness as a predictor of degree of hearing loss and discomfort levels has been assessed (e.g. Preves and Orton, 1978; Lower, 1980). It turns out not to be a very accurate predictor of threshold. Patients with similar stapedius reflex thresholds can have very different audiometric thresholds. However, it can be used to measure the gain of a hearing aid by comparing the aided and unaided stapedius reflex thresholds. Furthermore, because the reflex is triggered by a subjectively loud sound, it bears some relationship to the patient's discomfort levels. If the gain and maximum output are correctly set the reflex thresholds should be well above the aided speech levels. The disadvantages of stapedius reflex testing are principally

- that behavioural thresholds are still required in order to specify the hearing aid gain in the first place; and
- that the reflex is simply not measurable for many patients, particularly those where there is conductive involvement or more severe degrees of hearing loss.

Brain stem evoked response testing

For very young or difficult to test children, the best estimate of the degree of hearing loss may come from evoked response testing (see Chapter 7). This information is not very frequency-specific and probably only serves to give an approximate measure of the degree of hearing loss in the 2–4 kHz region. Aided and unaided ABR measurements have been explored as a means of measuring the gain of a hearing aid objectively. Unfortunately, the reliability of ABR testing is very dependent on the integrity of the stimulus, and some of this integrity is lost when the stimulus is processed by a hearing aid. However, there is some recent evidence (Kiessling, 1982; Thornton, Yardley and Farrell, 1987) that the growth in amplitude of the ABR waveform is related to the degree of recruitment and so the loudness discomfort levels. Work currently under way in this area may enable us to predict objectively to some extent the required maximum output settings of a hearing aid.

Probe tube microphone measurements

One of the frequently discussed difficulties in the area of hearing aid fitting is that of relating hearing aid data (either taken from manufacturer's specifications or measured directly in a coupler) to what happens when the aid is worn on a real ear. For adults, real-ear aided and unaided thresholds can be used to measure the real-ear performance of the aid (but see Dillon and Murray, 1987; Green, 1987). However, the process is time consuming and on young children not always accurate. The recent innovation of probe tube measurement involves the insertion of a thin flexible probe microphone into the ear canal, either with or without the hearing aid/earmould, in order to measure the soundfield in the ear canal either aided or unaided. This procedure has the advantage that we can concentrate on using the cooperative spells of a behaviourally reluctant child to obtain unaided thresholds which are as accurate as possible. This then leads to a prescription for hearing aid gain and so aid selection, which can be checked using probe tube measurement *without* the child's active cooperation. They are again required only to sit still.

While this technique has considerable potential it also has some pitfalls which should be clearly understood before this technique is incorporated too uncritically into the clinic. Also, it does not supplement the need for behavioural aided thresholds as soon as these become possible. This is partly because probe microphony only measures what is happening in the ear canal while we are fitting aids to the whole child. We still do not know enough about what happens to the sound between canal and cortex. Also the importance of demonstrating aid benefit to the parents is often vital and this is done more impressively if they can see their child responding to quieter sounds when the aid is worn.

Final comments

While this chapter has concentrated on the hearing aid, it is important to realize that there is much more going on in hearing aid sessions than just matching an aid to a patient. The whole process can be an anxious one for parents. They may still be at the stage of trying to come to terms with the diagnosis of deafness, and have many unasked questions about its consequences. The hearing aid sessions should therefore be used to impart all necessary information to them and to allow them time to ask these questions. It is even a good idea for the clinician to have a check list, just to make sure that all important points have been covered. There is far more to impart than can be done in one session, and a coordinated approach to this provision of information by the whole team of people involved with the child is the ideal.

Parents should be given clear information about:

- the nature of the child's loss;
- the probable cause of the loss;
- the possibility of the loss being progressive;
- genetic considerations (is there a need for genetic counselling?);
- the justification for the hearing aid system fitted (e.g. why two aids are fitted, why a body-worn aid is recommended);
- where appropriate, possible alternatives (e.g. cochlear implants/bone-anchored hearing aids);
- myths and legends (e.g. 'He's deaf – he'll never talk', 'She's deaf – why bother with an aid?' 'Hearing aids bring back normal hearing', 'She's not deaf enough for an aid').

Parents need good working knowledge of the following:

- how to insert the mould;
- how to fit the aid relative to the mould;
- how the aid works (microphone/amplifier/receiver/tubing/mould/on–off/volume/battery);
- battery life;
- when to wear the aid;
- how to clean the aid/mould;
- how to prevent feedback;
- where to go for help;
- how to create good listening conditions (e.g. by getting rid of background noise and moving close to the child).

It should be clear from this chapter that an audiologist working with the hearing-impaired child needs to be a versatile member of the rehabilitation team. He or she must understand in detail the acoustical performance of the hearing aids that are being used and must know how to relate these performance characteristics to the psychoacoustics of the patient that is being fitted. He or she must be sensitive to the feelings of the child and their family. The aid itself provides a door through which that child can enter a hearing world, but every child needs to be helped through the door. For that to happen, the audiologist must work in close liaison with parents, teachers, doctors and all other caregivers involved with the child. Only then will the child be provided with his or her best chance of overcoming the handicap of deafness.

References

Bamford, J.M., Wilson, I.M., Atkinson, D. and Bench, R.J. (1980). Pure tone audiograms from hearing-impaired children. A statistical approach to summarizing audiogram information. *Scandinavian Audiology* 9, 195–200.

Berger, K., Hagberg, N.S. and Rane, R.L. (1977). *Prescription of Hearing Aids*. Kent, OH: Herald Publishing.

Byrne, D. (1983). Theoretical prescriptive approaches to selecting the gain and frequency responses of a hearing aid. *Monographs in Contemporary Audiology* 4, 1.

Byrne, D. and Dillon, H. (1986). The National Acoustic Laboratories' (NAL) new procedure for selecting the gain and frequency response of a hearing aid. *Ear and Hearing* 7, 257–265.

Byrne, D. and Tonisson, W. (1976). Selecting the gain of hearing aids for persons with sensorineural hearing impairments. *Scandinavian Audiology* 5, 51–59.

Cox, R.M. (1983). Using ULCL measures to find frequency/gain and SSPL90. *Hearing Instruments* 34, 17–21.

Dillon, H. and Murray, N. (1987). Accuracy of twelve methods for estimating the real ear gain of hearing aids. *Ear and Hearing* 8, 2–11.

Green, R.J. (1986). An investigation into the efficacy of hearing aid selection procedures. PhD Thesis, University of Salford.

Green, R.J. (1987). The uses and misuses of speech audiometry in rehabilitation. In: Martin, M. (Ed.), *Speech Audiometry*. London: Taylor and Francis.

Green, R.J. (1988). The relative accuracy of coupler and behavioural estimates of the real ear gain of a hearing aid. *British Journal of Audiology* 22, 35–45.

Kamm, C.A., Dirks, D.D. and Mickey, M.R. (1978). Effect of sensorineural hearing loss on loudness discomfort level and most comfortable loudness judgements. *Journal of Speech and Hearing Research* 21, 668–681.

Kiessling, J. (1982). Hearing aid selection by brain stem audiometry. *Scandinavian Audiology* 11, 269.

Lower, M.C. (1980). Measuring the real ear response characteristics of hearing aids. PhD Thesis, University of Southampton.

Northern, J.L. and Downs, M.P. (1984). *Hearing in Children*, 3rd edn. Baltimore: Williams and Wilkins.

Preves, D. and Orton, J.F. (1978). Use of acoustic reflex impedance measures in hearing aid fitting. *Hearing Instruments* 29, 22–24, 34–35.

Rintelmann, W.F. and Bess, F.H. (1977). High-level amplification and potential hearing loss in children. In: Bess, F.H. (Ed.) *Childhood Deafness – Causation, Assessment and Management*, pp. 267–293. New York: Grune and Stratton..

Seewald, R. and Ross, M. (1988). Amplification for young hearing impaired children. In: Pollack, M. (Ed.) *Amplification for the Hearing Impaired*, 3rd edn. New York: Grune and Stratton.

Seewald, R.C., Ross, M. and Spiro, M.K. (1985). Selecting amplification characteristics for young hearing-impaired children. *Ear and Hearing* 6, 48–53.

Thornton, R., Yardley, L. and Farrell, G. (1987). A preliminary report of an objective estimation of loudness discomfort levels using auditory brainstem evoked response. In: Baker, C. and Blum, T. (Eds), *Evoked Potentials III: The Third International Evoked Potential Symposium* London: Butterworth.

Tucker, I. and Nolan, M. (1984). *Educational Audiology*. Beckenham: Croom Helm.

Turner, C.W. and Holte, L.A. (1983). *Clinical evaluation of FM amplification systems based upon the speech spectrum*. Paper presented at the annual meeting of the American Speech–Language–Hearing Association.

Wallenfels, H.G. (1967). *Hearing Aids on Prescription*. Springfield, IL: C. C. Thomas.

Watson, N.A. and Knudsen, V.O. (1940). Selective amplification in hearing aids. *Journal of the Acoustical Society of America* 11, 406–419.

Chapter 12
Earmoulds

MICHAEL NOLAN

Introduction

Over the last few years there has been an increasing awareness of the importance of the earmould as an integral component of a wearable hearing aid. On the one hand, it is now possible to manipulate the entire frequency response of the hearing aid by attention to parameters of the earmould (Libby, 1985; Nolan, 1985; Coehorst, 1986) but on the other, there has been an ever-increasing lobby of opinion expressing total dissatisfaction with basic earmould provision, particularly for children (Booth and Nolan, 1985; National Deaf Children's Society, 1985). This lobby is understandable when one considers that all the potential benefits for linguistic development of early detection of hearing loss and an appropriate habilitative educational programme may be frustrated by an inadequate earmould service.

Earmould requisites

Responding to the needs of the hearing aid user

The primary role of the earmould in the amplification chain is one of linking the hearing aid to the hearing-impaired child, facilitating efficient transfer of acoustic energy to the tympanic membrane. However, in satisfying this role the earmould must respond to certain demands of the user. It must be comfortable to wear, easy to fit and remove (with young children this will be relevant to the parents), have a good cosmetic appearance, be easy to keep clean and facilitate a good acoustic fit in the meatus. Should any of these factors not be satisfied, then the likely outcome will be ineffective use of residual hearing via the hearing aid fitting. This may be because the quality of acoustic fit of the earmould is such that the aid cannot be set at the desired gain level without acoustic feedback howl. Alternatively, a child may continually remove the earmould if it is uncomfortable and this in turn will generate stress and frustration within the family. Professionals responsible for such families must be able to respond quickly and positively to overcome such situations.

Earmould materials

The choice of material is very important. It must be reliable and robust so as to be able to stand up to the wear and tear that it will inevitably get from a lively young child. It must be such that it does not generate an allergy in the child's external auditory meatus. There is little point in providing an earmould that splits after a few days use (e.g. a soft skeletal mould) – so choice of earmould configuration is equally important.

The ears of young children grow rapidly. Although it is difficult to specify how long a good fitting earmould is likely to last before the 'growth factor' will deem it unsatisfactory, it is unlikely to be longer than 2–3 months. This means, therefore, that hearing-impaired children are regularly presenting for new earmoulds. An additional professional 'want' must therefore be a quick processing time.

Earmould fabricators are continually on the look out for new materials that facilitate ease of working, with a quick processing time and precise definition. The panacea as far as children are concerned must be an instant or direct earmould. However, at present the vast majority of hearing-impaired children use two-stage or indirectly processed earmoulds. This is not to say that instant earmould materials are unavailable; rather that the system of earmould provision is geared around the indirect approach. It will be instructive to examine the two possible approaches to earmould fabrication in a little more detail and consider the strengths and weaknesses for the child user.

Earmould fabrication

Direct or instant approach

In the direct or instant method of earmould fabrication, the ear impression acts as the final earmould. There are obvious advantages to such an approach, particularly for children:

1. There is minimal delay in the making and fitting of a new mould.
2. A technician is able to repeat the process immediately should a mould prove unsatisfactory.
3. The process is cost effective when compared to indirect approaches.
4. The inaccuracies intrinsic to an indirect process are reduced (Brooks and Nolan, 1984).

Modern-day instant earmoulds are silicone-based polymers that cure at room temperature in the ear without exotherm (Tucker, Nolan and

Colclough, 1978; Insta Mould, 1979: Booth and Nolan, 1985). The major weaknesses of such materials were recognized during development as their relatively low shear strength and an inability to support a conventional lock spring ring for pocket aid use. Such problems have, however, been effectively overcome by improvements in the mechanical strength of the polymers, by careful use of fillers, by use of composite structures and by use of novel designs for the ring clip.

The primary reason today for the infrequent use of instant earmoulds, particularly in the NHS, results from limitations on technician time and training opportunities. Yet recent research has demonstrated that the direct approach using high-quality silicone rubber is the most accurate process thus far used in earmould fabrication (Nolan and Combe, 1987).

It is of relevance to note that there is evidence of a renewed interest in direct earmoulds in the paediatric sector, particularly in the larger special schools for the hearing impaired. This has in part been triggered by the reported success of large-scale earmould development projects based in developing countries (Commonwealth Society for the Deaf, 1987; Nolan and Tucker, 1988). The direct process was the only practical approach that could be used in these projects. A training video on the successful process was produced and this is now available together with earmould making kits from the author.

Although instant or direct earmoulds have potential for child usage, it is important not to lose sight of the fact that the process is vulnerable to one particular point. This may be best described as the 'skill of the fabricator' factor. Clearly an unskilled technician will not produce accurate earmoulds regardless of the materials provided for use. If a direct process is to be adopted, then the technician will require basic handling skills, good training and time to complete the job in hand. One may estimate that an instant earmould will take 15 min of actual handling time to fabricate. However, it is desirable from a cost effective viewpoint to parallel process a batch rather than work completely through individual earmoulds.

The procedures involved in the direct earmould process – from the investment of the material into the ear to the drilling and finishing of the earmould, are common in many respects with those used in the indirect approach. They will therefore be discussed in detail during the description of this alternative method of earmould fabrication.

Indirect or two-stage approach

The alternative category of earmould fabrication is the indirect or two-stage. This approach is applied with the vast majority of hearing aid users. It may be best understood by reference to Table 12.1.

The basic difference between the two approaches lies in the role of

Table 12.1 Two-stage earmould fabrication procedure

1. Ear impression taken in clinic
2. Ear impression trimmed and boxed
3. Order form filled in giving instructions on earmould configuration, type of material and special modifications
4. Ear impression despatched to laboratory
5. Ear impression received and numbered
6. Ear impression trimmed and wax dipped (optional)
7. Ear impression invested in plaster or an alternative model making medium
8. Model packed with earmould material
9. Earmould material cured
10. Cured earmould processed
11. Final earmould returned to clinic
12. Patient recall and earmould fitting

the ear impression. In the two-stage approach the impression does not act as the final earmould. Rather it acts as a former upon which a replica is fabricated. Two-stage earmoulds are usually made in specially equipped laboratories. These are normally some distance from the clinic and it is therefore necessary to transmit the impression by post which may lead to delay in the fitting of the earmould to the child. Table 12.2 contains a listing of the most commonly used two-stage earmould materials.

Surveys into earmould provision

Numerous surveys into earmould provision have been reported. Interestingly, all were based on services for hearing-impaired children. Perhaps the most disturbing aspect of these surveys is that they span a 20-year period and continue to report the same basic problem areas (Boothroyd, 1965; Huntington and Powell, 1973; Nolan and Tucker, 1977; Nolan et al., 1978, 1986; Reidner, 1978; Huntington, 1979; Martin et al., 1980; Grier and McVey, 1983; National Deaf Children's Society, 1985). Table 12.3 summarizes the areas that have been identified as contributing to poor and inadequate earmould provision.

Table 12.2 Two-stage earmould materials

Hard acrylic
Soft tip acrylic
All soft acrylic
Vinyl
Silicones
Vulcanized rubber
Light curing resins

Table 12.3 Factors contributing to inadequacy of earmould provision

1. A lack of awareness on the part of professionals of available resources, ear impression and earmould materials
2. Restricted range of ear impression and earmould materials from which to choose
3. A lack of realization that the earmould is a customized prosthesis specific to an individual hearing aid user
4. A lack of skilled professionals to take accurate ear impressions
5. Inappropriate ear impression making procedure – including lack of appropriate tools, poor interaction with patient, wrong technique of investment of impression material into the ear, use of unstable impression materials, delay in transmitting the impressions to the earmould laboratory
6. Inaccurate earmould making procedure – including inappropriate wax build-up of impression, poor trimming of impression prior to casting, failure to vacuum mix plaster – leading to poor finish on final mould, over-polishing of acrylic moulds, under curing of mould materials, use of poor quality tubing, failure to drill the sound tube to the limits defined by the earmould, poor workmanship on earmould plumbing, an unacceptably long delay in the provision of the earmould – thus lessening the chance of a satisfactory acoustic fit in a rapidly growing ear
7. Inappropriate choice of earmould configuration
8. Inadequate acoustic fit leading to feedback howl – desired gain from hearing aid unattainable
9. Earmould uncomfortable to wear

Given the point that the earmould has the potential to effectively nullify the benefits afforded by an appropriate hearing aid fitting, it would seem desirable to examine how professionals working in this field can act to provide an efficient and effective service. To this end, Table 12.1 will be traced step by step, so that potential pitfalls inherent in the two-stage process can be identified and appropriate management strategies adopted. Some of the points raised in the following discussion will have relevance for the one-stage process as well.

Providing an efficient and effective earmould service

Ear impression taking

The claim that earmoulds are badly fitting and uncomfortable to wear as a direct result of the poor quality of the ear impression (Blue, 1977, 1979; Babington, 1979; Mahon, 1984) highlights the vital importance of this element of the earmould fabrication procedure. It is absolutely imperative that an accurate replica of the requisite parts of the external ear is obtained if there is to be any chance whatsoever of obtaining a satisfactory earmould. An accurate ear impression is therefore fundamental to an effective earmould service. There is a simple practical process involved in obtaining an accurate impression of a child's ear. The process is based on:

- a fundamental knowledge on the part of the clinician of the anatomical landmarks of the external ear relevant to the earmould;
- a knowledge of the technique to use in obtaining an accurate impression of the ear;
- a knowledge of ear impression materials;
- an ability to interact positively with the child and parents.

The soft texture of a child's pinna demands a syringe investment approach for the impression material (Brooks and Nolan, 1984; Tucker and Nolan, 1986; British Society of Audiology, 1987). In the case of very young children this is best achieved with the baby lying on its side along its mother's lap. The process is very easy if the baby is asleep. From about 6 months of age the baby should be sitting side-saddle on the parent's knee with the head held against the parent's chest (Figure 12.1).

A confident, straightforward approach is essential when working with young children. Both parents and child will be somewhat apprehensive about the impression taking, particularly early after diagnosis.

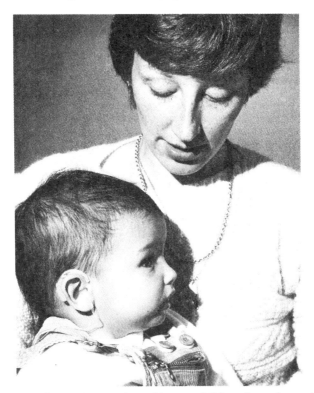

Figure 12.1 Set-up for ear impression taking on children from 6 months of age.

If the situation is well organized and relaxed these apprehensions will soon evaporate and subsequent impression-taking sessions can turn into a fun exercise. Clinicians should gain the trust of the child by playing for a short while before taking the impression (Figure 12.2).

The room where the impressions are to be taken should be clean, with the necessary tools including toys tidily laid out. A clear explanation of the job in hand should be given to the parents. Included in this should be details of how they can best help in getting the job done quickly and effectively.

Once a child has settled in the clinic the first job is to examine the external auditory meatus with a good auriscope. The canal should be free from debris and healthy. Small deposits of wax are of no consequence. However, should the canal be full of wax, obstructed by a foreign body or show evidence of disease, then the assistance of the GP or ENT specialist must be sought. The auriscope should be used by bracing one's hand against the side of the child's head so that any sudden movements from the child do not result in the instrument penetrating deep into the ear canal.

Following this examination, the ear canal must then be blocked by a suitably sized tamp made in either pre-expanded foam or cotton wool. The commercially available foam 'ear blocks' are very convenient yet generally too big for the ears of pre-school children. They must be pruned to a suitable size that facilitates a snug fit in the meatus and it is advisable to prune to a cone shape. There are still clinicians who

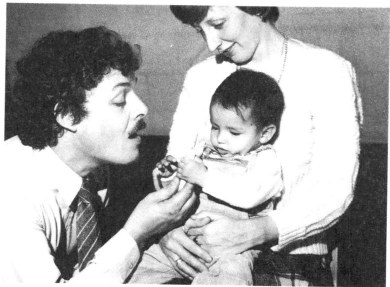

Figure 12.2 Child-oriented approach in ear impression taking – here the light pen is being used as a candle for the child to 'blow' out.

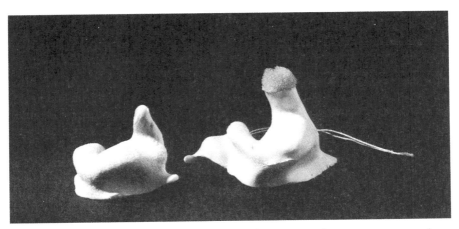

Figure 12.3 Examples of ear impressions from tamped versus no-tamped ear canals.

neglect to tamp the canal. Such a practice is both dangerous to the child and inevitably leads to a poorly defined meatal portion on the impression (Figure 12.3).

A knowledge of the anatomical landmarks of the external ear helps in siting the tamp at the 'target' spot in the meatus. This is at the junction of the cartilaginous and bony canal (Figure 12.4). It is not desirable for the tip of the final earmould to extend beyond the cartilaginous portion. If it does, then it is likely to prove uncomfortable to wear, difficult to fit and retain in the ear and, from an acoustical viewpoint, it will act to reduce the relative intensities of the higher speech frequencies (Nolan, 1985). The tamp should therefore be placed at the target spot sitting squarely in the meatus. The attached thread should be in the middle of the back of the tamp and run out of

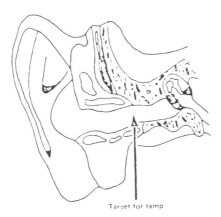

Target for tamp

Figure 12.4 Target for the tamp in the external auditory meatus.

the ear and hang freely down the side of the cheek (Figure 12.5). The tamp should be placed in position by means of a dedicated ear light or light pen, this being used in the same manner as the auriscope with the hand braced against the side of the child's head.

Once the tamp is in position the next job will be to prepare and then invest the impression material into the child's ear. The material must be invested in such a way that no distortion of the aural tissues occurs. Furthermore, the pinna must be in the 'wearing position', i.e. in the position relative to the head that it will take when the hearing aid is worn. This is an important point to note, particularly when children wear ear-level aids that may distort the pinna's position relative to the unaided situation. It is therefore recommended that the post-aural aid be placed in position before investment of the material in the ear (Figure 12.6).

The impression material must be invested into the ear by means of a syringe or 'gun' dispenser. Hand feeding of impression material, whereby the material is mixed, rolled into the shape of a carrot and forced into the ear by finger and thumb pressure, is no longer seen as an acceptable way of taking an accurate ear impression.

The choice of syringe for investment of the impression material is extremely important. Audiological syringes (Figure 12.7) are readily available from major outlets but they are only suitable for babies if supplied with the narrow 2 mm bore nozzles. It must be possible to place the syringe head adjacent to the tamp before investment of the material into the child's ear, otherwise the material tends to fall short in the

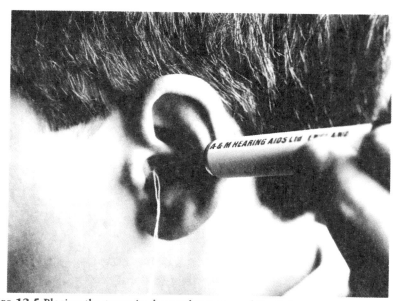

Figure 12.5 Placing the tamp in the ear by means of the light pen.

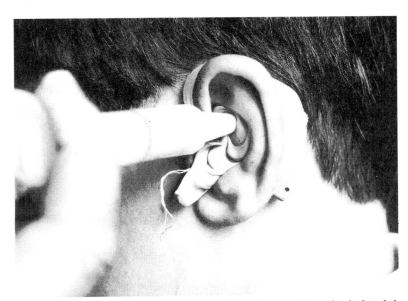

Figure 12.6 Investing the impression material in the ear. Note the behind-the-ear aid in position.

canal with resultant poor definition of the meatal projection of the impression. The diameter of the nozzles of the standard audiological syringes tends to be too wide and precludes placement at the desired position in the canal. Recent research has shown that the Impregum syringe (Figure 12.8) (available from dental wholesalers) is very effective for this purpose (Nolan et al., 1986). This syringe has a curved disposable nylon nozzle that can be cut to any desired diameter.

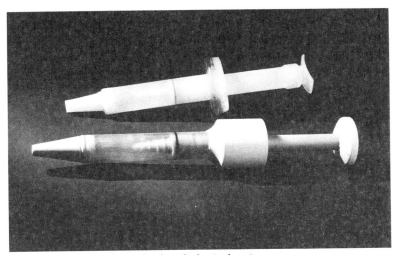

Figure 12.7 Examples of standard audiological syringes.

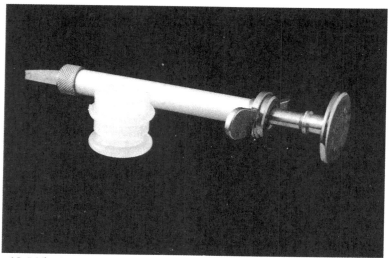

Figure 12.8 The Impregum syringe.

Nowhere can the need for a stable ear impression material be more apparent than in the fabrication of earmoulds for a child. In such a case one is dealing with an ear that is growing at an erratic rate. The earmould manufacturer can only fabricate to the accuracy inherent in the impression and any manufacturing ploys adopted to try to 'improve' upon the quality of the impression will inevitably lead to problems at fitting. Research into the properties of impression materials (McHugh and Purnish, 1984; Nolan and Combe, 1985; Combe, 1986) has clearly shown that alginates and acrylic based materials, such as Audalin, are totally unsuited to modern day needs, being unstable and showing massive shrinkage.

Clinicians who feel secure in the use of 'silicone' based materials should beware. The commonly used audiological silicones, whilst having improved properties over the alginates and acrylics, are not stable (Harcourt, 1978; Williams, Jackson and Bergman, 1984; Nolan and Combe, 1985). They belong to the condensation family of silicones. A new family of silicones – addition curing elastomers (vinyl polysiloxanes) has been developed. These materials find widespread use in dentistry because their dimensional accuracy is superb. Manufacturers have now introduced this material for audiological use (e.g. Dreve – Otoform A/K; 3M Health Care – Express Vinyl Polysiloxane) and it is strongly recommended that it be used with children.

It is vitally important for clinicians when working with impression materials to follow the manufacturer's mixing instructions to the letter. Having said that, one of the biggest criticisms of many ear impression manufacturers is the paucity of user instructions, particularly on mixing times and ratios. This is in stark contrast to the situation in dentistry where all materials have batch numbers and clearly written user instructions. Clinicians should seek the advice of their supplier should they be at all uncertain about the correct handling of impression materials.

Interestingly, manufacturers appear to be responding to the above criticism, the addition silicones having good user instructions. Measuring syringes for the two-component Otoform A/K system are available. The 3M Express system offers a quite novel means of ear impression taking. The two components are contained in twin barrels of a dispenser pack. This pack is loaded onto a special gun not unlike the mastic guns used in the building trade. When the trigger of the gun is pressed the two materials are automatically mixed via a disposable clip-on adapter through which they pass prior to investment into the ear (Figure 12.9). This approach has a number of advantages over the usual syringing technique. It removes the need for measuring out and mixing of the constituents. It speeds up the process considerably, particularly when dealing with groups of children. However, the basic problem at the present time is the cost per unit impression which makes the process uneconomical. Subsequent discussion will therefore centre on the more traditional syringing approach.

Sufficient impression material should be measured out to do one ear at a time. It should be thoroughly mixed to a uniform colour, not candy striped or blotchy. The syringe should then be loaded with sufficient material to fill the constituent parts of the child's ear. The syringe head should be placed adjacent to the tamp in the meatus and the material then smoothly invested, slowly withdrawing the syringe head but keeping it below the surface of the material. Particular attention

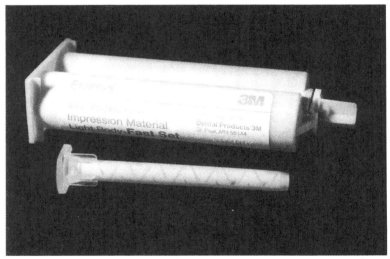

Figure 12.9 Components of the 3M Express system showing the twin barrel dispenser of addition cured silicone and the disposable mixing nozzle.

should be paid to the helix and a full concha bowl. The material should then be allowed to cure. Light pressure with a finger nail on the back of the impression will leave no mark when the impression has cured. The impression should then be very carefully removed by a rocking motion to avoid any undue stress or strain. It should be inspected for flaws and discarded if unsatisfactory. If all is well then the impression should be left to stand on a clean laboratory tile for 15 min to allow for complete polymerization.

Trimming and boxing of the ear impression

The meatal tip of the impression should be trimmed to the desired length with a scalpel. It should be cleaned to remove any deposits of cerumen etc., and then carefully packed in a strong box. On no account should the impression be placed in a tight plastic bag or be distorted by the lid of the box or accompanying paper work. Modern ear impression materials are pseudoplastic rather than elastic and will not recover their original shape following prolonged distortion. It is advisable to pin or glue the impression to the bottom of the box.

Choice of earmould material, configuration and special modifications

Before the earmould is despatched to the laboratory it will be necessary to advise the earmould contractor as to the required material, configuration and of any special modifications that are to be made. Table 12.2 lists the most commonly used earmould materials. It should be noted however, that not all of these will necessarily be available from any one laboratory. The acrylics will certainly be available but silicones and vinyl may not be. If earmoulds are provided via normal NHS channels then choice of materials will depend on which laboratory is allocated to a particular area. This is why some areas have adopted different arrangements of earmould provision for children and adults. The children's moulds are obtained from a private contractor in soft textured materials, e.g. high temperature vulcanized silicone rubber (Sneyd, 1986), vinyl (Dawson, 1977), while the adults are supplied through normal NHS channels.

Clearly, the choice of material for the earmould will depend on what is available. However, a wealth of research has demonstrated that paediatric services must have access to soft textured materials if the service is to be effective. In particular, heat cured vulcanized rubber, molloplast B denture soft lining material, soft acrylic and vinyl are cited as having advantages in terms of comfort, acoustic fit and in reducing the risk of damage to the external ear by play, in comparison with hard acrylic (Allen, 1973; McDonough, 1979 (unpublished MSc dissertation, University of Salford); Nolan, 1982; Brooks and Nolan, 1984; Roberts,

1984; Nolan et al., 1986; Sneyd, 1986). Yet despite this evidence and the earlier mentioned critical surveys into earmould provision where hard acrylic was found to be the most commonly used material, one still sees this material in widespread use with children today. Services must therefore take steps to organize supplies of soft textured earmoulds if they are to meet the demands of the majority of hearing-impaired young children.

The format of the final earmould will depend upon the type of hearing aid fitted (Figure 12.10). In the case of body-worn hearing aids a solid earmould with a lock ring in the backplate will be necessary. It is recommended that nylon rather than metal rings are used as they preclude the problem of the earphone nub being worn away by repeat insertion and removal from the earmould. If unchecked, this can result in acoustic feedback howl and eventually in the earphone continually falling from the ear.

With post-aural hearing aids a shell rather than skeletal format is desirable because the latter tend to crack after a relatively short time, particularly in the soft format. With very young children below 6 months of age, a hollow shell format in soft acrylic (Nolan et al., 1986), seems to be most appropriate.

In-the-ear hearing aids are packaged within the earmould. The custom ear or concha version is the most appropriate for use with young children. The shell or casing into which the electronic components are packed is produced in a very high quality acrylic format at the hearing aid manufacturer's premises. There is no choice of material with reference to texture with this type of hearing aid because of the nature of the prosthesis (Figure 12.11).

It was mentioned at the beginning of this chapter that it is technically possible to manipulate the entire frequency response of a hearing aid by attention to the earmould and associated plumbing. Attention to

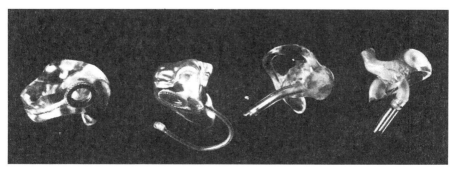

Figure 12.10 Earmould configurations. Left to right: solid mould for pocket use; solid mould with an ear hanger to support the mould in situ in the ear; skeletal mould for post-aural aid use; shell mould for post-aural aid use having a plastic elbow in the backplate.

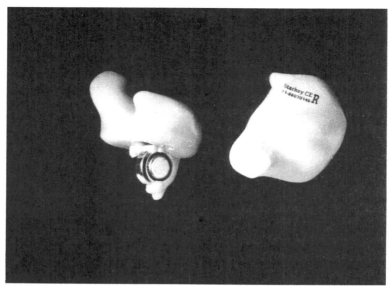

Figure 12.11 Custom ear and in-the-ear hearing aid.

the length and diameter of the sound tube (Nolan 1985), the use of earmould venting (Figure 12.12; Grover, 1984; Macrae, 1984; Nolan, 1985), open or no-mould fittings (Grover and Martin, 1979), damping elements and acoustic horn systems (Siemens, 1982; Ewens, 1984; Libby, 1985) can all quite separately and independently be used to manipulate the frequency response of the hearing aid in discrete frequency regions. Table 12.4 contains a summary of the possible manipu-

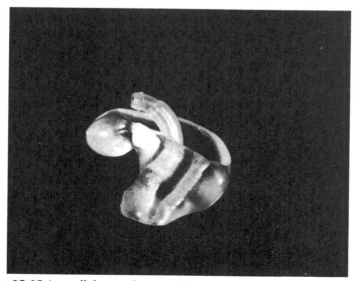

Figure 12.12 A parallel vented earmould.

Table 12.4 Possible earmould manipulations and anticipated influence on the hearing aid frequency response

Manipulation	Anticipated influence on frequency response
Bore diameter change	High frequency reduction as diameter is reduced (above 1 kHz)(Figure 12.13)
Meatal tip length change	1. A longer tip length produces a relative reduction in the higher speech frequencies (above 1 kHz)
	2. A longer tip increases the overall sound pressure level at the tympanic membrane (Figure 12.14) (+6 dB with a cavity size reduction of one half; Jirsa and Norris, 1976)
	3. Shortening the tip can act to reduce the 'barrel' or 'tunnel' effect about which subjects sometimes complain with respect to voice quality
Venting	1. A second bore is drilled through the mould either parallel or inclined into the sound tube – parallel venting is desirable. The result is de-emphasis of low frequencies below 1 kHz. The length and diameter of vent influences the frequency where roll off occurs. Increasing vent diameter or shortening its length increases attenuation of low frequencies
	2. Increased risk of acoustic feedback. 35 dB of gain is the maximum to expect with a vented earmould – compared to 60/65 dB with a well-fitting version
Damping	1. Facilitated by fused mesh elements or sintered metal pellets that fit snugly into the ear hook or earmould tubing
	2. Used to reduce the resonance effects in the sound transmission channel of post-aural aids resulting in a smoothing of frequency response. Effective in the 1–3 kHz region. Dampers are colour coded for different frequency bands
Horning	1.Facilitated by drilling of a stepped bore configuration through the earmould or by fitting of a precast plastic horn
	2. Provides the potential for extending the frequency response to the limits of the output transducer
	3. Increased risk of condensation in the sound tube

lations of the earmould and their anticipated effects on the frequency response of the hearing aid. It should be emphasized, however, that these effects must not be assumed to occur. The resulting changes to the frequency response must be formally assessed on individual patients by use of sound field or probe microphone measures (Pedersen, 1985).

This non-electronic tuning of the frequency response may be used to effect a more satisfactory quality of fit to a hearing-impaired individual.

However, it may do the opposite and generate more problems. As far as young children are concerned, specific difficulties arise because, for example, of the available space in which to work. This can make venting and horning difficult. Furthermore, the earmoulds of many hearing-impaired children are naturally vented anyway by a slit vent between the canal wall and the surface of the earmould. This is why feedback is often a real handicap and prevents the child using the hearing aid to maximum effect.

Clinicians ought to have the necessary tools, knowledge, skill and training to facilitate the modifications mentioned above when the need arises. A good-quality model-maker's drill, a selection of dental drill bits, damping elements, acoustic horns and tubing should be on hand in the clinic. The starting point should be an accurate earmould to which modifications may then be made.

A few general points of note may be made with reference to Table 12.4. For the vast majority of young children no modifications will be necessary and the aim will be to fit the hearing aid at the desired gain level without feedback. However, clinicians should check that the diameter of the sound tube has been drilled to its limits so as to minimize the filtering effects of narrow bores on the frequency response of the hearing aid above 1 kHz (Figure 12.13). It is vitally important to provide a child with as favourable an experience of the higher speech frequencies as possible (Pascoe, Miemoller and Miller, 1973; Triantos and McCandles, 1974). If there is scope for a wider bore and the material is amenable to manipulation (vinyl and silicones are difficult to work) then the bore should be widened and the tip flared.

Despatching the earmould

Once the ear impression has been taken the objective must be to fabricate the final earmould in as short a time as possible. Any unnecessary delay will increase the risk of the mould proving inadequate in terms of acoustic fit. A maximum turn-round of 8 days must be achieved with children's earmoulds. One potential problem of the two-stage process is the time taken to get the product to and from the laboratory. Some services have made special arrangements for children's earmoulds, having courier delivery of the impression and the final earmould. This has reduced the turn-round to a few days and also helped to improve the working relationship of the clinic and contractor.

Earmould fabrication

Over the last few years there has been a marked improvement in the quality control procedures as applied to earmould contractors supplying the NHS. This has resulted from the adoption of British Standard

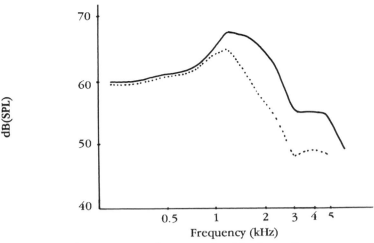

Figure 12.13 The mean sound pressure level in the auditory meatus as a function of the bore diameter of the earmould ($n = 4$, sound tube length 30 mm) ——2mm; ······1mm.

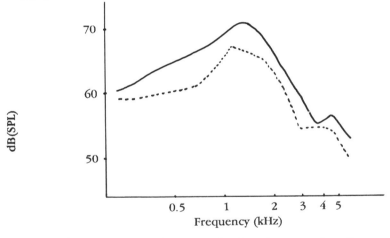

Figure 12.14 The mean sound pressure level in the external auditory meatus as a function of the length of the earmould sound tube ($n = 4$, sound tube diameter 2 mm). ——40 mm; ······30 mm.

5750, Part 2 (BSI, 1979). In addition, improvements in production procedures such as routine use of vacuum investing apparatus for plaster mixing (which precludes the problems of blow-holes and other surface blemishes on the earmould) have contributed to a more efficient earmould service.

Earmould manufacturers are continually striving to improve and extend their product range. Most of the new developments come from dentistry and one example, the light curing resins (Combe, 1986), appear to have exciting prospects for audiological application. At the present time, however, the soft textured silicones, acrylics and vinyl should be the materials of choice for children.

Earmould management

Parents must be given careful guidance on how to clean and dry the earmould and how to check and replace the tubing. Practice on insertion and removal of the earmould should be part of the programme of introduction to the hearing aid system.

It will be necessary for parents to obtain new earmoulds for their child quite frequently in the early years of life. It is not possible to put a time span on the life of an earmould because there are many factors that will be influencing the situation. What is certain, however, is that an open referral arrangement for new ear impressions must operate. Rigidly arranged appointments made at the time of the previous impression session, e.g. 'we'll see you in three months time', are a waste of time and will inevitably mean that many young children will be penalized in terms of effective use of their residual hearing. Parents must be informed that they should go for new impressions immediately there is any problem in setting the aids at the desired gain level. If this is a fortnight after the previous session then so be it. Parents must not be made to feel that they are being a nuisance if they persist in trying to maintain effective earmoulds for their child.

On odd occasions children present in the clinic as earmould nibblers. These are children who may habitually chew the tips of their earmoulds or on some occasions bite the tips completely off. This may be purely habit and if so the child should be dissuaded from doing it. However, it may be because the mould is uncomfortable to wear, perhaps because the tip is too long.

Professionals and parents should be on the look out for allergy to the earmould material. Dry, flaking skin or itching of the concha and meatus are clearly signs of this problem. Use of an alternative material, for instance, vulcanite, and referral to the GP are essential in such cases.

Parents must be alerted to the potential problem of condensation in the sound tubes of post-aural aids that can lead to intermittency of sound. The problem is easily overcome by detaching the mould from the aid and blowing the moisture out with a puffer. It is of interest to note the recent introduction of a new type of tubing – Stay-Dry, which the manufacturers claim will help overcome this problem (Takinishi and Itedan, 1984; Libby, 1985).

Acoustic feedback

Acoustic feedback or the characteristic high pitched whistle (howl) that can be sometimes heard emanating from children's hearing aids is one

Table 12.5 Factors contributing to acoustic feedback – management strategies.

Problem 1
Sound leakage from an acoustically poorly fitting earmould
Solution 1
Provide accurate earmoulds in soft textured materials; adopt a child-centred management programme

Problem 2
Sound leakage from the ear as a result of the earmould being incorrectly fitted. This usually occurs when the helix of the mould is not located behind the crus of the helix of the pinna
Solution 2
Instruct the parents and child on how to put the earmould in and how to remove it from the ear

Problem 3
Sound leakage from the coupling point between receiver and spring ring in body worn aids
Solution 3
Use nylon rings; replace the plastic washer on the receiver with a thin layer of blue tac'

Problem 4
Sound radiating from the tubing in post-aural aids
Solution 4
Use a thick walled tube (1 mm) especially with high power post-aurals. This strategy may require the use of a nylon insert in the back of the earmould rather than a bonded tube (Tucker and Nolan, 1986)

Problem 5
Sound radiating from tube connections and other plumbing connections in post-aural aids
Solution 5
Ensure that all connections are tight, that tubing is replaced regularly and not allowed to dry out, that the thread on the elbow of the hearing aid is not worn and the connection with the aid housing tight. Check the integrity of the plumbing by blocking the end of the mould with the thumb and listening for feedback howl. Should it occur then seek to isolate the problem by systematically reducing the sound path, i.e. remove the earmould and check again with thumb over the end of the elbow of the aid. Then remove the elbow and check again with thumb over the end of the output portal on the aid casing

Problem 6
Sound radiating from the ear as a result of an increase of sound pressure level in the ear canal. This may be due to a temporary conductive episode or impacted wax
Solution 6
Examine the ear canal for wax, arrange for an impedance measurement to be made and seek the opinion of an ENT specialist. This factor is often missed by clinicians who persist in making repeat earmoulds

of the most frustrating factors for both parents and professionals. It is by definition the return of some of the energy of the output signal from the hearing aid earphone receiver to the input transducer (the microphone). This leakage or feedback of sound initially causes colorations in the sound, followed by a noticeable ringing on transients with deterioration in sound quality, progressing to a howl or the characteristic high pitched whistle when the aid reaches oscillation point and a continuous saturation output is produced for no input (Nolan, 1983). The result of this condition is gross distortion of any processed signals and a totally unacceptable amplification system. The temporary cure for howl is reduction in the gain of the hearing aid because howl occurs when the gain exceeds the attenuation present in the feedback path. The unfortunate consequence of this action for a hearing-impaired child could be totally ineffective amplification because of inadequate usable gain.

Table 12.5 summarizes the main factors that contribute to acoustic feedback in modern conventional hearing aids together with suggested solutions for overcoming them. Feedback can result from factors other than acoustical. Electrical and mechanical feedback may arise (De Boer, 1963) although such factors should have been effectively dealt with by design engineers. It is of interest to note from Table 12.5 that feedback is not only caused by a poorly fitting earmould. Professionals should therefore adopt a logical procedure of investigation into the reason for a feedback problem particularly when the earmould appears to be satisfactory.

Concluding remarks

It is evident that an increasing number of hearing-impaired children are presenting for management in the first year of life. If these children are to benefit in terms of linguistic development from an early intervention programme, then it is vital that effective amplification is fitted immediately following diagnosis. This demands an efficient earmould service.

It should be apparent from the above discussion that the earmould is an integral component of a wearable hearing aid. It has the potential to make or break a habilitative programme for a hearing-impaired child. There is no excuse today for children being furnished with inadequate earmoulds. Research has shown the way for all professionals to achieve a satisfactory earmould service.

References

Allen, G.H. (1973). Report on the use of molloplast B for earmoulds. *Talk* **70**, 31–32.

Babington, A.G. (1979). Technology of the individual earmould. *Hearing Aid Journal* **32**, 22, 24.

Blue, V.J. (1977). Help us to help you! A good earmould is the key to a successful fitting. *Hearing Aid Journal* 30, 41–42.

Blue, V.J. (1979). Four keys to quality custom earmoulds. *Hearing Aid Journal* 32, 42–43.

Booth, C.L. and Nolan, M. (1985). *Compilation of a Bibliography on Earmoulds*. London: DHSS.

Boothroyd, A. (1965). The provision of better earmoulds for deaf children. *Journal of Laryngology and Otology* 79, 320–335.

British Society of Audiology (1987). Recommended procedure for taking an aural impression. *British Journal of Audiology* 20, 315–317.

British Standards Institution (1979). *Quality systems Part 2. Specification for manufacture and installation*. London: British Standards Institution.

Brooks, D.N. and Nolan, M. (1984). Good fitting earmoulds. In: Wald, M., Harris, G., Ewens, S. and Grover, B. (Eds), *The Earmould, Current Practice and Technology*, pp. 4–10. Reading: Hearing Aid Audiology Group, British Society of Audiology.

Coehorst, R. (1986). *Influencing Acoustic in the Fitting of Hearing Aids*. Eindhoven: Product Info. Hearing Aids, Philips.

Combe, E.C. (1986). *Notes on Dental Materials*, 5th edn. London: Churchill Livingstone.

Commonwealth Society for the Deaf (1987). *Report of the Madras Working Party*. London: The Commonwealth Society for the Deaf.

Dawson, F. (1977). Earmould production in vinyl – the end of feedback. *Journal of the British Association of Teachers of the Deaf* 1, 209–212.

De Boer, B. (1963). Avoiding feedback in hearing aids. *Morerate Akustik* 2, 122–125.

Ewens, S. (1984). Earmould plumbing. In: Wald, M., Harris, G., Ewens, S. and Grover, B. (Eds), *The Earmould, Current Practice and Technology*, pp. 13–19. Reading: Hearing Aid Audiology Group, British Society of Audiology.

Grier, A.M. and McVey, E. (1983). A survey of 3392 earmoulds in Scottish schools by the Scottish Association for the Deaf. *Health Bulletin* 41, 305–309.

Grover, B. (1984). Venting. In: *The Earmould, Current Practice and Technology*, pp. 10–13. Reading: Hearing Aid Audiology Group, British Society of Audiology.

Grover, B. and Martin, M.C. (1979). Physical and subjective correlates of earmould occlusion. *Audiology* 18, 335–350.

Harcourt, J.K. (1978). A review of modern impression materials. *Australian Dental Journal* 23, 178–186.

Huntington, A. (1979). How near is the end of feedback? *Journal of the British Association of Teachers of the Deaf* 3, 123–127.

Huntington, A. and Powell, C.A. (1973). Research into the practical efficiency of earmoulds worn by hearing-impaired school children. *British Journal of Disorders of Communication* 8, 72–73.

Insta Mold Prosthetics Inc. (1979). *Insta-mold Silicone for Earmoulds*. Philadelphia: Insta Mold Prosthetics Inc.

Jirsa, R. and Norris, T.W. (1976). *Relationship of performance characteristics in hearing aids to cavity volume*. Paper read at American Audiology Society Meeting, Las Vagus, NV.

Libby, E.R. (1985). Earmould modification by special bores and dampers, particularly in relation to the mid and high frequency range. *Audiology in Practice* 11, 5–7.

McHugh, E.R. and Purnish, H.A. (1984). Evaluating the accuracy of earmould impression materials. *Hearing Instruments* 35, 12, 15, 60.

Macrae, J. (1984). Earmould venting. *Audiology in Practice* 1, 7–8.
Mahon, W.J. (1984). Earmould remakes: The bottom line causes. *Hearing aid Journal* 37, 7–10.
Martin, M.C., Grover, B.C., Wright, V., Brooks, G. and Johnson, J. (1980). *Hearing Aids and Earmoulds at Heathlands School*. London: Royal National Institute for the Deaf.
National Deaf Children's Society (1985). Earmoulds: Fitting problems undermine the work of the hearing aid. *Talk* 117, 14–17.
Nolan, M. (1982). *Modern Developments in Earmould Technology: Implications for the Profoundly Deaf*. Paper presented at the 16th International Congress of Audiology, Helsinki, Finland.
Nolan, M. (1983). Acoustic feedback – causes and cures. *Journal of the British Association for Teachers of the Deaf* 7, 13–17.
Nolan, M. (1985). The earmould: variations in the transmission curve of a hearing aid as a result of changes in the sound bore diameter and length, and venting. *Audiology in Practice* 11, 1–4.
Nolan, M. and Combe, E.C. (1985). Silicone materials for ear impressions. *Scandinavian Audiology* 14, 35–39.
Nolan, M. and Combe, E.C. (1987). *Dimensional Accuracy and Stability of Materials and Techniques Associated with Audiology*. London: DHSS.
Nolan, M. and Tucker, I.G. (1977). A simple method of improving the acoustic seal of an earmould. *Journal of the British Association for Teachers of the Deaf* 1, 74–77.
Nolan, M. and Tucker, I.G. (1988). A project to develop services for hearing-impaired children in Ethiopia. In: Taylor, I.G. (Ed.), *The Education of the Deaf: Current Perspectives*, Volume 4, pp. 94–97. London: Croom Helm.
Nolan, M., Elzemety, S., Tucker, I.G. and McDonough, D.F. (1978). An investigation into the problems involved in producing efficient earmoulds for children. *Scandinavian Audiology* 7, 231–237.
Nolan, M., Hostler, M., Taylor, I.G. and Cash, A. (1986). Practical considerations in the fabrication of earmoulds for young babies. *Scandinavian Audiology* 15, 21–27.
Pascoe, D.P., Miemoller, A.F. and Miller, J.D. (1973). *Hearing aid design and evaluation for a presbycusis patient*. Paper presented at the eighty-sixth meeting of the Acoustical Society of America.
Pedersen, B. (1985). Fitting hearing aids using insertion gain measurements. *Audiology in Practice* 11, 3–4.
Roberts, A.C. (1984). *An Investigation into New and Advanced Prosthetic Materials and Techniques for Earmoulds*. London: DHSS.
Reidner, E.D. (1978). Monitoring of hearing aids and earmoulds in an educational setting. *Journal of the American Audiological Society* 4, 39–43.
Siemens (1982). *Some Possibilities to Vary the Transmission Curve of BTE Hearing Aids by Using Additional Acoustic Elements*. Erlangen: Siemens Electroacoustic Sector.
Sneyd, A. (1986). *EMTEC Earmould Handbook*. Letchworth, Herts: Emtec Labs.
Takinishi, K. and Itedan, I. (1984). A new earmould tubing to reduce moisture problems. *Hearing Instruments* 35, 32, 60.
Triantos, T.J. and McCandles, G.A. (1974). High frequency distortion. *Hearing Aid Journal* 27, 38.
Tucker, I.G. and Nolan, M. (1986). *Educational Audiology*. London: Croom Helm.

Tucker, I.G., Nolan, M. and Colclough, R.O. (1978). A new high efficiency earmould. *Scandinavian Audiology* **7**, 225–229.

Williams, P.T., Jackson, D.G. and Bergman, W. (1984). An evaluation of the time dependent-dimensional stability of eleven elastomeric impression materials. *Journal of Prosthetic Dentistry* **52**, 120–125.

Chapter 13
Cochlear implants

SARAH SHEPPARD

Introduction

Cochlear implants are a relatively new form of assistive device for the profoundly deaf who receive little, if any, benefit from conventional acoustic hearing aids. The development of cochlear implants has enabled the direct electrical stimulation of remaining auditory nerve fibres thus bypassing non-functional or absent hair cells in the cochlea. The electrically induced nerve impulses are transmitted to the auditory centres of the brain to produce a sensation of hearing (Figure 13.1).

The history of cochlear implants can be traced back to Volta's experiment in 1800, in which he applied electric current to his own ears, and is described in more detail by Luxford and Brackmann (1985), House and Berliner (1991) and Mecklenburg and Lehnhardt (1991). Modern research into cochlear implants was inspired by Djourno and Eyries (1957), who placed electrodes on the auditory nerve of a patient undergoing a cholesteatoma operation. When a small electric current was passed through these electrodes, some auditory sensation was evoked. William House and his colleagues developed the first clinical cochlear implant in the early 1970s in the USA (House et al., 1976). This device had a single active electrode which was sited inside the cochlea and has been used widely in both adults and children (House, Berliner and Eisenberg, 1983). Clark and his colleagues contributed significantly to the field of cochlear implantation by developing the Nucleus 22 multichannel device (Clark et al., 1987; Clark, Tong and Patrick, 1990). This implant is currently the most extensively used device for children. A different design of multichannel implant was developed alongside the Nucleus device in the USA and is known as the Ineraid (formerly Richards or Utah) cochlear implant (Eddington et al., 1978; Parkin and Stewart, 1988). Technology in the area of cochlear implants is advancing rapidly and several other research teams have developed a variety of other implant systems throughout Europe, the USA and Australia, some of which are commercially available although

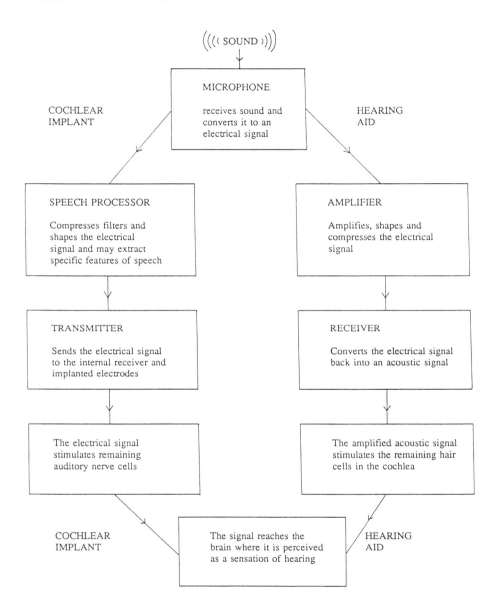

Figure 13.1 Diagrammatic representation of the components of a hearing aid and a cochlear implant, illustrating their function.

others are still at the experimental stage. Lance de Foa and Loeb (1991) have summarized the implant systems available and those in the development stage. Cochlear implantation had a late start in the UK but implants are now accepted as an appropriate treatment for suitable profoundly deaf children (Rosen, 1990; McCormick, 1991).

Cochlear implant design

All cochlear implant systems function in a broadly similar way. Externally the microphone, which is usually housed in a case similar to a miniature post-aural hearing aid, picks up sound and converts this acoustic signal into an electrical signal. The speech or sound processor is usually body worn and is connected to the microphone via a lead. A single-channel implant system has, however, recently been developed with a post-aural processor which also incorporates the microphone (Hochmair-Desoyer, Hochmair and Klasek, 1991). Speech processors modify the incoming signal into an appropriate form to be delivered to the internal implanted electrodes so that auditory neurones are stimulated to produce a sensation of hearing (Figure 13.2).

Cochlear implant systems vary in terms of the number and position of electrodes, the type of signal processing and the method of communicating information from the external to the internal parts of the device.

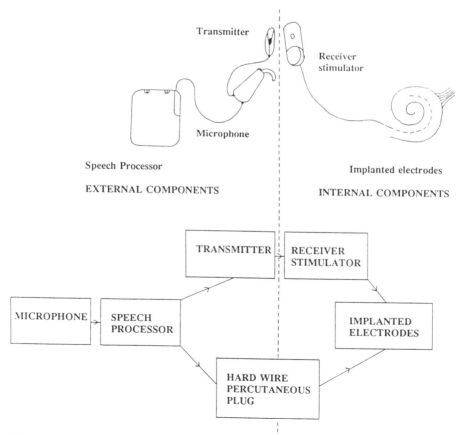

Figure 13.2 The external and internal components of cochlear implant systems.

Signal transfer from external to internal parts of implant

Transfer of the signal to the implanted electrodes may be achieved transcutaneously (across the skin), or via a percutaneous plug through the skin.

In transcutaneous systems an external transmitter connected via a lead to the speech processor transmits the signal by electromagnetic means through the intact skin to an implanted receiver. The transmitter and receiver are often magnetized to keep the transmitter in the correct position. Some systems use a percutaneous plug through the skin to allow transfer of the signal via a direct wire connection to the internal electrode array. Transcutaneous systems may be restricted in the implementation of future processing strategies but most paediatric implant programmes use transcutaneous systems because of the increased risk of damage and infection around the pedestal of percutaneous systems. Young children have, nevertheless, been successfully implanted with percutaneous implant systems (Montandon, Kasper and Pelizzone, 1991).

Electrodes

In order for an electric current to flow there must be an active electrode (or positive pole) and an inactive electrode (or negative pole). Charge flows from the active to the inactive electrode, thus inducing an electric current. The inactive electrode is sometimes called the *reference electrode*. In *monopolar* systems the active and reference electrodes are positioned remotely; for example, the active electrode may be inside the cochlea and the reference electrode embedded in muscle tissue outside the cochlea. If the active and reference electrodes are in close proximity, for example situated adjacently inside the cochlea the system is *bipolar*. Monopolar systems require less current because the current spreads over a wider area. Bipolar stimulation activates more discrete groups of nerve fibre and can be advantageous if different groups of nerve fibres are to receive different information, but more current is required because fewer fibres are stimulated around the electrode.

Location of electrodes

Cochlear implants may be extracochlear or intracochlear, terms which refer to the location of the active electrodes: *extracochlear* electrodes are placed on the promontory or round window; *intracochlear* electrodes are inserted inside the cochlea, necessitating the surgeon drilling into the cochlea, and therefore causing some damage to it and hence any residual hearing (Boggess, Baker and Balkany, 1989). No damage to the cochlea occurs with extracochlear placement of electrodes but higher current levels may be required because the active electrode is further away from the auditory nerve tissue.

Number of electrodes

The terms *multi-electrode, multichannel, single electrode* and *single channel* are often used to describe implant systems: multi or single electrode refers to the number of electrodes that the implant has; multi- or single channel describes the number of active electrodes through which different information is sent. In a single-channel system a single electrode or several electrodes may convey the same information. Occasionally more than one electrode is implanted but information is sent only through one active electrode: such a system would be described as multi-electrode but single channel.

If several electrodes are implanted, usually intracochlearly, and different information is conveyed through different electrodes the device is described as *multichannel*. Extracochlear multichannel systems have been used (Hortman et al., 1989) but have not shown the same promise as intracochlear multichannel systems which mimic the tonotopic organization of the cochlea.

Signal processing

Cochlear implant systems also vary in the type of signal processing that they employ. The electric current may be presented to the implanted electrodes as a continuous analogue waveform or as a series of short fast pulses. Pulsatile stimulation comprises series of pulses representing a digitized sample of the original waveform, which may affect the timing clues within the speech signal more than an analogue system but prevents interaction between channels in multichannel systems. Perceived loudness increases with increasing current level and duration of each pulse.

Processing of the signal from the microphone is necessary because the acoustic dynamic range is much wider than the electrical dynamic range (Clark and Tong, 1982). Information must therefore be compressed to be represented within the narrow electrical dynamic range. Signal processing strategies have varying philosophies but all aim to allow the implantee to discriminate speech to some degree. Most single-channel devices use a broad-band analogue signal which is compressed, filtered and then delivered to a single active electrode (Cooper et al., 1989; Hochmair, Hochmair and Zierhofer, 1990).

The Ineraid cochlear implant is a multichannel analogue system which transmits different frequency bands of the filtered spectrum to different channels. Other multichannel devices (such as the Nucleus

22-channel implant) employ a more vigorous approach to speech processing by extracting the formant frequencies of speech, that is the fundamental frequency F0, first formant F1, and second formant F2, which are important for speech intelligibility.

The most widely used coding strategy presently used with the Nucleus implant is known as MULTIPEAK. For this strategy the formants F1 and F2 are extracted from the speech signal together with three high-frequency bands of information which are transmitted to different electrodes. The fundamental frequency, F0, or the voice pitch is approximated by the pulse rate (von Wallenberg and Battmer, 1991).

Speech processing strategies are continually evolving. A new continuous interleaved sampling (CIS) processing technique allows different channels of filtered information to be presented in short fast pulses interleaving between electrodes at a very fast pulse rate (Wilson et al., 1991). Interactions between different channels that are stimulated simultaneously, and may give unpredictable fluctuations in loudness and pitch, are eliminated using the CIS processing method with the Ineraid implant – this may be one factor contributing to improved performance with CIS. Variations in the pitch perception of Ineraid implantees using standard analogue frequency band processing have been reported by Dorman et al. (1990). A new processing strategy is being developed for the Nucleus implant, which selects six peaks from the speech frequency range and presents these stimuli at 250 pulses/s to electrodes at positions selected on the basis of the spectral frequencies. This new processing method is still under investigation but is showing some improvements over previous speech feature extraction strategies (McKay et al., 1991). Combinations of broad-band analogue and feature-extraction pulsatile strategies delivered to different channels in the same implant are under investigation (von Wallenberg, Hochmair and Hochmair-Desoyer, 1990). New implants that are adaptable to different processing strategies are also being developed (Peeters, Officiers and Marquet, 1990; Shindler and Kessler, 1992).

Selection of a cochlear implant for use with children

Children implanted at an early age will need to use their implants for many years. The safety and efficacy of implant systems is therefore of great importance. Before using cochlear implants with children, sufficient time is needed to show proven benefit from the same implants in adults with acquired deafness and it is advisable to examine adult performance data with a particular device. This will not, however, guarantee success in the paediatric population because young children may have little or no memory of spoken language and will have different rehabilitation requirements than adults. House and Berliner (1986) reported results on the safety and efficiency of the House/3M device. Issues surrounding the biocompatibility and safety of implants have been addressed in detail by Shepherd, Franz and Clark (1990) with particular reference to the Nucleus device. This is the only cochlear implant currently used which has the full approval of the Food and Drug Administration of the USA for use with children.

Effects of chronic electrical stimulation

The effects of chronic electrical stimulation have been investigated in animal studies (Dodson et al., 1986). There is some suggestion that low levels of electrical stimulation have a beneficial effect on neuronal survival (Miller, 1991). Examination of the temporal bones of deceased implantees has shown that fibrous tissue develops around the drilled areas of the cochlea: there was, however, no difference in the ganglion cell population of the implanted ears compared with non-implanted ears, except for a small loss of ganglion cells in those who were using the Ineraid implant which has a deeply inserted electrode array (Terr, Sfogliano and Riley, 1989; Linthicum et al., 1991).

Long-term use of cochlear implants in humans has not shown any signs of deterioration in patient responses as a result of chronic electrical stimulation (Parkin and Randolph, 1991; Waltzman, Cohen and Shapiro, 1991). However, the full effects of electrical stimulation of auditory nerve tissues in humans over decades of cochlear implant use are as yet unknown.

Long-term support

Once a patient has been implanted they will need access to external equipment compatible with the implanted electrode array. Manufacturers of cochlear implants should ensure their commitment to existing implantees to allow for maintenance of implant systems and should, as far as possible, allow existing implantees to take advantage of new developments in speech processing and external hardware design. To provide this type of back-up support, cochlear implant manufacturers will, of course, need a high level of financial stability.

Ergonomics

Ergonomic features such as unpluggable leads are important for children, where damage to leads is more likely. If the leads do not unplug the whole headset needs to be changed if a lead is damaged. The external equipment needs to be durable but not too heavy or bulky for the child to wear.

Choice of device

Paediatric cochlear implant programmes may use more than one type of cochlear implant to best suit individual needs. In the case of ossified cochlea following meningitis (Hinojosa, Douglas Green and Marion, 1991; Nadol and Hsu, 1991) the surgeon may wish to use an extra-cochlear implant, whereas with other children a multichannel intra-cochlear implant would be preferred. Paediatric cochlear implant centres need to keep a good stock of spare equipment for each type of device used. If too many different devices are used greater resources will be involved in programming equipment and stocks of spare equipment. Once a child has been implanted it is important that the implant programme is able to supply and replace equipment quickly in the event of a breakdown so that the child can consistently use the implant.

The cochlear implant team

In order to provide a good service to implantees and to enable them to achieve the maximum benefit from their implant, many skilled professionals are involved from the stage of initial assessment through to long-term follow up. By using a team, all having input into the management of individual patients, the various skills are brought together to provide a cohesive service. Worldwide, team approaches have produced the best results for patients (Gersdoff, 1991)

The composition of a cochlear implant team is discussed by Fraser (1991). The requirements of a paediatric team differ from those of an adult programme: ideally it should comprise professionals experienced in working with young deaf children (Archbold, 1992).

The Department of Health in the UK has stimulated the development of specialized cochlear implant teams by directly funding a limited number of centres for a fixed period of time. This allows for the development of expertise in implantation and for more uniform data collection on the benefits of implantation (Rosen, 1990).

Although the composition of individual implant teams varies there should be a core of medical, audiological and rehabilitation personnel, usually otologists, audiological scientists, teachers of the deaf and speech and language therapists. The team also needs input from, or access to, the specialties of radiology, medical physics and educational psychology. All team members will use their skills in different pre-implant assessments and will contribute during the implantation and rehabilitation phases. An interactive approach is required among team members to decide which candidates are suitable for implantation, to maximize progress and resolve any problems following implantation. In most teams one member of the team also takes on a coordinating role.

Assessment of candidates for implantation

Audiological assessment

A significant but small proportion of children with sensorineural hearing loss will be suitable for cochlear implantation. The process of selection for implantation should be regarded in the wider context of determining the best form of help for the hearing-impaired child rather than a 'pass or fail' scenario. The implant team should be prepared to offer recommendations (and in some cases practical assistance) about the best form of help for each child, whether this is an implant, a change of hearing aid, consideration of tactile aids or other management. A schedule for the assessment of potential paediatric candidates for implantation is shown in Figure 13.3.

Cochlear implants can be effective for children with profound hearing losses but at present the performance of implanted children is no better than that of children fitted with conventional hearing aids who demonstrate good aided thresholds across the speech frequency range (Miyamoto et al., 1991; Osberger et al., 1991a). For this reason, and because cochlear implants are invasive and expensive, careful audiological assessment of candidates is essential to determine their responses with hearing aids.

The audiological assessment consists of testing the child's auditory sensitivity with and without hearing aids. Pure tone audiometry and unaided sound-field testing using conditioning techniques with vibrotactile stimulation provide measures of the degree of hearing loss. Auditory brain stem electric response measurements and sometimes also electrocochleography are routinely used to confirm objectively the degree of hearing loss (these techniques are described in detail in Chapter 7). Late cortical auditory potentials have been investigated in terms of their use before and after surgery with cochlear implant patients (Brix and Gedlicka, 1991). In order for accurate aided testing to be carried out the hearing aids should be appropriate models and settings for the child's hearing loss and should be tested for satisfactory functioning. Well-fitting earmoulds are a necessity.

Assessment of adults for cochlear implantation usually involves tests of speech discrimination to determine whether the patient derives any benefit from conventional hearing aids (King, 1991). For young children a speech discrimination test such as the McCormick Toy Discrimination Test may be used (McCormick, 1977; Ousey et al., 1989). However, many young profoundly deaf children have little or no memory of speech and it is therefore necessary to record sound-field aided measurements using frequency-specific stimuli such as warble tones to assess potential aided benefit (Miyamoto et al., 1991).

Middle ear fluid is common in young children and should be treated

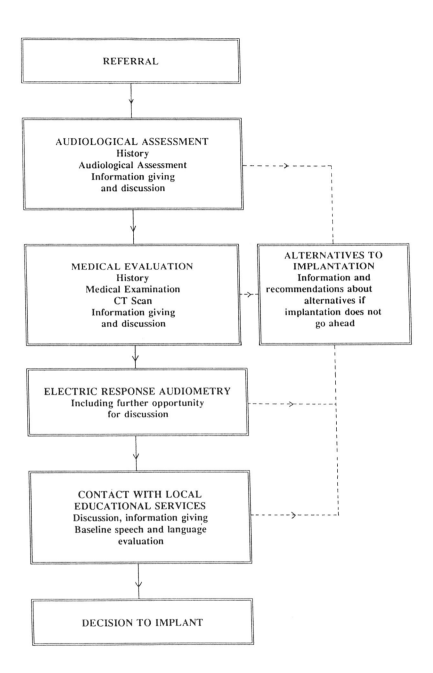

Figure 13.3 A sample schedule for assessing the suitability of hearing-impaired children for cochlear implantation.

before audiological assessment, to exclude the effect of any conductive overlay in the assessment of aided responses. Otoadmittance measurements should therefore be included in the audiological assessment of candidates. The absence of stapedial reflexes is consistent with a sensorineural hearing loss where there is no conductive element. Evoked otoacoustic emissions can be measured as a test of cochlear dysfunction in an ear where middle ear function is normal (Lutman et al., 1989). The absence of emissions is indicative of at least some cochlear dysfunction.

Most current paediatric programmes use the Nucleus 22-channel implant, which requires considerable postoperative testing using play audiometry techniques. The child must therefore demonstrate at pre-implant assessment the ability to carry out play audiometry and must be willing to cooperate in extended testing. If a child is not developmentally ready to complete the assessment some practice with conditioning games may be helpful before reassessment. If a child is inappropriately fitted with hearing aids suitable aids should be fitted without delay. A trial period of several months with new hearing aids should be carried out under the observation of the child's audiologist or teacher of the deaf to assess any additional benefit before reassessing the child with the new hearing aid. Reports from professionals locally involved with the child and observations by the parents can be useful when aided benefit is reassessed. In order to proceed with further cochlear implant assessment no significant benefit should be afforded by conventional hearing aids used consistently over a period of months. A guideline of aided responses worse than 70 dB (A) across the speech frequency range of 500 Hz to 4 kHz is widely accepted for justifying implantation assessment. The techniques used for audiological assessment of children for cochlear implantation are also widely used in paediatric audiology generally and have been described in Chapters 4, 5 and 6.

Auditory nerve function

A cochlear implant is thought to require at least some functioning auditory neurones to give the sensation of hearing. The number required is still under investigation but research so far suggests that even those with few surviving neurones will gain some benefit from a cochlear implant (Terr, Sfogliano and Riley, 1989; Nadol and Hsu, 1991). The measurement of evoked otoacoustic emissions or electrocochleography address this issue to some extent in that the presence of a response in either of these tests would indicate good cochlear function and any hearing loss is likely to be neural in origin. In adults, round window and promontory stimulation have been used in the belief that they measure the degree of neurone survival (Shipp and Nedzelski, 1991).

An electrode is placed on the promontory or in the round window to measure auditory percept and carry out psychophysical measurements. Positive results are felt to be predictive of auditory perception with a cochlear implant, but a negative response does not necessarily mean that the patient will not respond when implanted. Assessment of the status of the auditory nerve has been reviewed by Abbas and Brown (1991). Given that this procedure would be distressing for children and could not be performed under sedation because the child would be required to give responses, it is not usually employed with young children. There is still difficulty in extracochlear recording of electrical auditory brain stem responses (EABR) because the response elicited at or near the round window may be weak (Kasper, Pelizzone and Montandon, 1991). A technique using a 'salt' electrode is less invasive and is being investigated (Burian, Hochmair-Desoyer and Eisenwort, 1988).

Radiological and medical evaluation

Radiological investigation of the temporal bones is required to give clues to the cause of the hearing loss and to identify deformity or pathological changes within the cochlea that could hinder the surgical approach. If the cochlea is absent or deformed implantation may not be possible (Gray et al., 1991). Ossification of the cochlea can occur in post-meningitic patients (who make up a significant proportion of children being considered for a cochlear implant). Balkany, Gantz and Nadol (1988) report that 14% of implant candidates show ossification; Harnsberger et al. (1987) report 28%. Ultra-high-resolution computed tomographic (CT) scanning can be used to detect ossification but new bone formation or soft tissue is not necessarily distinguishable. It can, however, be seen using magnetic resonance imaging (MRI) (Yune, Miyamoto and Yune, 1991). MRI is becoming more widely used as a medical imaging technique and may become the preferred method of investigation. It is important to note that MRI cannot be used after implantation because of the effect of the magnetic field and radio frequency pulses on the implant (Portnoy and Mattucci, 1991).

The outcome of the radiological investigations will affect the decision of which ear to implant, which type of device to use and whether cochlear implantation is feasible at all. Usually only one ear is implanted to leave the other ear available for future more sophisticated implants (and also because of resource implications). Some intra-cochlear electrodes (such as the ball electrodes of the Ineraid device) are more difficult to insert into a deformed or partially ossified cochlea than others (such as the Nucleus device, which is a smooth electrode array of platinum rings). If ossification is present some surgeons advocate the use of an extracochlear single-channel system (Gray et al.,

1991). In the USA the Nucleus device is the only device currently available for children and some surgeons opt to drill through the ossification as far as possible and insert a few electrodes of the multichannel system (Balkany, Gantz and Nadol, 1988).

The child also undergoes a general medical examination to determine whether they are fit to undergo the surgical procedure. The risks are the same as those associated with any operation requiring general anaesthesia and may include skin flap infection or wound breakdown, compression or incorrect positioning of electrodes, weakness of the facial nerve, stimulation of the facial nerve, altered taste and transient dizziness (Cohen and Hoffman, 1991).

Educational requirements

Before implantation consideration should be given to the implanted child's educational needs. Professionals in the child's local educational setting should be willing to cooperate with the implant team because they will play a major role in the day-to-day rehabilitation. Although children from oral/aural, signing and total communication backgrounds can all be considered for implantation there should be a commitment to promoting the use of the auditory sensations provided by the implant. Baseline assessments of language status before implantation are important for future comparisons after implantation, and in guiding parental expectations (Archbold, 1992).

A profile for the selection of children for implantation has been devised by Hellman et al. (1991) and discusses further some of the issues in assessing suitability for implantation. Throughout the assessment process, members of the cochlear implant team will be required to provide information to parents, teachers of the deaf and other professionals. Parents should not feel rushed into making a decision about implantation for their child and adequate time for discussion is necessary. It is important to promote realistic parental expectation about cochlear implants so that they can appreciate that, while the benefits may be considerable, rehabilitation is a slow process requiring a high level of commitment (Downs and Owen Black, 1985; Quittner, Thompson Steck and Rouiller, 1991). Usually families find it helpful to meet other families with implanted children or to see videos of implanted children. They may also wish to meet adult implantees or families who opted against an implant. If at all possible, the child itself should be involved in the decision: this is not feasible with very young children but picture books and play activities can be used to inform young children about the implantation process. Members of the cochlear implant team will decide jointly whether a child is suitable for implantation but it is the child and family who ultimately decide whether to go ahead.

Cochlear implant surgery

The surgery required to insert the electrode array and receiver/stimulator varies according to which device is used. Accounts of the techniques used may be found in the manufacturers' surgical manuals. Details descriptions of surgical techniques are given by Burian, Hochmair-Desoyer and Klasek (1986), Webb et al. (1990), Clark et al. (1991) and Graham (1991).

Surgical procedure

Children are usually admitted to hospital for 4–5 days. After general anaesthesia is administered the hair is shaved behind and above the ear to be implanted.

- An incision in the shape of a C or a U is made in the shaved area to expose the section of the skull in which the receiver/stimulator will be embedded or where the plug of the percutaneous system will be anchored. The skin flap is fairly large so that sutures are remote from the receiver/stimulator package, which minimizes the risk of skin flap complications.
- In order to gain access to the cochlea the mastoid bone, which lies behind the ear, is drilled to form a cavity.
- A bed is created in the skull in which to seat the receiver/stimulator package and a groove to house the electrode lead wire.
- Holes are drilled for the Dacron ties that will be used to secure the receiver/stimulator in position.
- In a single-channel extracochlear device the active and reference electrodes are positioned appropriately outside the cochlea.
- For intracochlear devices the electrode array is inserted into the scala tympani via the round window niche, which may have been enlarged slightly by drilling or via a hole drilled in the bone directly over the scala tympani. The electrode array is inserted gently into the cochlea. Ideally the whole electrode array is inserted but this may not be possible if there is some ossification or soft tissue which may impede the electrode array as it curves round the cochlea. Although complete insertion of the electrode array is preferred not all electrodes have to be used and benefit may be gained from partial insertion (Balkany, Gantz and Nadol, 1988).
- The receiver/stimulator is secured in position and the entrance to the cochlea sealed around the electrode wire.
- The wound is sutured and a bulky pressure dressing applied.
- The surgical procedure takes about 3–4 hours to complete.

Objective measurements of auditory responses

Towards the end of the operation objective measurements can be carried out to give an indication of which electrodes can produce an auditory sensation. These measurements also provide an indication of the dynamic range for future stimulation. In the author's programme electrical stapedial reflex threshold (ESRT) measurements are carried out after the implant has been positioned but before the middle ear is closed. The implant is stimulated and the surgeon observes the contraction of the stapedius tendon via the operating microscope. The lowest level of stimulus at which the tendon is consistently observed contracting is the ESRT for that channel with the particular stimulation parameters used. ESRT can be obtained from about 10 electrode channels of the Nucleus 22-channel device in approximately 15 min using this technique. Other groups have recorded ESRT using admittance meters to detect the response contralaterally (Battmer, Laszig and Lehnhardt, 1990; Stephan, Welzi-Muller and Stilbrumer, 1991). The ESRT relates more closely to the maximum comfortable level but is well above the initial upper limit of stimulation.

Electrically evoked auditory brain stem response (EABR) measurements can be recorded when the implant is in position (described in detail in Chapter 7; see also Shallop et al. (1990)). Auditory responses in the brain stem are elicited by electrical stimulation of the electrodes of the implant. Measurements can be carried out on several electrodes while the surgeon is suturing the wound and need not prolong the period under anaesthesia. EABR thresholds have been related to the upper level of the initial dynamic range of stimulation (Shallop et al., 1991) and also to the threshold for electrical stimulation (Mason et al., 1993) but these differences probably reflect different recording parameters. EABR measurements are useful in showing that an electrode is functioning and also in determining the initial level to begin stimulation. Both EABR and ESRT measurements give some reassurance immediately after surgery that an auditory sensation can be elicited via the implant.

Surgical complications and reimplantation

Complications following implantation requiring surgery or hospital treatment have been reported in 5% of Nucleus implantees and 7.8% of Ineraid implantees (Cohen and Hoffman, 1991). The same study showed 18% of minor complications for the Ineraid device, all of which were due to mild or moderate pedestal inflammation (minor complication rate for the Nucleus device was 7%). Parisier and Chute (1991) reviewed the implant failure rate for the 3M/House single-channel implant (which is no longer available) and the Nucleus device, for which they found a 3% failure rate in one study and a higher failure rate of 12% in their own study.

Facial nerve stimulation has been reported in 12 of 82 implantees within 2 years of activation of the implant (Niparko et al., 1991) in both Nucleus and Ineraid multichannel systems where, if the problem did not resolve spontaneously, it was possible to deactivate the electrode responsible for the problem. Facial nerve stimulation was also reported in the 3M/Vienna single-channel implant but was resolved either spontaneously or by lowering the current output.

Case studies have reported specific problems. Daspit (1991) reported one case of meningitis after surgery, which was treated and the implantee is now successfully using the implant. Hoffman et al. (1991) have reported two cases of extrusion. In one patient the whole (Nucleus) device extruded through the skin after a period of bulging under the skin – this patient refused reimplantation. In a second case the electrode array gradually migrated out of the cochlea, during which time the patient's ability to discriminate speech declined – the electrode array was successfully repositioned and the patient was restored to his best preoperative level of performance.

Replacement of one Nucleus implant with another has been carried out successfully with no reduction in performance. Vienna single-channel implants have been removed and replaced with similar electrodes (Hochmair-Desoyer and Burian, 1985). Single-channel implants have been successfully replaced by multichannel implants (Gantz, Lowder and McCabe, 1989; Chute et al., 1992). Single-channel users reimplanted with multichannel devices usually, but not always, show an improvement in performance (Parisier et al., 1991).

Fitting and programming the speech processor

The external components of the implant system (the transmitter coil, microphone and speech processor) can be fitted 3–4 weeks after implantation, when the child has recovered fully from surgery (Figure 13.4). The speech processor is programmed or tuned to determine the characteristics of the electrical signal required to provide an auditory percept for each individual. First, the threshold of electrical stimulation (the lowest current density that produces an auditory sensation) is measured, then the maximum current level that the patient can tolerate without discomfort, sometimes referred to as the 'comfort level', is determined. The difference between the threshold and the upper level of stimulation is the *dynamic range*. Threshold and comfort levels vary between patients and between electrodes of multichannel systems. Lower thresholds and large dynamic ranges have, however, been associated with a greater percentage of surviving auditory neurones

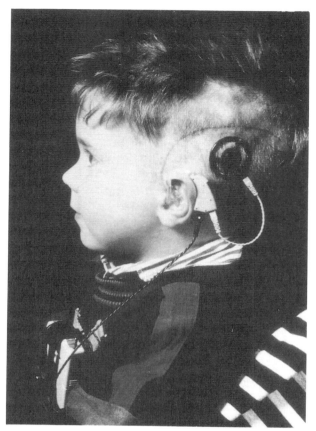

Figure 13.4 A young child, newly fitted with the external components of a Nucleus 22-channel cochlear implant: the microphone, speech processor, transmitter coil and connecting leads.

(Pfingst, Spelman and Sutton, 1980). Using the measurements of dynamic range the speech processor can be set so that speech and other sounds will be delivered through the implant within the audible range of stimulation but not so high as to cause discomfort.

Different implant systems utilize a variety of units of current which may be electrical decibels, units of current amplitude or arbitrary number values relating to current density. The measurements of dynamic range vary according to the processing strategy employed. For frequency-equalized single-channel systems measurements of threshold, most comfortable loudness and loudness discomfort level are made at several frequencies (Hochmair-Desoyer, 1986). For the Nucleus multichannel system threshold and maximum comfort levels are found for each electrode (Beiter, Staller and Dowell, 1991). Equipment specific to each device is required for programming the speech processor. This usually comprises some form of interface controlled by a computer. Speech processors may be set with hand-operated switches or may have a microchip memory which stores the stimulation parameters – sometimes referred to as a map.

With young children this is a lengthy and sometimes difficult process. Two testers are needed to carry out programming with young children: one operates the programming equipment while the other works closely with the child (Figure 13.5). Information from EABR and ESRT measurements is very helpful during the first programming session to determine levels appropriate to establish conditioned responses from the child.

Pre-training

Some groups advocate pre-training of on/off or big/small discrimination with vibrotactile or visual stimuli before initial stimulation through the implant (Mecklenberg et al., 1990). This may be advantageous but must be balanced against the tasks used becoming tedious for the child. The stimulus provided by the implant will be different from the pretraining stimuli and further conditioning to respond to the stimuli through the implant will be required at the initial programming session.

There is clearly some benefit in allowing the child to see, handle and become familiar with the speech processor and headset before initial stimulation, so that any fear of wearing the equipment is overcome. Parents should be prepared for a wide variety of responses to initial stimulation, ranging from no outward response to great distress at even minimal stimulation. Most children, however, adapt very quickly and begin to enjoy sounds that they can quite quickly associate with objects. For this reason the author's programme alternates tuning or programming sessions with rehabilitation sessions that encourage the child to use their processor and to experiment with sound.

Threshold measurements

Threshold measurements are carried out using conditioned response techniques in which the child is conditioned to respond to a stimulus by carrying out a play activity. This type of performance test or play audiometry technique is widely used in paediatric audiology and has been described in Chapters 4 and 6. With the Nucleus multichannel device up to 22 thresholds must be found and a wider variety of activities will be required to maintain the child's concentration than with audiometric testing. Many children may require several sessions to obtain thresholds for all the electrode channels.

Threshold levels often change over the first few months of stimulation as the child becomes more experienced with the implant and should therefore be remeasured at subsequent tuning sessions.

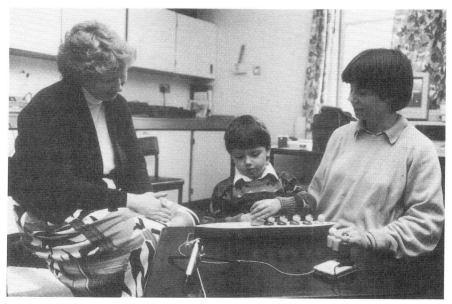

Figure 13.5 A young child undergoing testing to program a Nucleus 22-channel cochlear implant.

Maximum comfortable level

Finding the upper level of the dynamic range is more difficult because young children are most unlikely to be able to indicate a level which is just below discomfort level (MacPherson et al., 1991). It is therefore necessary to observe the child while gradually increasing the level of stimulation. Any sign of blinking, flinching, touching or attempting to remove the headset should be taken as a sign of discomfort. Clinicians must, however, be vigilant because some children may tolerate unpleasant sensations in order to please the clinician or because they feel that this is something that they have to endure: stilling or unusual quietness can thus also be a sign of discomfort. During the initial stimulation period it is advisable to set a very small, conservative dynamic range thus not allowing a discomfort level to be reached. Over subsequent tuning sessions the dynamic range can be increased gradually to reach the maximum comfortable levels.

Children aged 7 years and older who have some experience using their implant can usually indicate whether a sound is quiet, loud or too loud. This ability may be used in games in which the child indicates the level of the sound and when they want the sound to stop. Most children need practice with this type of task before reliable results can be obtained.

Additional measurements for the Nucleus device

The Nucleus 22-channel device is currently the most commonly used device with young children and it is also one of the most complex to programme. In addition to measurements of threshold and comfort levels, balancing of electrodes to check for comparable loudness growth on different channels and pitch ranking tests is advised (Roberts, 1991). These measurements may be difficult to obtain for adults and it is not possible to obtain meaningful results from this type of procedure with young children or inexperienced implant users.

With the Nucleus device it is also necessary to select the coding strategy that determines the nature of the feature extraction to be used and the stimulation mode, which will be one of several quasi-bipolar or bipolar modes of stimulation. Factors such as ease of finding faulty electrodes, the number of active electrodes and the value of the maximum comfortable stimulations are taken into account when choosing stimulation mode and coding strategy.

Several tuning sessions will be required in order to fully tune the processor. Minor changes to the map for the processor may be made for a year or more after initial stimulation. All children require some time to adapt to changes in the map, particularly older children and those who are experienced with their implants, because they may be less adaptable to a new signal.

Tuning checks

Implanted children require regular checks of the tuning of their implant systems to ensure that all components are functioning and to make any adjustments to the map for the speech processor that may be required. Children cannot always be expected to report faults with their equipment or to accurately describe the nature of the problem. For this reason parents and teachers should be advised to check any lights on the processor and to carry out a daily simple sound detection or discrimination task wherever possible. Liaison with rehabilitation officers and audiological staff regarding changes in a child's performance and behaviour at home or school may be suggestive of equipment malfunction. The implant clinic must stock sufficient spare equipment so that new equipment can be programmed and used to replace faulty equipment.

Interchange of information about children's progress with their implants between the team's audiological scientist tuning the speech processor and the teacher of the deaf and speech and language therapists will give valuable assistance in programming the device and reactions to map changes.

Rehabilitation

For the child to receive the maximum benefit from the implant the speech processor must be effectively programmed. The signal through the implant cannot, however, produce the same sensation as normal hearing. In addition, implanted children may have little or no memory of speech. Rehabilitation is the process of helping the implanted child to learn to integrate and interpret the new sound sensation received via the implant in order to communicate effectively and achieve their maximum potential. There should be considerable interaction between members of the implant team and local teachers and parents, to promote the development of listening and interpreting sound sensations from the implant (Selmi, 1985; Moog and Geers, 1991; Archbold, 1992). Many rehabilitation methods appropriate for young hearing-aid users are applicable to implanted children (Tait, 1986; Wood et al., 1986). Parents and class teachers need to be given information about simple checks of the functioning of the implant system and how to change batteries and leads if they suspect any problems. They should also be aware of any changes in the child's behaviour or responsiveness.

Expectations of the implanted child's auditory capabilities must be modified because the child has acquired hearing, having experienced a long period of very little (if any) hearing. An implant may give useful high-frequency hearing, which is unusual in profoundly deaf hearing-aid users: the rehabilitation programme devised for each child therefore needs to include reinforcement of this new sensation.

Initially, play with sound makers and musical instruments will help the child to enjoy using their device. Early responses to environmental sounds may be observed and the child alerted to the source of the sound. Pre-verbal skills such as eye contact, turn-taking and auditory processing are established first (Tait, 1987; Tait and Wood, 1987). Implanted children need to be reinforced and rewarded in learning to distinguish loud and soft, single and repeated, short and long, high and low pitched sounds. Discrimination of environmental and speech sounds should then be developed in a more structured way. Considerable input is required in speech and language therapy to develop the child's language skills further. Individual implanted children have widely different language abilities at the time of implantation and it is important to use materials and methods that will produce communication but which will be appropriate to the child's language status and chronological age so that he or she has a realistic chance of success at each task but is also sufficiently interested in the activity to participate. Practical rehabilitation ideas for young implanted children are discussed further by Mecklenburg et al. (1990), Archbold, Lloyd and Tait (1991) and Somers (1991a).

Evaluation of progress in auditory perception and in speech and language development is essential to highlight specific strengths and weaknesses and to ensure that children are achieving their potential. Measures appropriate to very young children require specific techniques not used in adult programmes. Video analysis techniques have been devised to investigate developing communication skills (Tait, 1987) and emerging spoken language (Osberger et al., 1991c). Other more formal tests can be used with older children (Geers and Moog, 1989; Osberger, 1989). The use of diaries, interviews and questionnaires such as the Meaningful Auditory Integration Scale (Robbins, Renshaw and Barry, 1991) can give valuable information about the child's longitudinal functioning at home and school (Archbold, 1992). Informing parents of changes in the child's use of the implant and auditory communication ability will encourage parents to continue to support their child throughout the rehabilitation process. Progress may appear slow to parents but they are often very pleased to see measured improvement in their child's functioning with the implant. Rehabilitation after cochlear implantation has been reviewed by Tucci, Lambert and Ruth (1990), whose study shows that the majority of implant programmes view rehabilitation as an important aspect of cochlear implantation. The same work revealed that paediatric programmes require considerably greater time and resources for rehabilitation than adult programmes.

Benefits of cochlear implants

Cochlear implants have been used for significant periods of time by adults. The lives of most implantees have been transformed and some multichannel implant users are able to carry out limited conversations on the telephone (Cohen, Waltzman and Shapiro, 1989; Dorman et al., 1991). Results from the Nottingham Paediatric Implant Programme revealed that of 19 implanted children all were aware of environmental sounds (11 responded to spoken language and 1 was able to understand speech with the aid of lipreading) immediately after initial stimulation through the implant. One year after implantation, of seven children, three could discriminate some speech sounds without lipreading and four could understand speech without lipreading (Gibbin 1992): before implantation none of these children showed any awareness of sound.

There is, however, a wide variation in the individual performance of implantees, which is potentially influenced by factors such as:

- age;
- duration of deafness;

- age of onset of deafness;
- mode of communication;
- degree of neuronal survival;
- type of device;
- cooperation of the implantee and the local service with the tuning of the device and rehabilitation.

It is, however, difficult for researchers to investigate individual aspects affecting the performance of implantees.

Multichannel and single-channel implants

High levels of word recognition without visual clues have been shown with the Vienna/3M cochlear implant (Tyler, 1988), which is a single-channel implant; but multichannel implantees may be more likely to obtain good results. Multichannel and single-channel cochlear implants were compared in a group study by Cohen, Waltzman and Fisher (1991): although some subjects with single-channel devices achieved good results in some speech and sound recognition tasks, multichannel implantees improved over a wider range of tests and to a greater degree – in no test did single channel users perform better than multichannel users. Similarly, Doyle, Pijl and Noel (1991) found improvements in speech and environmental sound recognition tests carried out on patients who had single channel implants replaced with Nucleus multichannel implants: the degree of improvement did, however, vary considerably between patients. Osberger et al. (1991c) compared speech and non-speech sounds uttered by children fitted with tactile aids, 3M/House single-channel implants and Nucleus multichannel implants using video analysis. More substantial improvements in speech production occurred with the multichannel implantees than with either single-channel implants or tactile aids. A case study of a patient in whom a single-channel implant has been replaced with a multichannel implant has shown that the multichannel improved performance (Pijl, 1991).

Gantz et al. (1988) compared the performance of five different implant systems and found comparable performance levels in two multichannel implants, the Ineraid and the Nucleus devices, in quiet conditions (in background noise the Ineraid device performed better). Further improvements in the speech processing strategy of the Nucleus device have resulted in better speech recognition in noise with this implant (von Wallenberg and Battmer, 1991). Teig et al. (1992) have specifically investigated the performance of implantees with the Ineraid and Nucleus devices (the two most widely used multichannel implants) which differ in their speech-processing strategies. Their results suggested better performance with the Ineraid, but only small numbers of implantees were studied and two of the Nucleus implantees were later discovered to have extensive nerve damage (which would have affected their performance with either device) and therefore definitive conclusions could not be reached. The pattern of performance of Ineraid and Nucleus implantees in another study (Tye-Murray et al., 1992) showed no significant difference during an 18-month postimplantation period.

Effect of nerve cell survival

Investigations have been carried out to assess the degree of survival of auditory neurones and the possible effect on performance with an implant. Studies with temporal bones from patients implanted 1–14 years before their death revealed little, if any, ganglion cell loss in the implanted ear compared with the non-implanted ear (Linthicum et al., 1991). In another report (Fayad et al., 1991) the temporal bones of two implanted ears were found to have only 10% of the normal number of spiral ganglion cells yet the performance of those two subjects on speech and sound recognition tasks had been as good as the average performance.

Variations in patient performance are, however, still felt by clinicians to be influenced by nerve cell survival (Lance de Foa and Loeb, 1991). This general view is supported by a case study in which a patient was implanted with a single-channel device in a recently deafened ear (Pijl,1991). Subsequent implantation of the other congenitally deafened ear with a Nucleus implant gave poor results. When the single channel implant was replaced with a second Nucleus implant the patient's performance improved dramatically. The author postulated that both peripheral and central neuronal elements may have been involved in the large performance differential observed.

Age of onset and duration of deafness

The age of onset of deafness and the duration of deafness are thought to influence performance after implantation. Parisier and Chute (1991) report that implantees aged 18 years and older who were either born deaf or deafened at an early age received less benefit than younger children. Only 29% of those over 18 years deafened at an early age demonstrated improved speech discrimination ability without lipreading: only 66% of this group used their implant all day, 21% used it for 1–3 h and 23% used their device less than 1 h each day. Better performances are reported with pre-adolescent implantees by Dowell et al. (1991). Waltzman, Cohen and Shapiro (1992) have shown that congenitally deaf children improved significantly in auditory and speech reception and perception skills, whereas congenitally deaf adults showed an increased awareness of sound but only minimal improvement in speech perception skills.

The performance of very young children using implants is, however, no different between those who acquired their hearing loss before the age of 3 years, and those who were congenitally deaf (Osberger et al., 1991d). Similarly, Somers (1991b) found no difference in the benefit received from an implant by a group of 4–8-year-old children who were deafened before the age of 3 years. Quittner and Thompson (1991) have, however, shown that later onset of deafness correlates positively to the meaningful use of sound.

Effect of rehabilitation and communication mode

Most implant teams invest considerable time in rehabilitation, which in itself may influence a child's performance. The effect of an intensive rehabilitation programme was investigated by Geers and Moog (1991), who compared potential implantees, currently using conventional aids but gaining little benefit from them, users of tactile aids and Nucleus implant users all participating in the same rehabilitation programme. Interestingly, all the children showed improvements but the speech perception of the implanted children improved faster than those using tactile or conventional aids. This clearly demonstrates the need for appropriate rehabilitation programmes to allow children to attain their maximum potential with any device used to assist hearing.

Some clinicians advocate a strong oral/aural mode of communication both before and after implantation (Tyler, 1990). Oral communication has been shown to correlate moderately with behavioural measures of the implanted child's use of sound (Quittner and Thompson, 1991). In another study of the spoken interactions of four children aged under 6 years and using the Nucleus implant (Hasenstab and Tobey, 1991), all were shown to improve in their spoken interactions regardless of their language status and communication mode at the time of implantation. Children using both oral and signed communication have been implanted in the author's programme. Although this programme emphasises auditory communication post-implantation to promote the use of the implant, children using oral or signed communication before implantation have achieved significant benefits from their implants.

Speech perception and production in implanted children

Much emphasis has been placed on the benefits of implantation in terms of speech perception and production in children because communication and language are so important for any child's education and quality of life. Improvements in speech perception have been well documented. In a study of 28 children who had used Nucleus implants for an average of 1.7 years (Osberger et al., 1991a), 61% were able to demonstrate some open-set speech recognition. Some of these children were able to carry out discrimination tasks using audition alone and a further 14% demonstrated closed-set recognition ability. Closed-set testing involves the subject selecting the correct response from a fixed set of items, whereas open-set testing provides no choices. Tyler (1990) reported significant speech perception abilities in five children implanted with the Nucleus device aged 6–10 years using open-set speech discrimination tasks without the aid of lipreading. A much larger group of 80 children with 1 year's experience using the Nucleus implant were assessed using age appropriate tests from a battery of 30 tests of sound detection and discrimination (Staller et al., 1991). Approximately two-thirds of these children showed improvements in closed-set tests and slightly less than half improved in open-set tests. In a study of speech production carried out on 61 children aged 2.4–17.8 years old using the Nucleus implant (Tobey et al., 1991), 77% improved in at least one-third of the speech production measures investigated.

The performance of cochlear implant users has been compared with that of tactile aid users and conventional hearing aid users demonstrating good aided thresholds, and considered to be effective hearing aid users (Miyamoto et al., 1991; Osberger et al., 1991b). Differences between conventional hearing-aid users, and multichannel Nucleus implantees were recorded in the lipreading and audition condition, not in the lipreading only condition and can therefore be attributed to the different information gained through each type of device. Multichannel implant users performed better than single-channel implantees but the conventional hearing-aid users performed better than the Nucleus implantees. It is acknowledged, however, that the hearing-aid users had been using their aids considerably longer than the implantees had been using their devices and it is therefore probable that the multichannel implantees will match the performance of the hearing-aid users given more experience. This work does however, demonstrate that careful selection of candidates is essential and that all possibilities of suitable fitting of conventional aids should be exhausted before implantation is considered.

Objective tests looking at brain activity in implanted patients also show auditory responses. Positron emission tomography has been used to record brain activity in the auditory cortices of patients when they were receiving stimulation through their implants (Ito et al., 1990). Comparisons of brain activity in the auditory cortex in the presence and absence of sound stimulation through the implant have shown objective responses in the central auditory system during electrical stimulation by a cochlear implant in both post- and prelingually deafened subjects (Herzog et al., 1991).

Other potential benefits of implantation

Cochlear implantation clearly gives significant benefit in terms of speech and language development, but the advantages of hearing environmental sounds should not be underestimated. The detection of traffic noise and warning signals is important for safety. Parents are often very encouraged by responses to environmental sounds and may report changes in their child's behaviour when they start using their implant systems (Cunningham, 1990). Positive psychological changes in adults following implantation have been reported by Knutson et al., 1991: after 18 months of implant use there was a significant reduction in depression, loneliness, social anxiety, social isolation and suspiciousness. Implantation has also been shown to relieve tinnitus in adults (Hazell, 1991; McKerrow et al., 1991). While many young deaf children do not indicate the presence of tinnitus, some children with acquired or progressive hearing losses may experience troublesome tinnitus. Alleviation of tinnitus is an additional potential benefit of implantation.

Since the ability to comprehend speech without lipreading has been shown to be possible with multichannel implants they have been used in patients with the dual sensory handicap of deafness and blindness (Martin et al., 1988). Provided that children fit all other assessment criteria and that they are able to carry out the test procedures required for programming the device and can participate in the rehabilitation programme they should be considered for implantation even if they have other disabilities.

Concluding remarks

Cochlear implants have developed considerably over the last 25 years from the first relatively simple single-channel implant to a variety of complex multichannel devices. In a questionnaire of implantees aged 14–66 years using five different implant systems (Tyler and Kelsay, 1990), the implantees were asked about the advantages and disadvantages of cochlear implants. Most implantees reported advantages in the following areas:

- speech perception with and without lipreading;
- environmental sound perception;
- psychological effects such as improved confidence and a reduction in the sense of isolation.

The disadvantages, expressed by fewer implantees, largely related to having to wear cumbersome equipment and breakdowns of different components of devices. Research into new implant designs is, however, very active in areas such as the size and sophistication of components and better signal processing techniques.

Cochlear implantation has progressed from an experimental procedure to an accepted form of treatment for both adults and children with profound hearing impairment. The benefits for adults are well documented. The implantees in Tyler and Kelsey's (1990) survey showed that on average implantees felt that they had achieved maximum benefit from their implants 7 months after initial stimulation. With young children many benefits are currently being reported but these children are continuing to improve in performance over periods of several years after implantation, given appropriate rehabilitative support. We may, therefore, see yet greater levels of achievement in young children using implants to develop speech and language. The challenge for clinicians will be to monitor the progress of such children and to apply the knowledge gained about improved implant designs, speech processing and rehabilitative procedures to helping implanted children reach their maximum potential.

References

Abbas, P.J. and Brown, C.J. (1991). Assessment of the status of the auditory nerve. In: Cooper, H. (Ed.), *Cochlear Implants – a Practical Guide*, pp. 109–124. London: Whurr.

Archbold, S.M. (1992). The development of a paediatric cochlear implant programme – a case study. *Journal of the British Association of Teachers of the Deaf* 16, 17–26.

Archbold, S., Lloyd, H. and Tait, M. (1991). *Rehabilitation: Young children with Cochlear Implants*. Booklet available from the Nottingham Paediatric Cochlear Implant Programme, General Hospital, Nottingham, UK.

Balkany, T., Gantz, B. and Nadol, J.B. (1988). Multichannel cochlear implants in partially ossified cochleas. *Annals of Otology, Rhinology and Laryngology* 97, 3–7.

Battmer, R.D., Laszig, R. and Lehnhardt, E. (1990). Electrically elicited stapedius reflex in cochlear implant patients. *Ear and Hearing* 11, 370–374.

Beiter, A.L., Staller, S.J. and Dowell, R.C. (1991). Education and device programming in children. *Ear and Hearing* 12, 25s–35s.

Boggess, W.J., Baker, J.E. and Balkany, T.J. (1989). Loss of residual hearing after cochlear implantation. *Laryngoscope* 99, 1002–1005.

Brix, R. and Gedlicka, W. (1991). Late cortical auditory potentials evoked by electrostimulation in deaf and cochlear implant patients. *European Archives of Otorhinolaryngology* 248, 442–444.

Burian, K., Hochmair-Desoyer, I.J. and Eisenwort, B. (1986). The Vienna cochlear implant programme. *Otolaryngology Clinics of North America* 19, 313–328.

Burian, K., Hochmair-Desoyer, I.J. and Klasek, O. (1988). Comparison of stimulation via transtympanic promontory electrodes, implanted electrodes and salt electrodes in the ear canal. In: Banfai, P. (Ed.), *Cochlear Implant: Current Situation*, pp. 157–160. Berman GMBH: Erhiters BD.

Chute, P.M., Hellman, S.A., Parisier, S.C., Tartter, V.C. and Ecouomou, A. (1992). Auditory perception changes after reimplantation in a child cochlear implant user. *Ear and Hearing* 13, 195–199.

Clark, G.M. and Tong, Y.C. (1982). A multiple channel cochlear implant; a summary of results for two patients. *Archives of Otolaryngology* 108, 214–217.

Clark, G.M., Tong, Y.T. and Patrick, J.F. (1990). *Cochlear Prostheses*. London: Churchill Livingstone

Clark, G., Franz, B., Pyman, B. and Webb, R. (1991). Surgery for multichannel cochlear implantation. In: Cooper, H. (Ed.), *Cochlear Implants – A Practical Guide*, pp. 169–200. London: Whurr.

Clark, G.M., Blamey, P.J., Brown, A.M., Gusby, P.A., Dowell, R.C., Franz, B. K-H., Pyman, B.C., Shepherd, R.K., Tong, Y.C., Webb, R.L., Hirshorn, M.S., Kuzma, J., Mecklenburg, D.J., Money, D.K., Patrick, J.F. and Seligman, P.M. (1987). The University of Melbourne–Nucleus multichannel cochlear implant. *Advances in Otology-Rhinology-Laryngology* 38.

Cohen, N.L. and Hoffman, R.A. (1991). Complications of cochlear implant surgery in adults and children. *Annals of Otology, Rhinology, Laryngology* 100, 708–711.

Cohen, N.L., Waltzman, S.B. and Shapiro, W.H. (1989). Telephone speech comprehension with use of the Nucleus cochlear implant. *Annals of Otology, Rhinology, Laryngology* 98, 8-11.

Cohen, N.L., Waltzman, S.B. and Fisher, S.G. (1991). Prospective randomized clinical trial of advanced cochlear implants. Preliminary results of a department of veterans affairs cooperative study. *Annals of Otology, Rhinology, Laryngology* 100, 823–829.

Cooper, H.R., Carpenter, L., Alesky, W., Booth, C.L., Read, T.E., Graham, J.M. and Fraser, J.G., (1989). UCH/RNID single channel extracochlear implant results in 30 profoundly deafened adults. *Journal of Laryngology and Otology* 18, 22–38.

Cunningham, J.K. (1990). Parents, evaluations of the effects of the 3M House cochlear implant on children. *Ear and Hearing* 11, 375–381.

Daspit, C.P. (1991). Meningitis as a result of a cochlear implant: case report. *Otolaryngology, Head and Neck Surgery* 105, 115–116.

Djourno, A. and Eyries, C. (1957). Prostheses auditive par excitation electrique a distance du nerf sensoriel a l'aide d'un bobinage inclus a demeure. *Presse Medicale* 35, 14–17.

Dodson, H.C., Walliker, J.R., Frampton, S., Douek, E.E., Fourcin, A.J. and Bannister, L.H. (1986). Structural alteration of hair cells in the contralateral ear resulting from extracochlear electrical stimulation. *Nature* 320, 65–67.

Dorman, M.F., Smith, L., McCandless, G., Dunnervant, G., Parkin, J. and Dankonski, K. (1990). Pitch scaling and speech understanding by patients who use the Ineraid Cochlear Implant. *Ear and Hearing* 11, 310–315.

Dorman, M.F., Dove, H., Parkin, J., Zacharchuk, S. and Danowski, K. (1991). Telephone use by patients fitted with the Ineraid Cochlear Implant. *Ear and Hearing* 12, 368–369.

Dowell, R.C., Dawson, P.W., Dettman, S.J., Shepherd, R.K., Whitford, L.A., Seligman, P.M. and Clark, G.M. (1991). Multichannel cochlear implants in children: a summary of current work at the University of Melbourne. *American Journal of Otology* 12, 137–143.

Downs, M.P. and Owen Black, F. (1985). Cochlear implants for children: Counselling the parents. *Seminars in Hearing* 6, 91–95.

Doyle, P.J., Pijl, S. and Noel, F.J. (1991). The cochlear implant: a comparison of single and multichannel results. *Journal of Otolaryngology* 20, 204–208.

Eddington, D.K., Dobelle, W.H., Brackmann, E.E., Mladejousky, M.G. and Parkin, J.L. (1978). Auditory prosthesis research with multiple channel intracochlear stimulation in man. *Annals of Otology, Rhinology, Laryngology* 87, 1–39.

Fayad, J., Linthicum, F.H., Otte, S.R., Galey, F.R. and House, W.F. (1991). Cochlear implants: Histopathology findings related to performance in 16 human temporal bones. *Annals of Otology, Rhinology, Laryngology* 100, 807–811.

Fraser, G. (1991). The cochlear implant team. In: Cooper, H. (Ed.), *Cochlear Implants – A Practical Guide*, pp. 84–91. London: Whurr.

Gantz, B.J., Lowder, M.W. and McCabe, B.F. (1989). Audiological results following reimplantation of cochlear implants. *Annals of Otology, Rhinology, Laryngology* 98, 12–16.

Gantz, B., Tyler, R.S., Knutson, J.F., Woodworth, G., Abbas, P., McCabe, B.F., Hinrichs, J., Tye-Murray, N., Lansing, C., Kuk, F. and Brown, C. (1988). Evaluation of 5 different cochlear implant designs: audiological assessment and predictors of performance. *The Laryngoscope* 98, 1100–1106.

Geers, A.E. and Moog, J.S. (1989). Evaluating speech perception skills: Tools for measuring benefits of cochlear implants, tactile aids and hearing aids. In: Owens, E. and Kessle, D.K. (Eds), *Cochlear Implants in Young Deaf Children*, pp. 227–256. Boston: Little Brown and Co.

Geers, A.E. and Moog, J.S. (1991). Evaluating the benefit of cochlear implants in an educational setting. *American Journal of Otology* 12, 116–125.

Gersdoff, M. (1991). Results of cochlear implants in children. *Acta Otologica-Rhinologica-Laryngologica Belgica* 45, 293–295.

Gibbin, K.P. (1992). Paediatric cochlear implantation. *Archives of Disease in Childhood* 67, 669–671.

Graham, J. (1991). Surgery for single channel cochlear implantation. In: Cooper, H. (Ed.), *Cochlear Implants – A Practical Guide*, pp. 155–168. London: Whurr

Gray, R., Evans, R.A., Freer, C.E.L., Szutowicz, H.E. and Maskell, G.F. (1991). Radiology for cochlear implants. *Journal of Laryngology and Otology* 105, 85–88.

Harnsberger, H. Ric., Dart, D.J., Parkin, J.L., Smoker, W.R.K. and Osborn, A.G. (1987). Cochlear implant candidates: Assessments with CT and MR Imaging. *Radiology* 164, 53–57.

Hasenstab, S.M. and Tobey, E.A. (1991). Language development in children receiving Nucleus multichannel cochlear implants. *Ear and Hearing* 12, 55s–65s.

Hazell, F. (1991). Electrical tinnitus suppression. In: Cooper, H. (Ed.), *Cochlear Implants – A Practical Guide*, pp. 355–369. London: Whurr.

Hellman, S.A., Chute, P.M., Kretschner, R.E., Nevins, M.E., Parisier, S.C. and Thurston, L.C. (1991). The development of a children's implant profile. *AAD/Reference* 136, 77–81.

Herzog, H., Lamprecht, A., Roden, W., Vosteen, K.H. and Fenendegen, L.E. (1991). Cortical activation in profoundly deaf patients during cochlear implant stimulation demonstrated by H_5 ^{15}O PET. *Journal of Computer Assisted Tomography* 15, 369–375.

Hinojosa, R., Douglas Green Jr., J. and Marion, M.S. (1991). Ganglion cell populations in labyrinthitis ossifications. *The American Journal of Otology* 12, 3-7.

Hochmair, E., Hochmair, I. and Zierhofer, C. (1990). Electronic circuits for cochlear implants. *Archiv für Elecktronic und Ubertagungstechnik (Electronics and Communication)* 44, 238–246.

Hochmair-Desoyer, I.J. (1986). Fitting of an analogue cochlear prosthesis – introduction of a new method and preliminary findings. *British Journal of Audiology* 20, 45–53.

Hochmair-Desoyer, I. and Burian, K. (1985). Reimplantation of moulded scala tympani electrode: impact on psychophysical and speech discrimination abilities. *Annals of Otology, Rhinology, Laryngology* 94, 65–70.

Hochmair-Desoyer, I., Hochmair, E. and Klasek, O. (1991). *New Vienna Cochlear Implant with postaural processor: Results*. Presentation at the annual conference of the German HNO Company May 1991 Aachen.

Hoffman, R.A., Cohen, N., Waltzman, S. and Shapiro, W. (1991). Delayed extrusion of the Nucleus multichannel cochlear implant. *Otolaryngology, Head and Neck Surgery* 105, 117–119.

Hortman, G., Pulec, J.L., Causse, J.B., Causse, J.R., Briend, C., Fontaine, J.P., Tetu, F. and Azena, B. (1989). Experience with the extracochlear multichannel implex system. In: Fraysse, B. (Ed.), *Cochlear Implant Acquisitions and Controversies*, pp. 307–317. Basel: Cochlear.

House, W.F. and Berliner, K.I. (1986). Safety and efficacy of the House/3M cochlear implant in profoundly deaf adults. *Otolaryngology Clinics of North America* 19, 275–286.

House, W.F. and Berliner, K.I., (1991). Cochlear implants: From idea to clinical practice. In: Cooper, H. (Ed.), *Cochlear Implants – A Practical Guide*, pp. 9–33. London: Whurr.

House, W.F., Berliner, K. I. and Eisenberg, L.S. (1983). Experiences with the cochlear implant in preschool children. *Annals of Otology, Rhinology, Laryngology* 92, 587–592.

House, W.F., Berliner, K., Crary, W., Graham, M., Luckey, R., Norton, N., Selters, W., Tobin, H., Urban, J. and Wexler, M. (1976). Cochlear implants. *Annals of Otology, Rhinology, Laryngology* 85, 1–93.

Ito, J., Sakakibara, J., Honjo, I., Iwrasaki, Y. and Yonekura, Y. (1990). Positron Emission Tomographic Study of Auditory Sensation in a patient with a cochlear implant. *Archives of Otolaryngology, Head and Neck Surgery* 116, 1437–1439.

Kasper, A., Pelizzone, M. and Montandon, P. (1991). Intracochlear potential distribution with intracochlear and extracochlear electrical stimulation in humans. *Annals of Otology, Rhinology, Laryngology* 100, 812–816.

King, A. (1991). Audiological assessment and hearing aid trials. In: Cooper, H. (Ed.),. *Cochlear Implants – A Practical Guide*, pp. 101–108. London: Whurr.

Knutson, J.F., Schartz, H.A., Tyler, R.S., Gantz, B.J. (1991). Psychological change following 18 months of cochlear implant use. *Annals of Otology, Rhinology, Laryngology* 100, 877–882.

Lance de Foa, J. and Loeb, G.E. (1991). Issues in cochlear prosthetics from an international survey of opinions. *International Journal of Technology Assessment in Health Care* 7, 403–410.

Linthicum, F.M., Fayad, J., Otto, S., Galey, F. and House, W. (1991). Inner ear morphological changes resulting from cochlear implantation. *The American Journal of Otology* 12, 8–10.

Lutman, M.E., Mason,. S., Sheppard, S. and Gibbin, K.P. (1989). Differential diagnostic potential of otoacoustic emissions: A case study. *Audiology* 28, 205–210.

Luxford, W.M. and Brackmann, D.E. (1985). The History of Cochlear Implants. In: Gray, R. (Ed.), *Cochlear Implants*, pp. 1–26. London: Croom Helm.

Martin, E.L., Burnett, P.A., Hunelick, T.E., Phillips, M.A. and Over, S.K. (1988). Speech recognition by a deaf-blind multichannel cochlear implant patient. *Ear and Hearing* 9, 70–74.

MacPherson, B.J., Effenbein, J.L., Schum, R.L. and Bentler, R.A. (1991). Thresholds of discomfort in young children. *Ear and Hearing* 12, 184–190.

Mason, S.M., Sheppard, S., Garnham, C.W., Lutman, M.E., O'Donoghue, G.M. and Gibbin, K.P. (1993). Application of intra-operative recordings of electrically evoked auditory brain stem responses in a paediatric cochlear implant programme. In: *Proceedings of the International Symposium on Cochlear Implants – New Perspectives, Toulouse, France, June 2nd–3rd, 1992*.

McCormick, B. (1977). The Toy Discrimination Test: An aid for screening the hearing of children above a mental age of 2 years. *Public Health* 91, 67–73.

McCormick, B. (1991). Paediatric cochlear implantation in the United Kingdom – a delayed journey on a well marked route. *British Journal of Audiology* 25, 145–149.

McKay, C., McDermott, H., Vandali, A. and Clark, G. (1991). Preliminary results with a six spectral maxima sound processor for the University of Melbourne/Nucleus multiple electrode cochlear implant. *Journal of the Otolaryngology Society of Australia* 6, 354–359.

McKerrow, W.S., Schreiner, C.E., Snyder, R.L., Merzenich, M.M. and Toner, J.G. (1991). Tinnitus suppression by cochlear implants. *Annals of Otology, Rhinology, Laryngology* 100, 552–558.

Mecklenburg, D. and Lehnhardt, E. (1991). The development of cochlear implants in Europe, Asia and Australia. In: Cooper, H. (Ed.), *Cochlear Implants – A Practical Guide*, pp. 34–57. London: Whurr.

Mecklenburg, D.J., Blamey, P.J., Busby, P.A., Dowell, R.C., Roberts, S. and Rickards, F.W. (1990). Auditory (re)habilitation for implanted deaf children and teenagers. In: Clark, G.M., Tong, Y.C. and Patrick, J.F. (Eds) *Cochlear Prostheses*, pp. 207–221. London: Churchill Livingstone.

Miller, J. (1991). Physiological measures of electrically evoked auditory system responsiveness: effects of pathology and electrical stimulation. *American Journal of Otology* 12, 28–36.

Miyamoto, R.T., Osberger, M.J., Robbins, A.M., Myres, W.A., Kessler, K. and Pope, M.L. (1991). Comparison of speech perception abilities in deaf children with hearing aids or cochlear implants. *Otolaryngology, Head and Neck Surgery* 104, 42–46.

Montandon, P., Kasper, A. and Pelizzone, M. (1991). A case study of a 4 year old perilingually deaf child implanted with an Ineraid multichannel cochlear implant. *Otorhinolaryngology* 53, 315–318.

Moog, J.S. and Geers, A.E. (1991). Educational management of children with cochlear implants. *AAD/Reference* 136, 69–76.

Nadol, J.B. and Hsu, W. (1991). Histopathological correlation of spiral ganglion cell count and new bone formation in the cochlea following meningogenic labyrinthitis and deafness. *Annals of Otology, Rhinology, Laryngology* 100, 712–716.

Niparko, J.K., Oviatt, D.L., Coker, N.J., Sutton, L., Waltzman, S.B. and Cohen, N.L. (1991). Facial nerve stimulation with cochlear implantation. *Otolaryngology, Head and Neck Surgery* 104, 826–830.

Osberger, M.J. (1989). Speech production in profoundly hearing impaired children with reference to cochlear implants. In: Owens, E. and Kessler, D.K. (Eds), *Cochlear Implants in Young Deaf Children*, pp. 257–282. Boston: Little Brown and Co.

Osberger, M.J., Robbins, A.M., Miyamoto, R.T., Berry, S.W., Myres, W.A., Kessler, K.S. and Pope, M.L. (1991a). Speech perception abilities of children with cochlear implants, tactile aids or hearing aids. *American Journal of Otology* 12, 105–115.

Osberger, M.J., Miyamoto, R.T., Zimmerman-Phillips, S., Kemink, J.L., Stroer, B.S., Firszt, J.B. and Novak, M.A. (1991b). Independent evaluation of the speech perception abilities of children with the Nucleus 22-channel cochlear implant system. *Ear and Hearing* 12, 665–805.

Osberger, M.J., Robbins, A.M., Berry, S.W., Todd, S.L., Hesketh, L.J. and Sedley, A. (1991c). Analysis of the spontaneous speech samples of children with cochlear implants or tactile aids. *American Journal of Otology* 12, 151–164.

Osberger, M.J., Todd, S.L., Robbins, A.M., Berry, S.W. and Miyamoto, R.T. (1991d). Effect of age at onset of deafness on children's speech perception abilities with a cochlear implant. *Annals of Otology, Rhinology, Laryngology* 100, 883–888.

Ousey, J., Sheppard, S., Twomey, T. and Palmer, A.R. (1989). The IHR/McCormick Toy Discrimination Test – description and initial evaluation. *British Journal of Audiology* 23, 245–251.

Parisier, S. and Chute, P. (1991). Cochlear implants: Indications and technology. *Medical Clinics of North America* 75, 1267–1275.

Parisier, S.C., Chute, P.M., Weiss, M.H., Hellman, S.A. and Wang, R.C. (1991). Results of cochlear implant reinsertion. *The Laryngoscope* 101, 1013–1015.

Parkin, J.L. and Randolph, L.J. (1991). Auditory performance with simultaneous intracochlear multichannel stimulation. *The Laryngoscope* 101, 379–383.

Parkin, J. and Stewart, B.E. (1988). Multichannel cochlear implantation: Utah-design. *Laryngoscope* 98, 262–265.

Peeters, S., Officiers, F.E. and Marquet. J.F.E. (1990). The Laura Cochlear Prosthesis: technical aspects. In: Sacritan, T., Alwares-Vicent, J.J., Bartual, J., Antole-Condela, F. et al. (Eds), *Proceedings of the XIV World Congress of Otorhinolaryngology, Head and Neck Surgery, Madrid, Spain. Otorhinolaryngology, Head and Neck Surgery*, pp. 1193–1202. Amsterdam: Kugler and Ghedini.

Pfingst, B.E., Spelman, F.A. and Sutton, D. (1980). Operating ranges for cochlear implants. *Annals of Otology, Rhinology, Laryngology* 89, 1–4.

Pijl, S. (1991). Single channel versus bilateral multichannel cochlear implant results: a case report. *Ear and Hearing* 12, 431–433.

Portnoy, W.M. and Mattucci, K. (1991). Cochlear implants as a contraindication to magnetic resonance imaging. *Annals of Otology, Rhinology, Laryngology* 100, 195–197.

Quittner, A.L. and Thompson, J. (1991). Predictors of cochlear implant use in children. *American Journal of Otology* 12, 89–94.

Quittner, A.L., Thompson Steck, J. and Rouiller, R. (1991). Cochlear implants in children: a study of parental stress and adjustment. *American Journal of Otology* 12, 95–104.

Robbins, A.M., Renshaw, J.J. and Barry, S.W. (1991). Evaluating meaningful auditory integration in profoundly hearing impaired children. *American Journal of Otology* 12, 144–150.

Roberts, S. (1991). Speech processor fitting for cochlear implants. In: Cooper, H. (Ed.), *Cochlear Implants – A Practical Guide*, pp. 201–218. London: Whurr.

Rosen, S. (1990). Cochlear implants: some consensus at last? *British Journal of Audiology* 24, 361–373.

Selmi, A. (1985). Monitoring and evaluating the educational effects of the cochlear implant. *Ear and Hearing* 6, 52s–59s.

Shallop, J.K., Beiter, A.L., Goin, D.W. and Mischke, R.E. (1990). Electrically evoked auditory brain stem responses (EABR) and middle latency responses (EMLR) obtained from patients with the Nucleus multichannel cochlear implant. *Ear and Hearing* 11, 5–15.

Shallop, J.K., Goin, D.W., Van Dyke, L. and Mischke, R.E. (1991). Prediction of behavioural threshold and comfort values for Nucleus 22 channel implant patients from electrical auditory brain stem response test results. *Annals of Otology, Rhinology, Laryngology* 100, 896–898.

Shepherd, R.K., Franz, B.K. – H.G. and Clark, G. (1990). The biocompatibility and safety of cochlear prostheses. In: Clark, G., Yong, Y.C. and Patrick, J.F. (Eds),

Cochlear Prostheses, pp. 69–98. London: Churchill Livingstone.

Shindler, R.A. and Kessler, D.K. (1992). Preliminary results with the Clarion cochlear implant. *The Laryngoscope* 102, 1006–1013.

Shipp, D.B. and Nedzelski, J.M. (1991). Round window versus promontory stimulation – assessment for cochlear implant candidacy. *Annals of Otology, Rhinology, Laryngology* 100, 889–892.

Somers, M. (1991a). Effects of cochlear implants in children: implications for rehabilitation. In: Cooper, H. (Ed.), *Cochlear Implants – A Practical Guide*, pp. 322–345. London: Whurr.

Somers, M. (1991b). Speech perception abilities in children with cochlear implants or hearing aids. *American Journal of Otology* 12, 174–178.

Staller, S., Beiter, A.L., Brimacombe, J.A., Mecklenburg, D.J. and Arnolt, P. (1991). Paediatric performance with the Nucleus 22 channel cochlear implant system. *American Journal of Otology* 12, 126–136.

Stephan, K., Welzi-Muller, K. and Stilbrumer, H. (1991). Acoustic reflex in patients with cochlear implants (analog stimulation). *American Journal of Otology* 12, 48–51.

Tait, M. (1986). Using singing to facilitate linguistic development in hearing impaired pre-schoolers. *Journal of the British Association of Teachers of the Deaf* 4, 103–108.

Tait, D.M. (1987). Making and monitoring progress in the pre-school years. *Journal of the British Association of Teachers of the Deaf* 11, 143–153.

Tait, D.M. and Wood, D.J. (1987). From communication to speech in deaf children. *Child Language Teaching and Therapy* 3, 1–17.

Teig, E., Lindeman, H.H., Floltorp, G., Tvete, O., Hanche-Olson, S. and Arntsen, O. (1992). Patient performance with two types of multiple electrode intracochlear implants. *Scandinavian Audiology* 21, 93–99.

Terr, L.I., Sfogliano, G.A. and Riley, S.L. (1989). Effects of stimulation by cochlear implant on the cochlear nerve. *The Laryngoscope* 99, 1171–1174.

Tobey, E.A., Angelette, S., Murchison, C., Nicosia, J., Sprague, S., Staller, S., Brimacombe, J.A. and Beiter, A.L. (1991). Speech production performance in children with multichannel cochlear implants. *American Journal of Otology* 12, 165–173.

Tucci, D.L., Lambert, P.R. and Ruth, R.A. (1990). Trends in rehabilitation after cochlear implantation. *Archives of Otolaryngology, Head and Neck Surgery* 116, 571–574.

Tye-Murray, N., Tyler, R.S., Woodworth, G.G. and Gantz, B.J. (1992). Performance over time with a Nucleus or Ineraid cochlear implant. *Ear and Hearing* 13, 200–209.

Tyler, R.S (1988). Open set word recognition with the 3M/Vienna single channel cochlear implant. *Archives of Otolaryngology, Head and Neck Surgery* 114, 1123–1126.

Tyler, R.S. (1990). Speech perception with the Nucleus cochlear implant in children trained with auditory/verbal approach. *American Journal of Otology* 11, 99–107.

Tyler, R.S. and Kelsay, D. (1990). Advantages and disadvantages reported by some of the better cochlear implant patients. *American Journal of Otology* 11, 282–289.

Von Wallenberg, E.L. and Battmer, R.D. (1991). Comparative speech recognition results in eight subjects using two different coding strategies with the Nucleus 22 channel cochlear implant. *British Journal of Audiology* 25, 371–380.

Von Wallenberg, E.L., Hochmair, E.S. and Hochmair-Desoyer, I.J. (1990). Initial results with simultaneous analog and pulsatile stimulation of the cochlea. *Acta Oto-Laryngologica Supplementum* **469**, 140–149.

Waltzman, S.B., Cohen, N.L. and Shapiro, W.H. (1991). Effects of chronic electrical stimulation on patients using a cochlear prosthesis. *Otolaryngology, Head and Neck Surgery* **105**, 797–801.

Waltzman, S.B., Cohen, N.L. and Shapiro, W.H. (1992). Use of a multichannel cochlear implant in the congenital and prelingually deaf population. *The Laryngoscope* **102**, 395–399.

Webb, R.L., Pyman, B.C., Franz, B.K.-H.G. and Clark, G.M. (1990). The surgery of cochlear implantation. In: Clark, G.M, Tong Y.C. and Patrick, J.F. (Eds), *Cochlear Prostheses*, pp. 153–180. London: Churchill Livingstone.

Wilson, B.S., Finley, C.C., Lawson, D.T., Wolford, R.D., Eddington, D.K. and Rabinowitz, W.M. (1991). Better speech recognition with cochlear implants. *Nature* **352**, 236–238.

Wood, D.J., Wood H.A., Griffiths, A.J. and Howarth, C.T. (1986). *Teaching and Talking with Deaf Children*. London: John Wiley & Sons.

Yune, H.Y., Miyamoto, R.T. and Yune, M.E. (1991). Medical imaging in cochlear implant candidates. *American Journal of Otology* **12**, 11–17.

Index